PHYSICAL MEDICINE & REHABILITATION
REVIEW QUESTIONS

PHYSICAL MEDICINE & REHABILITATION
REVIEW QUESTIONS

Shanti Ganesh, MD, MPH, MS

Staff Physiatrist Huntington, WV VAMC
Clinical Assistant Professor,
Department of Orthopedic Surgery,
Marshall University
Huntington, WV

Danielle Zelnik, MD

Staff Physiatrist
Absentee Shawnee Tribal Health System
Norman, OK

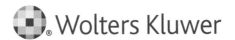

Philadelphia • Baltimore • New York • London
Buenos Aires • Hong Kong • Sydney • Tokyo

Acquisitions Editor: Kate Heaney
Editorial Coordinator: Lauren Pecarich
Marketing Manager: Rachel Mante Leung
Production Coordinator: Sadie Buckallew
Design Coordinator: Holly McLaughlin
Manufacturing Coordinator: Beth Welsh
Prepress Vendor: Absolute Service, Inc.

9 8 7 6 5 4 3 2 1

Printed in China

Library of Congress Cataloging-in-Publication Data

Names: Ganesh, Shanti, author. | Zelnik, Danielle, author.
Title: Physical medicine & rehabilitation review questions / Shanti Ganesh,
  Danielle Zelnik.
Other titles: Physical medicine and rehabilitation review questions
Description: Philadelphia : Wolters Kluwer, [2019] | Includes bibliographical
  references and index.
Identifiers: LCCN 2018011122 | ISBN 9781451151763 (pbk.)
Subjects: | MESH: Physical and Rehabilitation Medicine | Rehabilitation |
  Examination Questions
Classification: LCC RM701.6 | NLM WB 18.2 | DDC 615.5076—dc23 LC record available at https://lccn.loc.gov
/2018011122

Preface

Keep Calm and Study On!

On a perfect sunny day in July 2010, a sense of dread sank into my stomach as I looked out the window of my plane descending over the Pacific Ocean waters. Regret and panic immediately flooded over me as the plane's wheels touched the ground on the runway in Honolulu. What was I doing here when my PM&R board exam was next month? Months ago, travel seemed like a great idea when the board exam seemed like a distant event. Now, the exam was a dark cloud looming over me, quickly obscuring the clear blue Hawaiian sky.

Flash forward to 4 days later . . . when I found myself staring out the open exit door of a Cessna plane 12,000 feet in the air. The man strapped to my back yelled "JUMP!!!" as I let go of the bar and went into free fall. The rapid acceleration was unlike anything I had ever experienced. Seconds seemed like minutes until I felt the jerk of the opened parachute snapping me back. The ocean and beach below seemed oddly serene as we dropped through the remaining clouds and drifted down to the landing area. In that moment, I let go completely of all fears. When I touched the ground, I again felt a strange sense of calm. The anticipation before the jump had been worse than the actual jump. It suddenly occurred to me: Could it be that the anticipation before the board exam was worse than the actual exam?

It turned out to be right. The fear and anxiety before the written portion of the American Board of Physical Medicine and Rehabilitation (ABPMR) examination was worse than the actual examination. When I was able to relax and let go of my fear, I ended up enjoying the rest of my trip to Hawaii. The next weeks back home, I focused on studying while reminding myself to remain as calm as possible. I went on to pass the test with no regrets!

Would I recommend skydiving to relieve preexamination stress? Well, it certainly isn't for everyone, but it certainly was a fun and unforgettable experience that gave me a new perspective on life (and the board exam). The lesson is in not letting the stress before this exam overpower you—test anxiety can be your worst enemy! Underpreparation is another enemy that can be easily overcome with a good study plan and ways to identify your strengths and weaknesses. Weak test-taking skill is the other enemy that is overcome by time management and practice answering multiple choice test questions.

Shanti and I thought up the idea for this Q&A book while studying together in the resident room. There were no organized question and answer books in print for the ABPMR written examination. You could buy mock examinations, but the questions were not organized by topic, so our study group ended up having to sort all the questions and organize them into categories in order to study. Our specialty obviously is unique in that our knowledge base is broad, overlapping with other medical specialties as well as that of the physical and occupational therapy disciplines. Studying all these areas can seem daunting unless the material is well organized. Our goal is to bring you an organized multiple-choice question and answer book covering the general competencies, core knowledge, and the common topics in Physical Medicine & Rehabilitation. This book is primarily designed for those studying for the Part 1 certification examination and for the maintenance of certification (MOC) examination. It can also be to refresh your knowledge of subject material in preparation for Part 2. Additionally, we included bonus material, according to our expertise. I wrote a set of more challenging electrodiagnostic medicine questions geared toward the American Board of Electrodiagnostic Medicine (ABEM) subspecialty examination. Shanti also compiled a comprehensive chapter covering biostatistics, research, health policy, and epidemiology questions ideal for MD/MPH students.

Use this question and answer book along with your own topic outlines, textbook notes, and other study guides to get a well-rounded review. The exciting news is that Wolters Kluwer publishing is working with us to format our book questions into a computer-based practice test program to further help you hone your test-taking skills before the big day! If you adopt a low stress outlook combined with good preparation and test-taking skills, you'll be sure to conquer the boards! Use this book to take your exam prep to the next level!

Best of luck,
Danielle and Shanti

Note: Our book is not affiliated with or endorsed by the American Academy of Physical Medicine and Rehabilitation (AAPM&R), the American Board of Physical Medicine & Rehabilitation (ABPMR), or the American Board of Electrodiagnostic Medicine (ABEM) in any way. We use the names of these boards only in reference to the examinations offered by these entities.

Contents

The Low-Down on the Physical Medicine and Rehabilitation Boards

The Test

The part 1 written examination is a 6-hour computer-based, closed book test with 325 questions. The test is divided into a 3-hour morning session with 165 questions and a 3-hour afternoon session with 160 questions. There is an optional 1-hour lunch break between the morning and afternoon sessions. You must apply for the examination through the ABPMR (abpmr.org). Once your application is approved, you will receive e-mail instructions to schedule your test at a Pearson testing center (pearsonvue.com). Once you pass part 1, you are then eligible to take part 2, which is the oral examination held once a year in Rochester, Minnesota.

The maintenance of certification (MOC) examination for primary certification in Physical Medicine and Rehabilitation is also a computer-based, closed book test consisting of 160 questions in a 5-hour session. The MOC (i.e., global knowledge assessment) examination fulfills the third part of a four-part certification requirement to be completed during a 10-year cycle. The MOC examination must be passed by the end of your 10-year certification cycle (eligible years 7 to 10). You must apply for the examination through the ABPMR (abpmr.org). Once your application is approved, you will receive e-mail instructions to schedule your test at a Pearson testing center (pearsonvue.com).

Further details, including qualifications, current exam fees, calendar dates, and most current examination statistics, are on the ABPMR Web site.

Approach to Studying

There is no perfect way to study for an examination; everyone has their own unique study style. The fundamental assumption is that you have built already an existing knowledge base through textbook readings, journal articles, and clinical experience during your residency training years. If you are reading this book while still in residency training, we advise you to set aside dedicated time every week for reading in order to build your knowledge base. Take notes and make outlines of the most important facts you learned from each session of reading. Save these notes to use later for study purposes. As you get closer and closer to the examination date, you should be relying less and less on textbook material and focusing more on using review materials that contain practice questions, charts, outlines, and high-yield testable information. A general approach to studying would consist of addressing the following areas: managing preexamination stress, reviewing existing knowledge base to identify strengths and weaknesses, remediating weaknesses, and improving test-taking skills.

Managing Preexamination Stress

Most of us have felt some degree of anxiety and stress before an upcoming board examination. That is a normal reaction to an important life event where we do not know the outcome. The anxiety becomes problematic if it has consistently interfered with test preparation or caused us to perform poorly on the day of the examination. It is no surprise that multiple studies of test-taking college and allied health professionals have demonstrated a significant association between high levels of test anxiety and lower test performance scores. If you believe that you are prone to a level of test anxiety that could negatively affect your test performance, it is a treatable condition. Two studies of moderate- to high-anxiety medical students (one being a randomized controlled trial) showed significant success by employing a combination of progressive muscle relaxation, cognitive behavioral therapy/psychoeducation, and systemic desensitization. Also, there are promising studies of lower quality evidence using mindfulness meditation (including mindfulness based stress reduction/MBSR), biofeedback, eye movement desensitization and reprocessing (EMDR), and emotional freedom techniques (WHEE, EFT). A small, uncontrolled study of nursing students also showed a potential benefit of aromatherapy using lavender and rosemary sachets in reducing test stress. If you need further assistance in deciding which treatment is best for you, it is best to consult with a behavioral health specialist who treats anxiety disorders. For those with a history of debilitating anxiety, it is also important to be evaluated for any possible underlying learning disabilities or serious health conditions that could cause similar symptoms.

For most of us, it is useful to schedule free time for exercise, leisure reading, playing with pets or kids, outdoor physical activity, and hobbies in order to achieve balance during this hectic time. It goes without saying that a balanced diet and healthy sleep patterns are integral to maintaining your health while studying for the boards.

Identify Strengths and Weaknesses

We advise this test preparation step should be taken early in the process (at least 9 months before the examination). Review the ABPMR examination content outline and pick out any subject material you are not familiar with. Make a list of these topics and dedicate adequate time toward building a knowledge base for each one by reading relevant text-book chapters or research studies pertaining to them. Next, make a list of topics you are less familiar with and go through the same process. Last, use board review materials to look over the topics you are most familiar with as a refresher. After these steps are complete, we advise you to take a timed self-assessment examination (SAE). Fortunately, more than 90 residency programs administer the American Academy of Physical Medicine and Rehabilitation (AAPM&R) Self-Assessment Examination for Residents (SAE-R) annually. There are also SAEs available for purchase for maintenance of certification (approved list available on the ABPMR website at abpmr.org/MOC/PartII/SelfAssessment). The most common purchased SAEs are AAM&R SAE-Ps (available via the AAPM&R online portal).

Remediating Weaknesses

Most SAEs provide feedback on the numbers and types of questions that were answered correctly or incorrectly. This information will guide you in remediating your knowledge base weaknesses well in advance of the ABPMR examination. We advise this step should be taken at least 6 months before the examination. Analyze the questions that were answered incorrectly for clues as to the deficiency. Did you initially answer the question correctly but then decided to change the answer at the last minute? If so, why did the incorrect answer choice appeal to you? What concept needs to be reviewed in order to answer the question correctly the next time? Make a list of all topics and concepts that need to be reviewed. Go back and systematically cover each topic and concept using board review material with an occasional quick textbook read if more background information is needed for further clarification.

We advise concentrating on materials strictly designed for board review the last 2 to 3 months before the examination (unless there are a few topics where the knowledge base is still very weak). We have learned the hard way about getting mired down in verbose textbook chapters and minute details that will almost never show up on any test. One exception would be someone who knows they are already in the highest percentile of test takers and wants to do a thorough read for advanced information to sweep the most difficult questions and get an added competitive advantage (unnecessary in most cases as the prestigious Earl Elkins scholarship award has been retired). Use your board review materials to cover all topics to refresh your memory. Read, review, and repeat. . . .

Improving Test-Taking Skills

Use this book to practice timed test taking. If the chapter has 50 questions, set the timer to 50 minutes (or less). As a general rule, try not to spend more than a minute on each question unless you are 100% sure you can make up the time on easier questions. Don't beat yourself up and stay on a question too long thinking, "I just read this yesterday! Oh man, I should know this; I did a whole presentation on it for the med students!" Pick the best answer choice to your knowledge, flag the question using a sticky tab page marker, and move on. Later, if you finish ahead of time, you can return to the question and mull over the choices.

Get a feel for the computer-based examination software by downloading the Pearson VUE tutorial for the ABPMR exam (available at pearsonvue.com/abpmr/). The tutorial will teach you to take advantage of many features of taking a computer examination! The first advantage of a computer test is the timer counting down the remaining minutes left in the question block. The second advantage is the counter that shows the number of questions answered as you go through the section. The third advantage is the most useful—there is a tab on the top right of the screen, Flag for Review, that you click on to mark any question to go back to once all the questions have been viewed. Once all questions are complete, you are able to click tabs at the bottom of the screen to review any incomplete or flagged questions. This use of flagging is essential for you to manage your time and identify questions you need to return to once you have gone through the section once.

Become familiar with identifying multiple-choice question distractors (those answer choices that are obviously wrong) and using process of elimination based on your knowledge of the subject material. The last 4 weeks before the examination, we advise you to go back and identify any topic chapters where you had knowledge gaps and reread the answer explanations and the board review points (i.e., "Pearls" section). Close these remaining gaps while continuing to review a board review book chapter and questions daily to keep the information fresh in the mind.

Preparing for the Big Day

Those who have prepared well ahead of time may have the luxury of taking the day and night off before the examination to relax. Others will be studying up to bedtime the night before and first thing in the morning. There is no right or wrong way, except please make sure you get enough sleep the night before. Make sure everything is packed the night before and laid out for you to grab. The next page will include a preexamination checklist you can tear out and bring with you. The week before the examination, plan your transportation to the testing center and the route you will take. Estimate the amount of time it will take you to arrive at the testing center and leave a large window of time to account for any unplanned events that could happen on the day of the examination (e.g., traffic accident). If you are driving to a local center, you could do a practice drive to the center to find the building and get a feel for the route to troubleshoot any potential issues such as road construction or limited parking. You should arrive at least 30 minutes before the examination. You are prohibited from bringing test study material into the building. You are also prohibited from bringing electronic devices, such as computers, tablets, or cellular phones into the building. Keys, wallets, lunch, and other small personal items will be stored in a locker. Be sure to dress comfortably in layers to allow for any type of temperature change. Please check all rules and restrictions in the Preparing for the Computer Based Examination document on the ABPMR Web site and contact Pearson directly with any further testing center questions.

My Board Exam Checklist Page

- ☐ Transportation: car keys, metro pass, taxi or car service information . . .
- ☐ Address of testing center and copy of testing center confirmation e-mail
- ☐ Government-issued ID (valid driver's license, passport, or state identification card)
- ☐ Secondary ID bearing your signature (credit card, etc.)
- ☐ Snacks, bag lunch, water
- ☐ Good luck charm (optional)

Breaking Down the Topics

Before you delve into this book, take a moment to download and review the ABPMR Part 1 Examination Online or the MOC Outline (both available through ABPMR.org). In reviewing the outlines, you will note that the highest percentage of tested information is in the categories of neurologic disorders and musculoskeletal medicine. The focus of the majority of the questions will be on patient evaluation, diagnosis, and management.

The specific test breakdown of subjects and percentages is available on the ABPMR Web site. Familiarize yourself with the prosed test examination content before beginning your studies.

Best of luck!

REFERENCES & SUGGESTED READINGS

Benor DJ, Ledger K, Toussaint L, Hett G, Zaccaro D. Pilot study of emotional freedom techniques, wholistic hybrid derived from eye movement desensitization and reprocessing and emotional freedom technique, and cognitive behavioral therapy for treatment of test anxiety in university students. *Explore (NY)*. 2009;5(6):338-340. doi:10.1016/j.explore.2009.

Duty SM, Christian L, Loftus J, Zappi V. Is cognitive test-taking anxiety associated with academic performance among nursing students? *Nurse Educ*. 2016;41(2):70-74. doi:10.1097 /NNE.0000000000000208.

Frierson HT Jr, Hoban JD. The effects of acute test anxiety on NBME Part I performance. *J Natl Med Assoc*. 1992;84(8):686-689.

Kang YS, Choi SY, Ryu E. The effectiveness of a stress coping program based on mindfulness meditation on the stress, anxiety, and depression experienced by nursing students in Korea. *Nurse Educ Today*. 2009;29(5):538-543. doi:10.1016/j.nedt.2008.12.003.

McCaffrey R, Thomas DJ, Kinzelman AO. The effects of lavender and rosemary essential oils on test-taking anxiety among graduate nursing students. *Holist Nurs Pract*. 2009;23(2):88-93. doi:10.1097/HNP.0b013e3181a110aa.

Powell DH. Behavioral treatment of debilitating test anxiety among medical students. *J Clin Psychol*. 2004;60(8):853-865.

Saravanan C, Kingston R. A randomized control study of psychological intervention to reduce anxiety, amotivation and psychological distress among medical students. *J Res Med Sci*. 2014;19(5):391-397.

Musculoskeletal Medicine

1. Of the following answer choices, which is the smallest structure in skeletal muscle?

   A. fascicle

   B. myofibril

   C. muscle fiber

   D. muscle belly

2. Which is true regarding sarcomere structure in skeletal muscle contraction?

   A. Each sarcomere spans from Z line to Z line.

   B. Myosin fibers are found in the I band.

   C. Actin fibers are thick filaments with cross-bridges.

   D. Myosin fibers contain troponin and tropomyosin.

3. Which is true regarding sarcomere function in skeletal muscle contraction?

   A. ATP is required for myosin cross-bridge uncoupling from actin.

   B. As resting length increases, tension decreases in a linear fashion.

   C. Calcium is released into the myofibril in the resting state.

   D. The highest resting force potential occurs when there is extreme overlap of actin and myosin filaments.

4. Which best describes the appearance of normal muscle tissue on ultrasound examination?

   A. hyperechoic

   B. hypoechoic

   C. anechoic

   D. isoechoic

5. Which type and speed of muscle action generates the most force?

   A. slow concentric

   B. fast concentric

   C. slow eccentric

   D. fast eccentric

6. Which of the following is a progressive resistive exercise where muscle changes length while contracting to overcome a fixed resistance at variable speed?

   A. isometric

   B. isokinetic

   C. isotonic

   D. isoneutral

7. An abnormal finding during aerobic exercise would be

   A. increase in heart rate.

   B. decrease in total peripheral resistance.

   C. increase in maximum oxygen consumption ($\dot{V}O_{2max}$).

   D. no change in systolic blood pressure.

8. Muscle grade 3/5 on manual muscle testing indicates

   A. active movement against gravity and resistance.

   B. active movement with gravity eliminated.

   C. active movement against gravity.

   D. trace contraction.

9. Your patient, a 43-year-old male corporate executive, is an avid distance runner training for a marathon who sustained a grade 1 quadriceps muscle strain yesterday. He reports mild pain walking and moderate pain running uphill and on level surfaces. Your examination shows moderate tenderness, mild soft tissue swelling over the muscle, and pain with full active knee extension. He wants to return to running as soon as possible. Your best recommendation is

   A. an initial period of rest, ice, compression, and elevation.

   B. downhill running to take pressure off the injured muscle.

   C. return to full training regimen and treat pain with high-dose nonsteroidal anti-inflammatory medication.

   D. prescribe plyometric home exercise program, including depth jumping.

10. The commonly prescribed muscle relaxant, cyclobenzaprine, has which of the following mechanisms of action?

   A. direct skeletal muscle relaxant

   B. γ-aminobutyric acid (GABA) agonist

   C. alpha-2 agonist

   D. central nervous system depressant

11. Which of the following finding(s) indicate an active myofascial trigger point on physical examination?

   A. palpable taut muscle band

   B. exquisite focal tenderness

   C. patient reports referred pain

   D. all of the above

12. Which of the following is used to activate platelet rich plasma (PRP)?

   A. c-reactive protein

   B. sodium chloride

   C. fibronectin

   D. thrombin

13. Which growth factor in platelet rich plasma (PRP) has function of synthesis and preservation of the extracellular matrix?

    A. platelet-derived growth factor (PDGF)

    B. insulin-like growth factor

    C. transforming growth factor-beta (TGF-β)

    D. vascular endothelial growth factor

14. Which answer choice best describes tendinopathy/tendinosis?

    A. characterized by chronic inflammation

    B. characterized by ischemic and myxoid degeneration

    C. appears hyperechoic on ultrasound examination

    D. shows no vascularity on ultrasound examination

15. All are risk factors for fragility fractures associated with low bone mineral density, EXCEPT

    A. smoking.

    B. hip fracture in mother or father.

    C. obesity.

    D. Caucasian race.

16. Which dual-energy x-ray absorptiometry (DXA) age-matched score compares the test subject's measured bone mineral density to that of adults of the same age?

    A. T-score

    B. X-score

    C. Z-score

    D. Fracture Risk Assessment Tool (FRAX®)

17. Which statement is true regarding fragility fracture epidemiology and bone mineral density (BMD) in older adults?

    A. Previous fragility fracture predicts likelihood of future fracture.

    B. Fracture risk is determined only by BMD score.

    C. The majority of fragility fractures occur in those with T-score −2.5 to 3.0.

    D. The Fracture Risk Assessment Tool (FRAX®) calculates the 1-year probability of hip or other major osteoporotic fracture.

18. Which exercise is most beneficial to a postmenopausal woman whose goal is to maintain and improve bone mass?

    A. swimming

    B. hand bike

    C. antigravity treadmill

    D. weight lifting

19. Which bone is primarily composed of trabecular bone?

    A. humerus

    B. tibia

    C. lumbar vertebrae

    D. radius

20. Primary malignant bone tumors most frequently involve which part of the long bone?

    A. epiphysis

    B. metaphysis

    C. diaphysis

    D. articular cartilage

21. Which is considered a synovial joint?

    A. acromioclavicular joint

    B. first sternocostal joint

    C. pubic symphysis

    D. skull

22. Which characteristic is most consistent with noninfectious inflammatory synovial fluid?

    A. high viscosity

    B. good mucin clotting

    C. 100% neutrophils/polymorphonuclear leukocytes (PMNs)

    D. 4,000 cells/mm³ leukocyte count

23. How does gout differ from pseudogout?

    A. Gout crystals are made from calcium pyrophosphate.

    B. Gout crystals have positive birefringence under polarized light.

    C. Gout has asymmetric joint involvement.

    D. all of the above

24. Which gout medication decreases the synthesis of uric acid?

    A. probenecid

    B. allopurinol

    C. colchicine

    D. indomethacin

25. Morning stiffness lasting at least _____ is most suggestive of rheumatoid arthritis.

    A. 10 minutes

    B. 30 minutes

    C. 45 minutes

    D. 60 minutes

26. Which joint is LEAST likely to be affected in rheumatoid arthritis?

   A. proximal interphalangeal joint

   B. distal interphalangeal joint

   C. metacarpal phalangeal joint

   D. metatarsal phalangeal joint

27. Which radiographic finding is most characteristic of rheumatoid arthritis (RA)?

   A. osteophyte formation

   B. subchondral bony sclerosis

   C. juxtaarticular osteopenia

   D. asymmetric joint space narrowing

28. The swan-neck deformity of rheumatoid arthritis involves

   A. flexion of the proximal interphalangeal joint.

   B. hyperextension of the distal interphalangeal joint.

   C. hyperextension of the metacarpal phalangeal joint.

   D. hyperextension of the proximal interphalangeal joint.

29. In rheumatoid arthritis, which of the following causes destruction of articular cartilage and other associated soft tissue structures?

   A. crystal deposits

   B. osteoblasts

   C. pannus

   D. bacteria

30. Regarding rheumatoid factor (RF):

   A. RF positive status predicts poor prognosis in rheumatoid arthritis (RA).

   B. RF needs to be positive to make a diagnosis of RA.

   C. RF in serum represents autoantibodies to synovial membrane proteins.

   D. RF is specific for RA only and is not positive in other diseases.

31. All are characteristic musculoskeletal structural complications associated with rheumatoid arthritis (RA), EXCEPT

A. protrusio acetabuli.

B. atlantoaxial instability.

C. equinovarus foot.

D. ulnar deviation of the metacarpophalangeal joints.

32. Which of the following types of exercise is beneficial for strengthening weak muscles in those with rheumatoid arthritis?

A. isometric

B. isotonic

C. isokinetic

D. all of the above

33. What would be the most appropriate monotherapy treatment for a patient with early rheumatoid arthritis of less than 6 months duration?

A. methotrexate

B. sulindac

C. etanercept

D. prednisone

34. A 70-year-old woman present with a 2-month history of morning stiffness and aching pain in her neck, bilateral shoulders, and bilateral hips. Review of systems is positive for morning stiffness lasting 45 to 60 minutes daily and recent 10-lb weight loss. She denies headache or vision changes. She brought with her laboratory tests she had done last week remarkable for erythrocyte sedimentation rate of 75 mm/h and c-reactive protein 6 mg/L. You prescribe her prednisone and book a referral rheumatology evaluation for her for the following week. She calls you the next day to tell you the prednisone is a "miracle" and you are "the best doctor ever." What is the most likely diagnosis?

A. polymyalgia rheumatica

B. psoriatic arthritis

C. systemic lupus erythematosus

D. scleroderma

35. Which is NOT commonly associated with the seronegative spondyloarthropathies?

A. Raynaud phenomenon

B. mucocutaneous lesions

C. enthesopathy

D. sacroiliitis

36. The L1 vertebral level of the spine forms how many joints with the level below it?

A. one

B. two

C. three

D. four

37. A 40-year-old male presents with a 1-month history of low back pain radiating down the posterior aspect of the left lower extremity to the bottom of his foot with associated plantarflexion weakness. The clinical history, physical examination, and needle electromyography (EMG) are consistent with the diagnosis of an acute left S1 radiculopathy secondary to disc herniation. The corresponding lumbosacral magnetic resonance imaging (MRI) study would most likely show

A. central disc herniation at L4-5 compressing the thecal sac.

B. left paramedian disc herniation at L5-S1 compressing the traversing nerve root.

C. left foraminal disc herniation at L5-S1 compressing the exiting nerve root.

D. left paramedian disc herniation at L4-5 compressing the traversing nerve root.

38. An interventional pain management physiatrist wants to perform radiofrequency ablation to target the innervation of the L4-5 and L5-S1 zygapophyseal joints. Which nerves should he or she target?

A. the medial branches of L4, L5, and S1

B. the medial branches of L3, L4, and the L5 dorsal ramus

C. the medial branches of L3 and L4

D. the medial branch of L4 and the L5 dorsal ramus

39. Which of the following is an example of a positive nerve root tension sign on physical examination?

A. Supine patient reports posterior thigh pain with elevation of affected lower limb to 10 degrees off the examination table.

B. Prone patient reports posterior thigh pain when examiner flexes the knee.

C. Patient sitting with spine flexed, arms behind back, and knee extended reports radiating pain down the arms when the examiner dorsiflexes the ankle and applies pressure to the neck.

D. Patient sitting reports reproduction of ipsilateral radiating pain into arm when examiner extends neck, rotates to affected side, and applies downward pressure on head.

40. Which of the following is a clinical or radiographic finding that could distinguish ankylosing spondylitis (AS) from diffuse idiopathic skeletal hyperostosis (DISH)?

A. AS has presence sacroiliac joint erosion.

B. AS has "flowing" ossification of anterior longitudinal ligament.

C. AS has limitation in spine mobility.

D. AS is associated with diabetes mellitus.

41. Cervical disc disease most often affects which level?

A. C4-5

B. C5-6

C. C6-7

D. C7-T1

42. Which syndrome, predominantly involving the lower extremities, is the most common lesion for cervical spondylotic myelopathy?

   A. transverse lesion syndrome

   B. motor system syndrome

   C. central cord syndrome

   D. Brown-Séquard syndrome

43. All the following are considered "red flags" in the assessment of low back pain, EXCEPT

   A. prolonged use corticosteroids.

   B. history of cancer.

   C. previous surgery.

   D. progressive pain at night.

44. What is the best nonoperative management for a patient with atlantoaxial instability?

   A. traction

   B. neck strengthening exercises

   C. sternal-occipital-mandibular immobilizer (SOMI) brace

   D. hard cervical collar

45. Which of the following spine orthoses is most ideal for a stable, uncomplicated lower thoracic vertebral compression fracture?

   A. Philadelphia

   B. Milwaukee

   C. Jewett

   D. Chairback

46. Which of the following muscles is NOT a hip flexor?

   A. sartorius

   B. pectineus

   C. tensor fasciae latae

   D. long head of the biceps femoris

47. What is the function of the iliofemoral ligament (a.k.a. the Y-ligament of Bigelow)?

   A. limit flexion, adduction, and internal rotation of the hip

   B. promote extension, abduction, and external rotation of the hip

   C. limit extension, abduction, and external rotation of the hip

   D. limit flexion, abduction, and internal rotation of the hip

48. Which type of hip fracture is LEAST likely to require surgical intervention?

   A. tension-side femoral neck stress fracture

   B. compression-side femoral neck stress fracture

   C. Garden type 2 femoral neck stress fracture

   D. intertrochanteric femur fracture

49. A positive dynamic ultrasound examination for snapping hip syndrome typically would show displacement of the

   A. gluteus minimus tendon over the greater trochanter.

   B. iliotibial band over the greater trochanter.

   C. iliopsoas tendon over the anterior inferior iliac spine.

   D. gluteus maximus tendon over the iliopectineal eminence.

50. Which of the following is true regarding hip dislocation?

   A. Anterior dislocation is more common than posterior dislocation.

   B. The clinical presentation of posterior dislocation is hip flexed, abducted, and externally rotated.

   C. Closed reduction is unsuccessful for hip dislocations.

   D. Sciatic nerve injury is a complication of posterior dislocation.

51. Which physical examination maneuver would best provoke symptoms of piriformis syndrome?

A. hip flexion, adduction, and internal rotation (FADIR)

B. hip flexion, abduction, external rotation, and extension (FABERE)

C. hip abduction and long axis traction

D. hip hyperextension in side lying position

52. Which pelvic structure is the most important determinant of pelvic stability following trauma?

A. pubic symphysis

B. ischial tuberosity

C. iliolumbar ligament

D. posterior sacroiliac ligaments

53. Which structure would be the most appropriate target for nerve block for presumed chronic pelvic pain from endometriosis?

A. pudendal nerve

B. superior hypogastric plexus

C. iliohypogastric nerve

D. lumbar sympathetic plexus

54. A 50-year-old male with a medical history significant for active alcoholism is referred to musculoskeletal medicine clinic by his primary care doctor for a 2-week history of severe left hip/groin pain of sudden onset without known injury and no recent illness. He tested negative for sexually transmitted infections on recent labs. He reports no previous history of hip problems and has no other joint pains. He is a nonsmoker and does not use recreational drugs. He is afebrile, normotensive, normal body mass index. He is most at risk for which condition?

A. osteoarthritis

B. osteonecrosis

C. rheumatoid arthritis

D. reactive arthritis

55. What is the most common direction of glenohumeral instability?

A. anterior inferior

B. anterior superior

C. posterior inferior

D. posterior superior

56. With abduction, the humerus naturally

A. pronates.

B. internally rotates.

C. externally rotates.

D. circumducts.

57. Medial scapular winging results from weakness of which muscle(s)?

A. trapezius

B. rhomboids

C. latissimus dorsi

D. serratus anterior

58. Which nerve is LEAST likely to be affected by a proximal humerus fracture?

A. ulnar

B. radial

C. median

D. axillary

59. A newborn infant's birth is complicated by shoulder dystocia. The infant is examined after birth and found to have right upper extremity weakness. The right upper extremity is found to be in a position of adduction, internal rotation, elbow extension, forearm pronation, and wrist flexion. Where is the injury?

A. upper trunk of the brachial plexus

B. middle trunk of the brachial plexus

C. lower trunk of the brachial plexus

D. both B and C

60. You are covering a football game where a 19-year-old male player was struck on the side of the neck during a tackle and complained of immediate burning pain, numbness, and tingling involving the right arm. You check on him 5 minutes later, and he is symptom free with full range of motion in neck and shoulders with no pain and full strength. What is true about his condition?

A. There is risk of symptom recurrence within 30 minutes.

B. He will require electrodiagnostic testing even if asymptomatic.

C. He can return to play if full strength and symptom free.

D. Treatment consists of anti-inflammatory medication.

61. Which structure would be torn in a high-grade superior labrum anterior posterior (SLAP) tear?

A. supraspinatus tendon

B. long head biceps brachii tendon

C. subscapularis tendon

D. coracoacromial ligament

62. A 50-year-old female swimmer complains of right lateral shoulder pain worse with overhead activity and lying on the affected side. There was no precipitating injury. She denies weakness or instability. Which physical examination maneuver is most likely to be positive?

A. O'Brien test

B. Gerber test

C. Speed test

D. Neer test

63. What is an indication for reverse shoulder arthroplasty?

A. rotator cuff tear in presence of arthropathy

B. glenohumeral osteoarthritis with intact rotator cuff

C. multidirectional instability

D. axillary neuropathy

64. A Hill-Sachs lesion most often occurs in association with

   A. proximal biceps tendon rupture.

   B. displaced distal clavicle fracture.

   C. acute nondisplaced one-part proximal humerus fracture.

   D. anterior shoulder dislocation.

65. The finding that distinguishes a type IV from a type III acromioclavicular joint shoulder separation is that a type IV injury has

   A. intact coracoclavicular ligament.

   B. buttonhole through trapezius fascia.

   C. inferior clavicle displacement.

   D. no widening of joint with weighted radiographs.

66. Cozen test is a provocative test primarily used in the evaluation of what condition?

   A. shoulder instability

   B. lateral epicondylitis

   C. carpal tunnel syndrome

   D. patellofemoral syndrome

67. All the following elbow injuries are typically associated with throwing, EXCEPT

   A. medial epicondylitis.

   B. valgus extension overload syndrome.

   C. lateral epicondylitis.

   D. ulnar collateral ligament sprain.

68. The most common site for ulnar nerve compression/entrapment is at the

   A. cubital tunnel.

   B. wrist.

   C. medial epicondyle.

   D. deep flexor aponeurosis.

69. Regarding elbow dislocation:

    A. Anterior is the most common direction of dislocation.

    B. Complications include loss of range of motion in flexion.

    C. Mechanism of injury is fall on outstretched hand.

    D. all of the above

70. What structure(s) is/are found in the sixth extensor compartment of the wrist?

    A. extensor carpi ulnaris

    B. abductor pollicis longus

    C. extensor pollicis longus

    D. extensor digiti minimi

71. The scaphoid fracture site with highest chance of nonunion and avascular necrosis (AVN) is

    A. proximal pole.

    B. waist.

    C. distal pole.

    D. tuberosity.

72. The anatomic pathology of which disorder involves injury to the terminal extensor tendon attachment to the distal phalanx?

    A. jersey finger

    B. swan-neck deformity

    C. mallet finger

    D. boutonnière deformity

73. Regarding diagnosis of carpal tunnel syndrome (CTS):

    A. Electrodiagnostic testing must be positive to make a diagnosis.

    B. It is a clinical diagnosis.

    C. Tinel test is the most sensitive test for diagnosis.

    D. Cross sectional median nerve area of 5 mm^2 measured by ultrasound is diagnostic.

74. Which of the following is NOT part of the triangular fibrocartilage complex (TFCC)?

A. extensor digiti minimi sheath

B. ulnar meniscus homolog

C. ulnar collateral ligament

D. triangular fibrocartilage

75. A 68-year-old male presents with right thumb pain with no known history of injury. Upon examination, his typical pain is reproduced by the examiner compressing and rotating the patient's thumb metacarpal against the trapezium while the examiner stabilizes the patient's thumb. He reports no pain when the examiner places the patient's thumb within the hand and bends the hand in exaggerated ulnar abduction. He also reports no pain with valgus stress of the metacarpophalangeal joint in 30 degrees of flexion. What is the most likely diagnosis?

A. De Quervain tenosynovitis

B. trigger thumb

C. ulnar collateral ligament (UCL) sprain

D. carpometacarpal (CMC) joint osteoarthritis

76. Which type of splint is most appropriate for a boxer's fracture?

A. thumb spica

B. ulnar gutter

C. sugar tong

D. all of the above

77. Which knee bursa is located between the tendons of the sartorius, gracilis, and semitendinosus muscles and the medial collateral ligament?

A. prepatellar

B. suprapatellar

C. lateral popliteus

D. pes anserinus

78. Continuous passive motion (CPM) after uncomplicated total knee arthroplasty (TKA)

    A. is a popular device used in the immediate postoperative period.

    B. has strong evidence for its effectiveness in reducing hospital stay.

    C. has strong evidence for its effectiveness in reducing deep venous thromboembolism.

    D. is a mobilization technique used by a trained physical therapist.

79. A small knee meniscus tear in which location is MOST likely to heal?

    A. outer periphery

    B. inner two-thirds

    C. inner one-third

    D. middle one-third

80. Which of the following conditions is a common cause of nontraumatic anterior knee pain in runners with symptoms during exercise, squatting, kneeling, and using stairs? The physical examination is normal in many cases. The condition typically responds to conservative treatment, especially physical therapy.

    A. popliteus strain

    B. patellofemoral pain syndrome

    C. iliotibial band syndrome

    D. pes anserine bursitis

81. Which injury or injuries can occur with a tear of the knee anterior cruciate ligament (ACL)?

    A. bone contusion

    B. medial collateral ligament tear

    C. medial meniscus tear

    D. all of the above

82. Your patient with medial compartment knee osteoarthritis is asking which type of orthotic can relieve pressure off her knee. You recommend

A. heel lifts.

B. medial wedge shoe insoles.

C. patellar tendon strap.

D. valgus brace.

83. Which physical examination maneuver tests for injury to the anterior cruciate ligament (ACL) of the knee?

A. Apley grind

B. posterior drawer

C. Lachman

D. McMurray

84. Your patient informs you that she wants to try glucosamine-chondroitin for her knee osteoarthritis (OA) because it helped a friend of hers and her dog. You inform her that

A. she should not pursue it as there are no studies that show it is effective.

B. the scientific evidence is conflicting, but it is generally safe to try.

C. intra-articular injections could be effective in mild OA with pain relief up to 24 weeks.

D. she is foolish to pursue this type of "voodoo medicine."

85. A 19-year-old male college cross-country runner presents with 6-month history of progressively worsening pain, numbness, and swelling in both his lower legs that occurs during exercise and resolves within 30 minutes of rest. The initial physical examination is completely normal in the office. You ask the patient to run around the building for 15 minutes and immediately run back to the exam room. When he returns, you notice the bilateral anterolateral shins are tense upon palpation with bulging of the tibialis anterior muscles. Which diagnosis is suggested by this vignette?

A. medial tibial stress syndrome

B. stress fracture of the tibia

C. chronic exertional compartment syndrome

D. tibialis anterior muscle strains

86. Injury to which ligament would be involved in a high ankle sprain?

A. calcaneofibular

B. anterior inferior tibiofibular

C. anterior talofibular

D. posterior talofibular

87. Which of the following is NOT an indication for obtaining an ankle x-ray after an acute sprain injury?

A. positive anterior drawer test

B. pain in malleolar region

C. bone tenderness posterior edge or tip of lateral and/or medial malleolus up to 6 cm

D. inability to bear weight immediately and in emergency room

88. Regarding Achilles tendon rupture:

A. It occurs more often in females than males.

B. It most commonly occurs at the insertion site of the tendon.

C. A positive Thompson test elicits plantarflexion when the calf is squeezed.

D. The main risk for nonsurgical treatment is increased rate of rerupture.

89. Acquired flatfoot deformity involves which tendon?

A. posterior tibialis

B. extensor hallucis longus

C. peroneus longus

D. flexor digitorum longus

90. Treatment for plantar fasciitis includes

A. night splint.

B. stretching of gastrocnemius and soleus.

C. footwear modification.

D. all of the above

91. Initial treatment for acute Jones fracture is most often

A. stiff-soled shoe.

B. non–weight-bearing cast.

C. external fixator.

D. walker boot.

92. An orthotic prescription for clawfoot deformity would ideally consist of

A. heel lift.

B. longitudinal arch support.

C. extra high toe box.

D. UCBL orthosis.

93. Which ballet dance foot overuse injury is often associated with a symptomatic os trigonum?

A. flexor hallucis longus (FHL) tendon dysfunction

B. posterior ankle impingement

C. sesamoid stress fracture

D. both A and B

94. The female athlete triad refers to

   A. a constellation of tendon overuse injuries that occurs in female throwing athletes.

   B. a structured training program to prevent anterior cruciate ligament, medial meniscus, and medial collateral ligament injuries in competitive female athletes.

   C. the presence of metabolic syndrome, polycystic ovarian syndrome, and thyroid disorder in female athletes between ages 15 and 21 years.

   D. the interrelationship among energy availability, menstrual function, and bone mineral density in female athletes.

95. The most prevalent type of primary headache is

   A. migraine.

   B. tension-type.

   C. cluster.

   D. exertional.

96. You see a patient referred to you for pain medication management who takes acetaminophen-codeine 4 to 6 times daily. The patient's initial urine drug test result is summarized below.

Test	Result
Morphine	Positive
Hydrocodone	Negative
Codeine	Positive
Hydromorphone	Negative
6-Monoacetylmorphine	Negative
Norhydrocodone	Negative

What can be determined from the above information?

   A. The patient is taking codeine.

   B. The patient is using heroin.

   C. The patient is taking codeine and morphine.

   D. The patient is taking codeine, morphine, and hydrocodone.

97. Which of the following is a risk factor for prescription opioid misuse?

    A. female sex

    B. increased medical complexity

    C. nonopioid substance abuse

    D. high pain visual analog score

98. In order to diagnose complex regional pain syndrome (CRPS),

    A. bone scan must be positive.

    B. erythrocyte sediment rate must be elevated.

    C. history and physical examination is necessary.

    D. sympathetic nerve block must be positive.

99. Which therapeutic approach for chronic pain management is based on the premise that changing a person's perspective on his or her pain can impact his or her pain-related and functional outcomes? It uses coping skills training, education and rationale, relaxation and imagery, goal setting, pacing, restructuring negative thoughts, and distraction as some of its tools.

    A. cognitive behavioral therapy

    B. psychodynamic psychotherapy

    C. Feldenkrais Method®

    D. biofeedback

100. All the following are considered first-line medications for neuropathic pain, EXCEPT

    A. gabapentin.

    B. duloxetine.

    C. oxycodone.

    D. capsaicin.

ANSWER KEY WITH EXPLANATIONS

1. The correct answer is B.

The myofibril is the smallest anatomic structure, and within each myofibril, the smallest contractile unit is the sarcomere. Structures from largest to smallest: The muscle belly contains fascicles; fascicles are bundles of muscle fibers (cells); muscle fibers contain myofibrils; myofibrils contain sarcomeres; sarcomeres contain actin and myosin filaments.

2. The correct answer is A.

The length of a sarcomere spans from Z line to Z line. Actin fibers are thin filaments that contain troponin and tropomyosin. Actin fibers only are found in the I band (from two adjacent sarcomeres), and they anchor to the Z line. Myosin fibers are thick filaments containing cross-bridges that bind with actin during muscle contraction. Myosin fibers are found in the H zone and anchor to the M-Line.

3. The correct answer is A.

ATP is both required for myosin cross-bridges to reach a high-energy, flexed configuration before actin binding and, also, for uncoupling of myosin from actin. Nerve action potential leads to calcium release from the sarcoplasmic reticulum into the myofibril to cause muscle contraction. The muscle relaxes when calcium is pumped back into the sarcoplasmic reticulum. The sarcomere length–tension relationship is an important concept in muscle physiology—the optimal resting length of muscle is demonstrated as the peak in a downward parabola graph (x axis = length and y axis = tension). At very short resting muscle length, there is low force potential due to excessive overlap of actin and myosin filaments and further tension from contraction cannot be generated. At very long resting muscle length, there is low force potential due to not enough myofilament overlap to create effective cross-bridges and generate tension. The "sweet spot" of resting muscle length is where there is optimal myofilament alignment that can generate the most cross-bridges and generate the most tension.

4. The correct answer is B.

Normal muscle tissue appears hypoechoic on musculoskeletal ultrasound examination with fine hyperechoic streaks, representing the septa (perimysium). Normal bone surface, ligament, and tendon have hyperechoic appearances.

5. The correct answer is D.

Fast eccentric muscle contractions generate the most force. Fast concentric contractions generate the least force.

6. The correct answer is C.

Progressive resistive exercise is isotonic; the muscle changes length at variable speed to overcome a fixed external resistance. Isometric exercise occurs at a constant muscle length with exertion against an immovable or static object; the external resistance is equal to the muscle's internal contractile force. Isokinetic exercise involves changing muscle length and occurs via use of specialized machines that ensure variable resistance at a constant velocity. There is no such thing as "isoneutral" exercise.

7. The correct answer is D.

During aerobic exercise, there is an increase in systolic blood pressure. The remainder of the answer choices are normal findings during aerobic exercise.

8. The correct answer is C.

Manual muscle testing: 0/5 = no movement, 1/5 = trace contraction, 2/5 = active movement with gravity eliminated, 3/5 = active movement against gravity, 4/5 = active movement against gravity and resistance, 5/5 = normal movement

9. The correct answer is A.

Initial management of acute phase muscle strain injuries is a period of RICE—rest, ice, compression, and elevation. Downhill running is not advised as it places significant strain on the quadriceps muscles due to eccentric concentrations that could cause further muscle damage. Continuing a regular, high-intensity training program, while masking pain with nonsteroidal anti-inflammatory drugs (NSAIDs) is not the best recommendation of the listed answer choices. It is too early in the rehabilitation course to be prescribing plyometrics such as depth jumping; they are typically added in once patient is pain free.

10. The correct answer is D.

Cyclobenzaprine is a central nervous system depressant with properties of a tricyclic antidepressant. Almost all prescription medications considered "muscle relaxants" do not have direct action on the skeletal muscle. An example of a GABA agonist is baclofen. An example of an alpha-2 agonist is tizanidine.

11. The correct answer is D.

All the answer choices were found to be reliable indicators of active myofascial trigger points.

12. The correct answer is D.

Thrombin and/or calcium chloride are commonly used to activate PRP. Presence of collagen can also activate PRP.

13. The correct answer is C.

All the answer choices represent PRP growth factors secreted from alpha granules after platelet activation. PDGF and TGF-β are the main growth factors in PRP. Among other roles, TGF-β has primary function of synthesis and preservation of the extracellular matrix. PDGF is the main mitogenic growth factor in PRP.

14. The correct answer is B.

Tendinopathy is characterized by ischemic and myxoid degeneration, not chronic inflammation. Tendinopathy appears with tendon thickening, hypoechoic appearing areas of tendon with focal loss of fibrillar echotexture. Neovascularity can be found in tendinopathy and will show up on ultrasound power or color Doppler.

15. The correct answer is C.

Low body weight is a risk factor for fragility fracture associated with osteopenia and osteoporosis, not obesity.

16. The correct answer is C.

The Z-score is age-matched to the population and considers sex and ethnicity in cases where adequate reference data exist. According to the International Society for Clinical Densitometry (ISCD), Z-score is useful in children, premenopausal women, and men younger than 50 years. Z-scores of −2.0 below standard deviation are considered "below expected range for age." For men older than 50 years and postmenopausal women, the T-score is preferred. T-score is the number of standard deviations that a subject's bone mineral density is above or below the reference value for a healthy young adult. T-score −1.0 to −2.5 is osteopenia. T-score −2.5 and less is osteoporosis.

The FRAX® combines clinical risk factors with or without femoral neck bone mineral density. There's no such thing as X-score.

17. The correct answer is A.

Previous fracture strongly predicts likelihood of future fracture. Both clinical risk factors and BMD score determine fracture risk. Most fragility fractures occur in those who meet BMD criteria for osteopenia (DXA T-scores between −1.0 and −2.5) because osteopenia is more prevalent in the population than osteoporosis. FRAX® calculates the 10-year probability of hip or other major osteoporotic fracture. Recent consensus statements have recommended treatment for osteoporosis in those men and postmenopausal women age 50 years or older with history previous fracture (hip or vertebral), osteopenia with FRAX® risk hip fracture of ≥3% with risk major osteoporotic fracture of ≥20%, or BMD −2.5 or less (femoral neck or spine). For more information, please refer to the "Suggested Readings" section for articles: "The Clinical Diagnosis of Osteoporosis: A Position Statement from the National Bone Health Alliance Working Group," "The Assessment of Fracture Risk," and "Clinician's Guide to Prevention and Treatment of Osteoporosis."

18. The correct answer is D.

Full weight-bearing exercise and muscle strengthening or resistance training would be more beneficial in maintaining and improving bone mass than cardiovascular, endurance, partial weight offloading, and exercise without resistance or weight.

19. The correct answer is C.

Vertebrae have a high proportion of trabecular bone compared to long bones.

20. The correct answer is B.

Malignant bone tumors, such as classic osteosarcoma most frequently involve the metaphysis of lone bones. Classic osteosarcoma is most common in the first to second decades of life and most commonly found in the femur and tibia. Benign bone tumors most often have geographic, well-circumscribed borders. Malignant tumors, on the other hand, are more likely to present with diffuse "moth eaten" or "permeative" appearances.

21. The correct answer is A.

The acromioclavicular joint is a synovial plane joint. The first sternocostal joint is a synchondrosis cartilaginous joint. The rest of the sternocostal joints are synovial plane joints. The pubic symphysis is a cartilaginous joint. The skull is a fibrous joint.

22. The correct answer is D.

Normal or noninflammatory synovial fluid typically has high viscosity, good mucin clotting, <2,000 leukocytes/mm^3, and less than 25% PMNs. In contrast, noninfectious inflammatory fluid typically has more than 2,000 leukocytes/mm^3, decreased viscosity, fair to poor mucin clotting, and 25% to 75% PMNs. Septic synovial fluid is typically opaque, low viscosity, poor mucin clotting, >80,000 leukocytes/mm^3, and >75% PMNs. Tables and information are found in *Current Diagnosis & Treatment in Orthopedics*, 3rd edition, and *DeLisa's Physical Medicine & Rehabilitation: Principles and Practice* (see "Suggested Readings" section).

23. The correct answer is C.

Gout crystals are monosodium urate with negative birefringence. Gout is known for asymmetric joint involvement, subcutaneous nodules (tophi), and erosion seen on radiographs. Pseudogout crystals are calcium pyrophosphate with positive birefringence, symmetric joint involvement, and chondrocalcinosis seen on x-ray.

24. The correct answer is B.

Allopurinol reduces the production of uric acid (inhibits xanthine oxidase). Probenecid inhibits reabsorption of urate in the renal tubules which induces urinary excretion (uricosuria). Colchicine, a medication commonly used for acute gout flares, is thought to act at the immune system level to mitigate the inflammatory enzymes produced by neutrophils and monocytes as well as inhibit microtubule assembly. Indomethacin is a nonsteroidal anti-inflammatory medication that inhibits prostaglandins and cyclooxygenase.

25. The correct answer is D.

Morning stiffness of at least 1 hour or greater is most suggestive of rheumatoid arthritis.

26. The correct answer is B.

The distal interphalangeal (DIP) joint is least likely to be affected in rheumatoid arthritis. DIP joints are most often affected in osteoarthritis. The other answer choices are joints commonly affected by rheumatoid arthritis.

27. The correct answer is C.

Marginal bone erosions and juxtaarticular osteopenia are radiographic findings characteristic of RA. The joint space narrowing in RA is more likely symmetric than asymmetric. The other answer choices are characteristic of osteoarthritis.

28. The correct answer is D.

The Swan-neck deformity of rheumatoid arthritis involves hyperextension of the proximal interphalangeal joint and flexion of the distal interphalangeal joint.

29. The correct answer is C.

A combination of the inflammatory pannus and enzymes released by immune cells in response to antigen-antibody complexes causes joint and soft tissue destruction. The pannus is thick, hypertrophic synovium containing activated immune cells, including monocytes. Osteoclasts (not osteoblasts) have been found to play a role in bone destruction in rheumatoid arthritis.

30. The correct answer is A.

RF positive status predicts poor prognosis in RA along with other factor (including but not limited to) rheumatoid nodules, erosive changes on radiographs, insidious onset, low education level. RF is autoantibody to a fragment of IgG molecules and is present in about 75% of patients with RA. Thus, there are people who meet the 2010 American College of Rheumatology (ACR) classification criteria for RA who test negative for RF. RF is not specific for RA and can be found in other diseases (e.g., hepatitis), but anti-citrullinated protein antibody is specific for RA.

31. The correct answer is C.

Planovalgus (pronation) foot deformities are well known to occur in those with RA in addition to forefoot complication, such as plantar subluxation of the metatarsal heads, hammertoes, and great toe hallux valgus. Protrusio acetabuli is intrapelvic protrusion of the acetabulum in the hip. In the upper cervical spine, atlantoaxial instability occurs from erosion of the alar and transverse ligaments. Ulnar deviation of the metacarpophalangeal joints is a characteristic deformity in the hands of those with RA.

32. The correct answer is D.

All these forms of exercise have shown some benefit for strengthening weak muscles in those with rheumatoid arthritis. The one rehabilitation caution to be aware of is not to perform these strengthening exercises on an acutely inflamed joint as research has suggested it may worsen symptoms (even in the case of isometrics which were previously thought to be safe during acute flares). Of all the choices, isometrics produce the least joint stress and could be started in subacute phase after flare-ups.

33. The correct answer is A.

The 2015 American College of Rheumatology (ACR) recommendation for rheumatoid arthritis treatment recommend a "treat-to-target" strategy for managing early disease because the goal is to slow disease progression and joint destruction. Methotrexate is a classic disease-modifying anti-rheumatic drug (DMARD) and would be most appropriate for monotherapy. Sulindac is a nonsteroidal anti-inflammatory medication that does not affect the progression of autoimmune disease. Etanercept is an example of a biologic agent (tumor necrosis factor inhibitor) recommended for those with moderate to high disease activity despite DMARD. If disease activity remains moderate or high despite DMARD or biologic therapy, consider a low-dose glucocorticoid. The full 2015 guidelines can be accessed (at time of print) at https://www.rheumatology.org/Portals/0/Files /ACR%202015%20RA%20Guideline.pdf.

34. The correct answer is A.

This clinical vignette is most consistent with the clinical features of polymyalgia rheumatica (PMR). This condition affects individuals age 50 years and older with peak from 70 to 80 years. PMR predominantly affects females and responds rapidly to corticosteroids, which are the mainstay of treatment. Notice that review of systems mentioned the clinician asked about headache or vision changes. That is because PMR is related to another vasculitis disorder, giant cell (temporal) arteritis.

35. The correct answer is A.

Raynaud phenomenon is associated with systemic sclerosis (scleroderma), which is not a type of spondyloarthropathy. The other three answer choices are commonly associated with seronegative spondyloarthropathies.

36. The correct answer is C.

The spine forms a three-joint complex with the level below it. It is composed of the two zygapophyseal (facet) synovial joints and the syndesmosis intervertebral joint.

37. The correct answer is B.

To answer the question, you will need to review anatomy of the lumbar spinal nerve roots to identify where the left S1 nerve root would be compressed by a disc herniation. At L5-S1 level, the L5 nerve roots are exiting out of the lateral foramina on each side. The bilateral S1 nerves are more medial in location, traversing inferiorly through the spinal canal to exit at the level below.

38. The correct answer is B.

The interventionalist will target the medial branches of L3, L4, and L5 dorsal ramus to cover the L4-5 and L5-S1 zygapophyseal joints. The medial branch and lateral branches are derived from the dorsal ramus at each level (if it is time to do quick anatomy review, see articles in the "Suggested Readings" section). Each facet joint receives innervation from the medial branches of two dorsal rami, from the one above and the one below. Thus, the L4-5 Z-joint receives innervation from the L3 and L4 medial branches. At the lumbosacral region, the L5 dorsal ramus runs a longer course than the other lumbar levels and is the most accessible target due to its anatomy. To target the L5-S1 Z-joint, the L4 medial branch and the L5 dorsal ramus are targeted.

39. The correct answer is D.

The correct answer describes Spurling neck compression test, which reproduces typical cervical radicular pain on the side tested. The straight-leg raise test for lower lumbar nerve root tension is positive between 30 and 70 degrees of supine leg elevation. The femoral nerve stretch test detects high lumbar disc herniation when prone patient reports anterior thigh pain in distribution of his or her usual symptoms when affected knee is flexed. The seated slump test for sciatica produces lower extremity pain on the side tested when the examiner dorsiflexes the extended ankle and applies forward pressure to the neck and upper back while patient flexes the spine with hands behind back.

40. The correct answer is A.

Erosions are a characteristic that distinguishes AS from DISH, along with ankylosis of the sacroiliac and zygapophyseal joints. DISH is characterized by "flowing" bridging ossifications of the anterior longitudinal ligament bridging at least three contiguous levels. Similar to AS, DISH has limitation in spine mobility and the presence of enthesopathies. Unlike AS, DISH is associated with diabetes mellitus (estimated 26% diabetics) and obesity. AS specifically has association with human leukocyte antigen (HLA) B27, and DISH does not.

41. The correct answer is B.

The C5-6 level is most often affected, followed by the C6-7 and C4-5 levels. This is thought to be because of increased segmental motion on this level.

42. The correct answer is A.

Transverse lesion syndrome is the most common presenting lesion of cervical spondylotic myelopathy. It predominantly involves the lower extremities from the spinothalamic, corticospinal, and posterior column tracts.

43. The correct answer is C.

The author's suggestive review of the common "red flags" that could suggest fracture, malignancy, severe neurologic injury, systemic disease, or infection. In addition to "red flags," there are "yellow flags" that suggest increased risk for prolonged course, "chronicization," and poor outcome from standard treatment.

44. The correct answer is C.

The SOMI is a three-poster cervicothoracic orthosis with chin and occipital supports that provides excellent restriction of flexion in the upper cervical segments. Therefore, it is ideal to use in atlantoaxial instability, which is primarily instability in direction of flexion. A standard hard cervical collar (e.g., Thomas-Type) will not provide enough flexion restriction. Traction is contraindicated in atlantoaxial instability. Neck strengthening exercise is probably not a good idea as immobilization is required if the spine is unstable.

45. The correct answer is C.

Of the listed answer choices, the Jewett is most ideal for a thoracic compression fracture. It is a thoracolumbosacral orthosis that best restricts flexion from T6-L1 levels. The Philadelphia is actually categorized as a head cervical orthosis, so it would not be useful for a thoracic compression fracture. The Milwaukee is a cervical thoracolumbosacral orthosis used for the treatment of scoliosis. The Chairback is a lumbosacral orthosis and would not provide motion restriction for lower thoracic region.

46. The correct answer is D.

The long head of the biceps femoris is not a hip flexor. It extends and adducts the hip. The primary hip flexor is the iliopsoas muscle complex. The other muscle that provide hip flexion are the sartorius, rectus femoris, pectineus, tensor fasciae latae, adductor brevis, adductor longus, adductor magnus, and gracilis.

47. The correct answer is C.
The function of the iliofemoral ligament (a.k.a. the Y-ligament of Bigelow) is to limit extension, abduction, and external rotation of the hip. It extends from the anterior inferior iliac spine to the intertrochanteric line. The ischiofemoral ligament extends from the ischium to the acetabular capsule. It functions to limit internal hip rotation. The pubofemoral ligament extends from the superior pubic ramus to the iliofemoral ligament and works to limit hip abduction.

48. The correct answer is B.
Compression-side (inferior) femoral neck stress fractures commonly are stable and are amenable to nonoperative management. Tension-side (superior, "transverse") femoral neck stress fractures have a high risk of progressing to displacement and typically undergo prophylactic fixation. Similarly, Garden type 2 (complete, nondisplaced) femoral neck stress fractures have risk displacement and are treated with fixation. Although intertrochanteric femur fractures can potentially be treated conservatively, surgeons opt for surgical fixation in the ambulatory patient who does not pose risk for surgical complication because early mobilization after fixation reduces rates of illness and mortality.

49. The correct answer is B.
In lateral snapping hip syndrome, either the iliotibial tract or the gluteus maximus is seen displacing over the greater trochanter when the patient reproduces the snap. In medial snapping hip syndrome, the iliopsoas tendon displaces over the iliopectineal eminence when the patient reproduces the snap.

50. The correct answer is D.
Sciatic nerve injury is present in 10% to 20% of those who have sustained a posterior hip dislocation. Posterior hip dislocation is more common than anterior. Posterior hip dislocation presents with hip adduction, internal rotation, and shortening of the affected limb. Closed reduction can be successful when performed in a timely manner and in the absence of acetabular fracture.

51. The correct answer is A.
FADIR is a provocative maneuver for piriformis syndrome. FABERE is a provocative maneuver for intra-articular hip disorders.

52. The correct answer is D.
The integrity of the posterior sacroiliac ligament complex is the most important determinant of pelvic stability following trauma, as the posterior pelvis provides most of the stability. Pelvic ring fractures involving two or more structures are unstable to varying degrees. Disruption to the weaker anterior sacroiliac ligaments and pubic symphysis and anteriorly displaced fractures results in rotational instability. Further disruption involving the posterior arch and sacroiliac ligaments would result in vertical instability as well.

53. The correct answer is B.

The superior hypogastric plexus receives sensory input from the pelvic viscera, and this nerve block is considered for endometriosis-related pelvic pain unresponsive to conservative treatment. Peripheral nerve blocks of the pudendal and iliohypogastric nerves are considered for neuropathic pain syndromes involving the specific distributions of these nerves. Lumbar sympathetic plexus blocks are most often used for those with complex regional pain syndrome involving the lower limb(s).

54. The correct answer is B.

Osteonecrosis or avascular necrosis (AVN) of the femoral head is most commonly associated with heavy alcohol consumption (20% to 40%) or corticosteroid use (20% to 40%) in the United States. Although the patient's age does increase risk of osteoarthritis, he is of male gender with a normal BMI. Although he is in age range for rheumatoid arthritis, the vignette does not supply any further information suggestive of increased risk rheumatoid arthritis (female, family history, smoking). Although is male and in the appropriate age range, he is apparently free of sexually transmitted infection and had no recent illness making reactive arthritis less likely. Human leukocyte antigen (HLA) B27 status was not provided, so this could not be factored in.

55. The correct answer is A.

The most common direction of instability is anterior inferior. External rotation and abduction of the arm can promote this movement. Complications can include injury to the axillary nerve. Posterior glenohumeral instability is less common and may occur in patients with seizure. Patients may also incur this type of instability after a fall on an arm that is adducted and flexed forward and can present with an internally rotated adducted arm. Multidirectional instability is even more rare and may be found in patients with generally hypermobile joints.

56. The correct answer is C.

The humerus naturally externally rotates with abduction.

57. The correct answer is D.

Medial scapular winging occurs due to weakness of the serratus anterior muscle. It presents as winging of the medial border of the scapula away from the ribs and is more obvious when the patient flexes his arms forward or pushes against a wall. The serratus anterior is innervated by the long thoracic nerve. Lateral scapular winging is due to weakness of the trapezius muscle, which is innervated by the spinal accessory nerve. It appears as a rotation of the scapula around the thorax. Trapezius strength can be tested by resistance to shrug (for the upper fibers of the muscle) and by a prone row for the middle and lower fibers of the muscle.

58. The correct answer is C.

The median nerve is the least likely to be affected significantly in a proximal humeral fracture. The axillary nerve may often be involved, and the radial and ulnar nerves are sometimes affected. Depending on the exact area of injury, there may be involvement of the axillary artery.

59. The correct answer is A.

This position is the classic "Erb palsy," "waiter's tip" position is associated with upper trunk brachial plexus injury (and also C5-6 nerve roots). Make sure you both memorize and conceptually understand the physical examination manifestations of brachial plexus injuries for the board examination.

60. The correct answer is C.

The vignette describes the classic presentation of "burner," "stinger" stretch injury (i.e., brachial plexus neurapraxia). In most cases, recovery is achieved within minutes without further complications or recurrence. The athlete can return to play as long as the cervical spine and shoulder examinations are normal, symptoms of brachial plexus neuralgia (burning pain, numbness, tingling) are absent, and sensorimotor examination is normal. The athlete should not return to play if symptoms remain, and residual symptoms can be referred for further medical work-up, including magnetic resonance imaging (MRI) and/or electrodiagnostic testing. Because symptoms are nerve-related, anti-inflammatories used for sprain/strain injury are not as useful in treatment.

61. The correct answer is B.

The anchor origin for the long head of the biceps brachii tendon is torn in a high-grade SLAP tear types 4 to 7. Type 1 SLAP injury is fraying of the superior capsulolabrum. Type 2 SLAP injury (most common) is detachment of the superior capsulolabrum from the glenoid. Type 3 SLAP is a bucket handle tear of the labrum. Type 4 SLAP is a bucket handle tear extending to the biceps tendon. Types 5 to 7 describe varying degrees biceps tendon and/or labrum separation.

62. The correct answer is D.

The clinical vignette is suggestive of subacromial rotator cuff impingement syndrome. The Neer impingement test is performed by passive flexion and internal rotation of the shoulder. A positive test will elicit typical pain symptoms. Gerber (lift-off) test is for subscapularis tendon tear. Speed test is for biceps tenosynovitis. O'Brien test is for superior labrum anterior posterior (SLAP) tear.

63. The correct answer is A.

"Cuff tear arthropathy" has been the classic orthopedic surgery indication for reverse shoulder arthroplasty, an irreparable rotator cuff tear associated with glenohumeral arthritis. In a reverse arthroplasty, the ball is embedded in the glenoid and the socket in the humerus. Traditional shoulder arthroplasty can be considered when rotator cuff is intact in uncomplicated cases of glenohumeral osteoarthritis. Multidirectional instability responds most often to nonoperative measures. Axillary neuropathy is a contraindication because intact deltoid lever muscle function is integral to the arthroplasty prosthesis function.

64. The correct answer is D.

The Hills-Sachs lesion refers to a compression fracture of the posterolateral humerus in setting of anterior shoulder dislocation.

65. The correct answer is B.

The type IV injury involves posterior clavicle displacement with buttonhole through the trapezius fascia. Both types III and IV injuries have complete tears of the acromioclavicular and coracoclavicular ligaments. Type II injuries have intact coracoclavicular ligaments and will not show displacement on radiographs. Type VI injury will involve inferior displacement of the clavicle.

66. The correct answer is B.

Cozen test is a provocative test primarily used for the evaluation of lateral epicondylitis (tennis elbow). This test involves the examiner holding the patient's elbow with the examiner's thumb just beyond the patient's lateral epicondyle. The examiner then resists the patient's movement of pronating the arm while extending the wrist with radial deviation with the hand clenched in a fist. The test can also be done with extension at the elbow. It is positive with pain at the lateral epicondyle to the resisted movement. Repeated wrist extension or forearm supination causes the injury.

67. The correct answer is C.

Repetitive or excessive valgus forces placed on the medial elbow in throwing are responsible for pathologic conditions, such as medial epicondylitis, valgus extension overload syndrome, and ulnar (medial) collateral ligament sprain. Lateral epicondylitis is associated with racquet sports, such as tennis where there is overload of the supinator and extensor tendons or in cases of activities where there is repetitive wrist extension.

68. The correct answer is A.

Although all the answer choices are potential sites, the cubital tunnel is the most common site of ulnar nerve compression/entrapment.

69. The correct answer is C.

Posterior is the most common direction of elbow dislocation. Mechanism of injury is fall on outstretched hand. Complications include loss of range of motion in extension (typically 5 to 10 degrees).

70. The correct answer is A.

The sixth extensor compartment of the wrist contains the extensor carpi ulnaris.

71. The correct answer is A.

Most of the blood flow to the scaphoid bone is distal. Therefore, fractures of the proximal pole have highest chance nonunion and AVN. The waist is located at the middle portion and has moderate chance nonunion and AVN. Distal fracture site, including the tuberosity have least chance of union and AVN.

72. The correct answer is C.

Mallet finger is disruption of the terminal extensor tendon insertion site at the distal phalanx. Jersey finger is disruption of the flexor digitorum profundus tendon at the base of the distal phalanx. Swan-neck deformity is injury or laxity of the volar plate at the proximal interphalangeal joint, resulting in unrestrained hyperextension. Boutonnière deformity is disruption of the central slip tendon insertion on the dorsal proximal phalanx.

73. The correct answer is B.

CTS is a clinical diagnosis, supported by electrodiagnostic test findings. Electrodiagnostic studies can be normal in patients with clinical CTS. Tinel test is NOT the most sensitive test for CTS (wrist compression and Phalen test are more sensitive). Actually, Tinel test has a low sensitivity of 25% to 44% and a high specificity of 94% to 98%. This is detailed in Malanga's *Musculoskeletal Physical Examination* book (see "Suggested Readings" section). Ultrasound is emerging as an accurate complimentary tool to support the clinical diagnosis by measurement of the cross-sectional area of the median nerve proximal to the level of the pisiform, ≥ 10 mm^2 is considered positive according to Jacobson's *Fundamentals of Musculoskeletal Ultrasound* (see "Suggested Readings" section).

74. The correct answer is A.

The extensor carpi ulnaris sheath, not the digiti minimi, is part of the TFCC. All the remaining answer choices are part of the TFCC.

75. The correct answer is D.

The vignette describes the thumb CMC grind test as being positive, indicating pain in this joint. The vignette describes negative Finkelstein and UCL testing, making these diagnoses less likely. There is no report of triggering or catching, making trigger thumb less likely.

76. The correct answer is B.

According to *Current Diagnosis & Treatment in Orthopedics*, the boxer's fracture involves the neck of the fourth or fifth metacarpal. In an uncomplicated metacarpal neck fracture (mild angulation), the hand should be splinted with metacarpophalangeal joint(s) in 70- to 90-degree flexion, proximal interphalangeal (PIP) + distal interphalangeal (DIP) in slight flexion, wrist in slight extension to prevent joint stiffness, ligament shortening, and contractures. The ulnar gutter splint immobilizes the metacarpals on the ulnar side of the hand. The thumb spica is obviously best suited for thumb injuries. Sugar tong splint is used to stabilize wrist and distal forearm fractures.

77. The correct answer is D.

The question describes the location of the pes anserinus bursa, one of the three medial bursae of the knee. The prepatellar bursa is superficial, under the skin of the anterior patella. The suprapatellar bursa is located between the femur and the quadriceps femoris muscle. There are three lateral bursae, two of which involve the popliteus muscle as an anatomic landmark.

78. The correct answer is A.

CPM is a popular device used in the immediate postoperative period following total knee arthroplasty. Despite its popularity, systematic reviews have shown no conclusive evidence that CPM should be a standard of care following uncomplicated TKA and has not been shown to reduce hospital stay. Similarly, in systematic reviews, CPM has no conclusive evidence that it reduces venous thromboembolism (VTE). For more information, see "Suggested Readings" section articles "Cochrane in CORR®: Continuous Passive Motion Following Total Knee Arthroplasty in People with Arthritis (Review)" and "Continuous Passive Motion for Preventing Venous Thromboembolism After Total Knee Arthroplasty."

79. The correct answer is A.
Small tears at the outer periphery of the meniscus are in the vascular (red–red) zone and are most likely to heal. Tears in the middle third (red–white) zone have intermediate potential to heal. Tears of the inner third of the meniscus are in the avascular (white–white) zone and are least likely to heal.

80. The correct answer is B.
Patellofemoral pain syndrome is a very common cause of anterior knee pain in runners and is thought to be caused by abnormal patellar tracking. Popliteus strain would cause posterior knee pain. Iliotibial band syndrome would cause lateral knee pain. Pes anserine bursitis would cause inferior medial knee pain.

81. The correct answer is D.
All the answer choices can occur simultaneously in the setting of an ACL injury. The "unhappy" O'Donoghue triad refers to ACL, medial meniscus, and medial meniscus tears occurring together in contact sports due to an active valgus force applied to a flexed and rotated knee. The "pivot shift" is a noncontact ACL injury (often seen in skiers and basketball players) due to rapid deceleration, also with valgus knee stress while the knee is flexed and rotated. When the ACL tears by way of the aforementioned forces, the lateral femoral condyle can impact the posterolateral tibial plateau, causing a bone contusion.

82. The correct answer is D.
A valgus (medial compartment offloading/unloading) brace relieves pressure off the knee with medial arthritis by external application of a valgus load that shifts pressure away from the medial compartment. Similarly, lateral wedge insoles are suggested as another way to alter tibiofemoral alignment to relieve pressure off the medial compartment. Conversely, a varus brace and medial wedge insoles would relieve pressure off the lateral compartment.

83. The correct answer is C.
Lachman test is used to test the ACL, which provides anterior stability to the knee. A positive test will demonstrate anterior displacement of the tibia on the femur with no firm endpoint. The anterior drawer test (not posterior drawer) also tests the ACL but is considered less sensitive. The McMurray and Apley grind tests are for meniscus injury.

84. The correct answer is B.
The evaluation and decision process whether or not to recommend supplements and other forms of complementary medicine is the same as evaluating any other medical treatment. One simplistic way to conceptualize risk–benefit analysis is to consider four categories: high safety + high efficacy, high safety + low efficacy, low safety + high efficacy, and low safety + low efficacy. In the case of glucosamine-chondroitin for OA, small studies have shown efficacy, but larger studies and meta-analyses have not shown conclusive evidence for its efficacy. It is generally safe; therefore, the risk is low for the motivated patient with a flexible budget to try it for a period of time to see whether or not she notices a benefit. Hyaluronic acid (not glucosamine-chondroitin) has evidence for relieving pain in less advanced cases of knee OA. Shaming a patient for wanting to try a supplement for her condition is never advised as the doctor–patient relationship should be collaborative and educational, not condescending or antagonistic.

85. The correct answer is C.

The vignette suggests clinical diagnosis of chronic exertional compartment syndrome because of the condition duration, symptoms triggered by exercise and relieved by rest, normal physical examination at rest, and tense posterolateral compartment with muscle herniation after exertion. The gold standard for diagnosis would be compartment pressure testing (an invasive manometric study). First, you would want to exclude other differential diagnoses. Medial tibial stress syndrome (MTSS) would be suggested by initial pain with exercise that decreases after warming up and then often symptomatic again after activity. Classic physical examination for MTSS is diffuse tenderness to palpation along the junction of the upper two-thirds and lower third of the medial tibia border. Stress fracture would present with focal pain and tenderness at the fracture site along the medial tibia border; pain becomes more severe as exercise continues and can occur at rest. Muscle strains are generally acute and not typically bilateral with finding muscle tenderness and pain with contraction of the muscle on physical examination.

86. The correct answer is B.

The anterior inferior tibiofibular ligament is a syndesmotic ligament. Syndesmotic (high) ankle sprains are considered a severe form of ankle sprain that takes longer to heal. The rest of the answer choices are lateral ankle ligaments that could potentially be injured in an inversion sprain.

87. The correct answer is A.

The other answer choices describe the Ottawa ankle rules for obtaining ankle radiograph series in acute ankle injury.

88. The correct answer is D.

Surgical treatment is recommended for athletes/active individuals. Nonsurgical treatment with cast immobilization is recommended for those who are sedentary or at high risk for surgical complications. Nonsurgical treatment runs higher risk of rerupture than surgical repair. Achilles rupture occurs more often in males than females (10:1 ratio). It most commonly occurs at the watershed area 3 to 6 cm proximal to tendon insertion. A negative Thompson test elicits plantarflexion when the calf is squeezed; a positive Thompson test is when there is no plantar movement with the calf is squeezed.

89. The correct answer is A.

Posterior tibialis tendon dysfunction is a cause of acquired flatfoot deformity.

90. The correct answer is D.

All the listed answer choices are treatment options for plantar fasciitis.

91. The correct answer is B.

The Jones fracture (zone 2) of the metaphyseal–diaphyseal junction at the base of the fifth metatarsal is most often non–weight-bearing cast for at least 6 weeks. These fractures take longer to heal than other metatarsal fractures and have higher rates of nonunion due to decreased vascularity in the region of the fracture. This is not to be confused with an avulsion fracture of the base of the fifth metatarsal (dancer's fracture) which initially can be treated with a walker boot.

92. The correct answer is C.

Clawfoot/claw toe deformity requires a shoe with an extra high toe box to prevent crowding and chafing of the toes. University of California, Berkeley (UCBL) orthosis and longitudinal arch supports are used in case of flatfoot deformity. Heel lift (in one shoe) is for leg length discrepancy and bilateral heel lifts are useful to unload plantar fascia and the Achilles tendon.

93. The correct answer is D.

FHL tendon dysfunction/entrapment/stenosing tenosynovitis "dancer's tendonitis" often occurs with a coexisting symptomatic accessory os trigonum. Posterior ankle impingement occurs with "en pointe" extreme plantarflexion position when the calcaneus and posterior tibia impact the posterior talus; this can entrap an os trigonum (look up the anatomy and it will all make sense).

94. The correct answer is D.

The female athlete triad refers to the interrelationship among energy availability, menstrual function, and bone mineral density in female athletes. Intentional or unintentional disordered eating (low energy availability) can lead to menstrual irregularities, such as amenorrhea, as well as low bone mineral density in female athletes.

95. The correct answer is B.

According to Bonica's *Management of Pain* (see "Suggested Readings" section), tension-type headache is reported at prevalence of as high as 69%. Migraine is reported at 16%. Cluster is reported at 0.1%. Exertional is reported at 1%.

96. The correct answer is A.

A common error in interpreting urine drug test results is not realizing that the active metabolite of codeine is morphine. If the patient is taking codeine, he or she will be positive for both codeine and morphine. If the patient is taking both codeine and morphine, he or she will also be positive for hydromorphone because morphine is metabolized to hydromorphone. If the patient is using heroin, 6-monoacetylmorphine will be positive. If the patient is taking codeine, morphine, and hydrocodone, norhydrocodone and hydromorphone will be positive.

97. The correct answer is C.

Studies have shown those with co-occurring substance disorders and mental health disorders are at highest risk for opioid misuse. Other potential risk factors include white males, younger age, and family history of substance abuse.

98. The correct answer is C.

The diagnosis of CRPS is clinical and requires presence of symptoms or physical examination findings of sensory, vasomotor, sudomotor/edema, and motor/trophic disturbances. Bone scans and sympathetic nerve blocks can corroborate the diagnosis but are not mandatory to make the diagnosis.

99. The correct answer is A.

Cognitive behavioral therapy (CBT) is the most studied therapeutic approach to chronic pain management and has the strongest scientific evidence to support its effectiveness. Psychodynamic psychotherapy uncovers the client's history of relationships and life development to process unconscious factors affecting the client's current life with emphasis on self-reflection and the therapist–client relationship to achieve this. Feldenkrais uses slow, gentle movements to promote body awareness through somatic education. Biofeedback is a technique using equipment to monitor physiologic parameters and training clients to master voluntary control over physiologic responses related to pain and stress. Clients are given feedback in real-time about physiologic response and taught relaxation techniques to change parameters.

100. The correct answer is C.

Opioids are second-line treatments for neuropathic pain. The remainder of answer choices are first-line medications.

Board Review Points ("Pearls") for Musculoskeletal Medicine

Exercise Science

The length–tension curve of a muscle sarcomere. The length–tension curve of a sarcomere demonstrates how the length of the muscle sarcomere influences its force production.

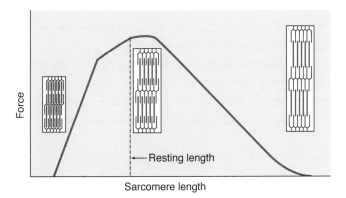

Reprinted with permission from Oatis CA. *Kinesiology: The Mechanics and Pathomechanics of Human Movement.* Baltimore, MD: Lippincott Williams & Wilkins; 2004.

- Fast eccentric muscle contractions generate the most force. Fast concentric contractions generate the least force.
- Rough estimate of maximal heart rate in healthy adults is 220 − age.
- Progressive resistive exercise is isotonic; the muscle changes length at variable speed to overcome a fixed external resistance

- Isometric exercise occurs at a constant muscle length with exertion against an immovable or static object; the external resistance is equal to the muscle's internal contractile force.
- Isokinetic exercise involves changing muscle length and occurs via use of specialized machines that ensure variable resistance at a constant velocity.

Bone Health

- Previous history of fracture due to low BMD predicts the greatest risk for future fracture. Most fractures occur in those who meet BMD criteria for osteopenia but not osteoporosis because osteopenia is more prevalent in the population.
- Vertebrae have a high proportion of trabecular bone compared to long bones.
- Malignant bone tumors, such as classic osteosarcoma, most frequently involve the metaphysis of lone bones.
- Classic osteosarcoma is most common in the first to second decades of life and most commonly found in the femur and tibia.

Rheumatology

- Rereview the pediatric rheumatology questions in the Pediatric Rehabilitation chapter.
- Normal or noninflammatory synovial fluid typically has high viscosity, good mucin clotting, <2,000 leukocytes/mm^3, and less than 25% PMNs. In contrast, noninfectious inflammatory fluid typically has more than 2,000 leukocytes/mm^3, decreased viscosity, fair to poor mucin clotting, and 25% to 75% PMNs. Septic synovial fluid is typically opaque, low viscosity, poor mucin clotting, >80,000 leukocytes/mm^3, and >75% PMNs. Information is from tables in *DeLisa's Physical Medicine & Rehabilitation: Principles and Practice* and Skinner's *Current Diagnosis & Treatment in Orthopedics*.
- Gout crystals are monosodium urate with negative birefringence. Gout is known for asymmetric joint involvement, subcutaneous nodules (tophi), and erosion seen on radiographs. Pseudogout crystals are calcium pyrophosphate with positive birefringence, symmetric joint involvement, and chondrocalcinosis seen on x-ray.
- Allopurinol reduces the production of uric acid (inhibits xanthine oxidase). Probenecid inhibits reabsorption of urate in the renal tubules which induces urinary excretion (uricosuria). Colchicine, a medication commonly used for acute gout flares, is thought to act at the immune system level to mitigate the inflammatory enzymes produced by neutrophils and monocytes as well as inhibit microtubule assembly. Indomethacin is a nonsteroidal anti-inflammatory medication that inhibits prostaglandins and cyclooxygenase.
- Marginal bone erosions and juxtaarticular osteopenia are radiographic findings characteristic of rheumatoid arthritis.
- In patients with polymyalgia rheumatica, also evaluate for signs and symptoms of giant cell (temporal) arteritis. These vasculitis disorders are related!

- Psoriatic arthritis (PA) is considered a spondyloarthropathy. PA changes in nails: pitting, grooves, subungual hyperkeratosis; PA changes in fingers: "telescoping" on clinical exam or "pencil in cup" appearance of DIP on x-rays.
- Fatigue is common barrier to rehabilitation in patient in systemic lupus erythematosus.
- Systemic sclerosis (scleroderma)–associated CREST syndrome (calcinosis, Raynaud phenomenon, esophageal dysmotility, sclerodactyly, and telangiectasia)
- The seronegative spondyloarthropathies are AS, Reiter syndrome, PA, and inflammatory bowel disease–related arthritis. All have increased likelihood in those with positive HLA-B27.
- Reiter syndrome associated with chlamydia, shigella, salmonella, yersinia, campylobacter

Sports, Spine, Neuromusculoskeletal Disorders

- Rereview the pediatric musculoskeletal questions in the Pediatric Rehabilitation chapter.

Spine

- Things to know: spinal anatomy and the courses of spinal nerves, intervertebral discs, types of spine orthoses, interventional procedures, stenosis, spondylolisthesis, spondylosis, DISH, and AS. Rereview the spinal fractures and spinal cord syndromes in the Spine Trauma and Spinal Cord Injury Medicine chapter.
- Note that cervical disc problems most commonly occur at the C5-6 level, followed by the C6-7 and C4-5 levels. This is thought to be because of increased segmental motion on this level.
- Transverse lesion syndrome is the most common presenting lesion of cervical spondylotic myelopathy. It predominantly involves the lower extremities from the spinothalamic, corticospinal, and posterior column tracts.
- Straight-leg raise test for lower lumbar nerve root tension is positive between 30 and 70 degrees of supine leg elevation. The femoral nerve stretch test detects high lumbar disc herniation when prone patient reports anterior thigh pain in distribution of his or her usual symptoms when affected knee is flexed. The seated slump test for sciatica produces lower extremity pain on the side tested when the examiner dorsiflexes the extended ankle and applies forward pressure to the neck and upper back while patient flexes the spine with hands behind back.
- DISH is associated with diabetes mellitus (estimated 26% diabetics) and obesity. AS has association with HLA-B27. (Reference: Olivieri I, D'Angelo S, Palazzi C, Padula A, Mader R, Khan MA. Diffuse idiopathic skeletal hyperostosis: differentiation from ankylosing spondylitis. *Curr Rheumatol Rep.* 2009;11:321-328. doi:10.1007/s11926-009-0046-9; and Wyatt LH, Ferrance RJ. The musculoskeletal effects of diabetes mellitus. *J Can Chiropr Assoc.* 2006;50[1]:43-50.)

Hip

- Things to know: Review anatomy of muscles and their attachments around the hip as well as pelvic floor muscles. Know what muscles and nerves are responsible for leg movement in different directions, the hip physical examination, hip disorders such as osteoarthritis, greater trochanter bursitis, other types of bursitis, various muscle strains (hamstring, piriformis), "snapping" hip, hip dislocation, hip fracture, AVN of the femoral head, avulsion fractures (ischial tuberosity, anterior superior iliac spine, anterior inferior iliac spine), adductor strain, osteitis pubis.
- The function of the iliofemoral ligament (a.k.a. the Y-ligament of Bigelow) is to limit extension, abduction, and external rotation of the hip. The ischiofemoral ligament limits internal hip rotation. The pubofemoral ligament limits hip abduction.
- Compression-side (inferior) femoral neck stress fractures commonly are stable and are amenable to nonoperative management. Tension-side (superior, "transverse") femoral neck stress fractures have a high risk of progressing to displacement and typically undergo prophylactic fixation.
- Sciatic nerve injury is present in 10% to 20% of those who have sustained a posterior hip dislocation. Posterior hip dislocation is more common than anterior.
- Review types of pelvic fractures and know that the integrity of the posterior sacroiliac ligament complex is the most important determinant of pelvic stability following trauma.
- AVN is bilateral in 60% to 70% of case, check the other hip! Review causes and risk factors (corticosteroid use, alcohol, HIV, autoimmune disease, etc.).

Shoulder

- Things to know: Review what muscles and nerves are responsible for shoulder movement in different directions, shoulder girdle anatomy including rotator cuff, acromioclavicular joint injury, glenohumeral joint injury, rotator cuff injury, shoulder osteoarthritis, biceps injury, supraspinatus injury, adhesive capsulitis, scapular winging, clavicular fracture, humeral fracture, the shoulder physical examination.
- When performing the Empty Can test to examine the supraspinatus muscle, you will need to internally rotate the arm to accurately perform testing by resisting a patient's flexed, abducted, internally rotated arm. Neer test involves stabilizing the scapula and passively flexing the arm overhead, eliciting pain around 90 degrees. In Hawkin test, the scapula is stabilized; the patient's arm is held horizontal from the body and internally rotated. Pain is felt if the supraspinatus tendon compresses against the coracoid ligament.
- The classic "Erb palsy," "waiter's tip" position is associated with upper trunk brachial plexus injury (and also C5-6 nerve roots). Lower trunk brachial plexus (and also C8-T1 nerve roots) would appear as arm supinated, elbow flexed, wrist extended. Make sure you both memorize and conceptually understand the physical examination manifestations of brachial plexus injuries for the board examination.

Wrist/Hand

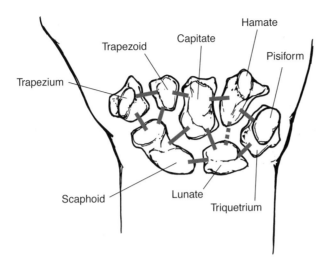

Reprinted with permission from Oatis CA. *Kinesiology: The Mechanics and Pathomechanics of Human Movement.* Baltimore, MD: Lippincott Williams & Wilkins; 2004.

- Things to know: Review wrist range of motion, the carpal bones, what muscles and nerves are responsible for wrist movement in various directions, common deformities (from injury, osteoarthritis, and rheumatoid arthritis), De Quervain tenosynovitis, ganglion cyst, osteonecrosis of the lunate, scaphoid fracture, hamate fracture, trapezium fracture, fracture of the distal radius. Review: bones of the hand, function of the tendons, digit range of motion, muscles and nerves responsible for finger movement, Dupuytren contracture, stenosing tenosynovitis (trigger finger), ligament injuries, injury of the flexor digitorum (jersey finger), mallet finger, common fractures of the metacarpals, CMC joint arthritis.
- Contents of the other wrist extensor compartments are
  - ☐ Compartment 1—abductor pollicis longus, extensor pollicis brevis
  - ☐ Compartment 2—extensor carpi radialis longus, extensor carpi radialis brevis
  - ☐ Compartment 3—extensor pollicis longus
  - ☐ Compartment 4—extensor digitorum communis, extensor indices proprius
  - ☐ Compartment 5—extensor digiti minimi
  - ☐ Compartment 6—extensor carpi ulnaris

Knee

- Things to know: Review what muscles and nerves are responsible for knee movement in different directions, joint compartments, bony prominences, ligamentous and meniscus anatomy, knee bursae, knee physical examination, knee disorders such as ACL/posterior cruciate ligament (PCL)/medial collateral ligament (MCL)/lateral collateral ligament (LCL) injury, meniscus and ligament injury, iliotibial band (ITB) syndrome, patellar dislocation, patellofemoral syndrome, osteoarthritis, chondrocalcinosis on x-rays, popliteal cyst.
- Medial osteoarthritis = varus deformity
- Lateral osteoarthritis = valgus deformity

Ankle/Foot

- Things to know: Review muscles and nerves responsible for ankle movement in different directions, bones and ligaments of the foot and ankle, ankle disorders including sprains in different areas of the ankle, Haglund deformity and how it contributes to insertional Achilles pain, symptomatic os trigonum, injuries to various tendons (peroneal, posterior tibial, tibialis anterior, Achilles), ankle and foot physical examination, plantar fasciitis, Morton neuroma, hammer toe/claw toe/mallet toe/hallux valgus, sesamoid bone pain.
- Lateral inversion ankle sprains (the anterior talofibular ligament [ATFL] is the weakest and will tear first):
  - Grade 1 = partial tear ATFL
  - Grade 2 = complete tear ATFL, partial tear calcaneofibular ligament (CFL)
  - Grade 3 = complete tear ATFL, CFL, partial tear posterior talofibular ligament (PTFL)
  - Dislocation = complete tears ATFL, CFL, PTFL
- High ankle sprains:
  - Anterior-inferior tibiofibular ligament (AITFL)
  - Posterior inferior tibiofibular ligament (PITFL)
  - Interosseous membrane
- Medial ankle sprains:
  - Deltoid ligament
- Posterior tibialis tendon dysfunction is a cause of acquired flatfoot deformity. Review treatment options.
- The Jones fracture (zone 2) of the metaphysial–diaphyseal junction at the base of the fifth metatarsal has high rates of nonunion due to decreased vascularity. The avulsion fracture of the base of the 5th metatarsal (zone 1) "dancer's fracture" can be treated with a walker boot and has better chance of healing than the Jones fracture.
- FHL tendon dysfunction/entrapment/stenosing tenosynovitis "dancer's tendonitis" and posterior ankle impingement often occurs with a symptomatic accessory os trigonum.

REFERENCES & SUGGESTED READINGS

Aletaha D, Neogi T, Silman AJ, et al. 2010 Rheumatoid arthritis classification criteria: an American College of Rheumatology/European League Against Rheumatism collaborative initiative. *Ann Rheum Dis*. 2010;69:1580-1588.

Buenaver LF, Campbell CM, Haythornthwaite JA. Cognitive-behavioral therapy for chronic pain. In: Fishman S, Ballantyne J, Rathmell JP, eds. *Bonica's Management of Pain*. 4th ed. Baltimore, MD: Lippincott Williams & Wilkins; 2010: chap 82.

Chaudhry H, Bhandari M. Cochrane in CORR®: continuous passive motion following total knee arthroplasty in people with arthritis (review). *Clin Orthop Relat Res*. 2015;473(11):3348-3354. doi:10.1007/s11999-015-4528-y.

Cosman F, de Beur SJ, LeBoff MS, et al. Clinician's guide to prevention and treatment of osteoporosis. *Osteoporos Int*. 2014;25:2359-2381. doi:10.1007/s00198-014-2794-2.

Cuccurullo S. *Physical Medicine and Rehabilitation Board Review*. 3rd ed. New York, NY: Demos; 2014.

Dommerholt J, Shah JP. Myofascial pain syndrome. In: Fishman S, Ballantyne J, Rathmell JP, eds. *Bonica's Management of Pain*. 4th ed. Baltimore, MD: Lippincott Williams & Wilkins; 2010: chap 35.

Drake GN, O'Connor DP, Edwards TB. Indications for reverse total shoulder arthroplasty in rotator cuff disease. *Clin Orthop Relat Res*. 2010;468(6):1526-1533. doi:10.1007/s11999-009-1188-9.

Frontera WR, Lexel J. Assessment of human muscle function. In: Frontera WR, DeLisa J, eds. *DeLisa's Physical Medicine & Rehabilitation: Principles and Practice*. 5th ed. Philadelphia, PA: Lippincott Williams & Wilkins; 2010:69-88.

Frost F, Najarian CR. Spinal orthoses. In: Campagnolo DI, Kirshblum S, eds. *Spinal Cord Medicine*. 2nd ed. Philadelphia, PA: Lippincott Williams & Wilkins; 2011:359-370.

Graham P, Adler RA, Bonner FJ, Kasturi G. The prevention and treatment of osteoporosis. In: Frontera WR, DeLisa J, eds. *DeLisa's Physical Medicine & Rehabilitation: Principles and Practice*. 5th ed. Philadelphia, PA: Lippincott Williams & Wilkins; 2010:979-1014.

Guo J, Pandey S, Doyle J, Bian B, Lis Y, Raisch DW. A review of quantitative risk–benefit methodologies for assessing drug safety and efficacy—report of the ISPOR risk–benefit management working group. *Value Health*. 2010;13(5):657-666.

He ML, Xiao ZM, Lei M, Li TS, Wu H, Liao J. Continuous passive motion for preventing venous thromboembolism after total knee arthroplasty. *Cochrane Database Syst Rev*. 2012;(1):CD008207. doi:10.1002/14651858.CD008207.pub2.

Hickey AH, Bajwa ZH. Neck and arm pain. In: Fishman S, Ballantyne J, Rathmell JP, eds. *Bonica's Management of Pain*. 4th ed. Baltimore, MD: Lippincott Williams & Wilkins; 2010: chap 68.

Inturrisi CE, Lipman AG. Opioid analgesics. In: Fishman S, Ballantyne J, Rathmell JP, eds. *Bonica's Management of Pain*. 4th ed. Baltimore, MD: Lippincott Williams & Wilkins; 2010: chap 78.

Jackson KC II, Argoff CE. Skeletal muscle relaxants and analgesic balms. In: Fishman S, Ballantyne J, Rathmell JP, eds. *Bonica's Management of Pain*. 4th ed. Baltimore, MD: Lippincott Williams & Wilkins; 2010: chap 79.

Jacobson JA. *Fundamentals of Musculoskeletal Ultrasound*. Philadelphia, PA: Saunders/Elsevier; 2007.

Joe GO, Hicks JE, Gerber LH. Rehabilitation of the patient with rheumatic diseases. In: Frontera WR, DeLisa J, eds. *DeLisa's Physical Medicine & Rehabilitation: Principles and Practice*. 5th ed. Philadelphia, PA: Lippincott Williams & Wilkins; 2010:1015-1074.

Lipetz JS, Lipetz DI. Disorders of the cervical spine. In: Frontera WR, DeLisa J, eds. *DeLisa's Physical Medicine & Rehabilitation: Principles and Practice*. 5th ed. Philadelphia: Lippincott Williams & Wilkins; 2010:811-836.

Malanga GA, Nadler SF. *Musculoskeletal Physical Examination: An Evidence-Based Approach*. Philadelphia, PA: Elsevier; 2006.

McGuirk BE, Bogduk N. Acute low back pain. In: Fishman S, Ballantyne J, Rathmell JP, eds. *Bonica's Management of Pain*. 4th ed. Baltimore, MD: Lippincott Williams & Wilkins; 2010: chap 71.

Moya-Angeler J, Gianakos AL, Villa JC, Ni A, Lane JM. Current concepts on osteonecrosis of the femoral head. *World J Orth*. 2015;6(8):590-601. doi:10.5312/wjo.v6.i8.590.

Negrini S, Zaina F, Romano M, Atanasio S, Fusco C, Trevisan C. Rehabilitation of lumbar spine disorders: an evidence-based clinical practice approach. In: Frontera WR, DeLisa J, eds. *DeLisa's Physical Medicine & Rehabilitation: Principles and Practice*. 5th ed. Philadelphia, PA: Lippincott Williams & Wilkins; 2010:837-882.

Olivieri I, D'Angelo S, Palazzi C, Padula A, Mader R, Khan MA. Diffuse idiopathic skeletal hyperostosis: differentiation from ankylosing spondylitis. *Curr Rheumatol Rep*. 2009;11: 321-328. doi:10.1007/s11926-009-0046-9.

Prentice WE. Impaired muscle performance: regaining muscular strength and endurance. In: Voight ML, Hoogenboom BJ, Prentice WE, eds. *Musculoskeletal Interventions: Techniques for Therapeutic Exercise*. New York, NY: McGraw-Hill; 2007:135-152.

Sanders TG, Medynski MA, Feller JF, Lawhorn KW. Bone contusion patterns of the knee at MR imaging: footprint of the mechanism of injury. *RadioGraphics*. 2000;20(suppl 1):S135-S151.

Santos Duarte Lana JF, Andrade Santana MH, Dias Belangero W, Luzo ACM. *Platelet-Rich Plasma: Regenerative Medicine: Sports Medicine, Orthopedic, and Recovery of Muscular Injuries*. New York, NY: Springer; 2014.

Schatman ME. Interdisciplinary chronic pain management: perspectives on history, current status, and future viability. In: Fishman S, Ballantyne J, Rathmell JP, eds. *Bonica's Management of Pain*. 4th ed. Baltimore, MD: Lippincott Williams & Wilkins; 2010: chap 105.

Sehgal N, Manchikanti L, Smith HS. Prescription opioid abuse in chronic pain: a review of opioid abuse predictors and strategies to curb opioid abuse. *Pain Physician*. 2012;15(3 suppl): ES67-ES92.

Sells P, Prentice WE. Impaired endurance: maintaining aerobic capacity and endurance. In: Voight ML, Hoogenboom BJ, Prentice WE, eds. *Musculoskeletal Interventions: Techniques for Therapeutic Exercise*. New York, NY: McGraw-Hill; 2007:153-164.

Shuang F, Hou S-X, Zhu J-L, et al. Clinical anatomy and measurement of the medial branch of the spinal dorsal ramus. *Medicine*. 2015;94(52):e2367. doi:10.1097/MD.0000000000002367.

Siris ES, Adler R, Bilezikian J, et al. The clinical diagnosis of osteoporosis: a position statement from the National Bone Health Alliance Working Group. *Osteoporos Int*. 2014;25(5):1439-1443. doi:10.1007/s00198-014-2655-z.

Skinner HB, McMahon PJ. *Current Diagnosis & Treatment in Orthopedics*. New York, NY: McGraw-Hill; 2014.

Stand P. The female athlete triad. *Med Sci Sports Exerc*. 2007;39(10):1867-1882.

Unnanuntana A, Gladnick BP, Donnelly E, Lane JM. The assessment of fracture risk. *J Bone Joint Surg Am*. 2010;92(3):743-753. doi:10.2106/JBJS.I.00919.

van Boekel MA, Vossenaar ER, van den Hoogen FH, van Venrooij WJ. Autoantibody systems in rheumatoid arthritis: specificity, sensitivity and diagnostic value. *Arthritis Res*. 2002;4(2): 87-93. doi:10.1186/ar395.

Vasiliadis HS, Tsikopoulos K. Glucosamine and chondroitin for the treatment of osteoarthritis. *World J Orthop*. 2017;8(1):1-11. doi:10.5312/wjo.v8.i1.1.

Wyatt LH, Ferrance RJ. The musculoskeletal effects of diabetes mellitus. *J Can Chiropr Assoc*. 2006;50(1):43-50.

Zamorani MP. Muscle and tendon. In: Bianchi S, Martinoli C, eds. *Ultrasound of the musculoskeletal system*. New York, NY: Springer; 2007:45-96.

Zhou L, Schneck C, Shao Z. The anatomy of dorsal ramus nerves and its implications in lower back pain. *Neurosci Med*. 2012;3(2):192-201. doi:10.4236/nm.2012.32025.

Electrodiagnostic Medicine

---

1. Spinal cord ventral horn cells give rise to

   A. unmyelinated afferent neurons.

   B. myelinated efferent neurons.

   C. unmyelinated efferent neurons.

   D. myelinated afferent neurons.

---

2. Motor nerve conduction studies are

   A. antidromic.

   B. orthodromic.

   C. both antidromic and orthodromic.

   D. neither antidromic nor orthodromic.

---

3. You are performing needle electromyography (EMG) on a patient who you highly suspect of having a left L4 radiculopathy based on clinical symptomatology, physical examination findings, and imaging studies. You are choosing additional L4 innervated muscles to test. All of the following muscles could be tested, EXCEPT

   A. iliopsoas.

   B. gracilis.

   C. tensor fasciae latae.

   D. gluteus minimus.

4. Needle electromyography (EMG) is expected to be normal in which of the following muscle diseases?

    A. myotonic dystrophy

    B. steroid myopathy

    C. fiber type disproportion

    D. nemaline myopathy

5. High-dose toxicity from which metal can cause an acute polyneuropathy that mimics Guillain-Barré syndrome?

    A. lead

    B. mercury

    C. arsenic

    D. gold

6. During voluntary skeletal muscle contraction, the first recruited motor units have which characteristic(s)?

    A. fast-twitch motor units

    B. type II motor units

    C. small motor units

    D. all of the above

7. Median nerve sensory innervation of digit 2 is derived from

    A. posterior cord and upper trunk of the brachial plexus.

    B. medial cord and lower trunk of the brachial plexus.

    C. lateral cord, upper trunk, and middle trunk of the brachial plexus.

    D. medial cord, middle trunk, and lower trunk of the brachial plexus.

8. Which mechanism contributes to maintaining a resting steady state nerve cell membrane potential in humans?

A. voltage-gated sodium channels

B. voltage-gated potassium channels

C. voltage-gated calcium channels

D. Na^+-K^+-ATP pump

9. The H reflex late response is described as

A. having a stable latency from one stimulus to the next.

B. a polysynaptic reflex.

C. obtained by supramaximal stimulation.

D. arising from a collateral axon sprout.

10. A 35-year-old store clerk struck the inside of his left elbow against the sharp edge of an open cash register till and presented to your office for an evaluation. Examination revealed skin laceration, extensive soft tissue swelling, and paralysis involving the ulnar innervated muscles of his left hand. Left ulnar motor nerve conduction studies were obtained 2 days postinjury showing normal compound muscle action potential (CMAP) waveforms at the wrist and below the elbow but an absent CMAP above the elbow. Repeat studies are performed at 3 weeks postinjury and record absent CMAP waveforms at all three stimulation sites. Based on the given information, what is the most likely type of nerve injury sustained by this patient?

A. partial conduction block

B. axonal injury

C. complete conduction block

D. demyelinating injury

11. A clinical feature of multifocal motor neuropathy (MMN) distinct from motor neuron disease is the presence of

A. diminished reflexes.

B. muscle fasciculations.

C. normal sensory examination.

D. weakness in peripheral nerve distributions.

12. You clinically diagnose a 23-year-old male semiprofessional football player with a right upper trunk brachial plexopathy. The physical examination could demonstrate

   A. diminished sensation over the medial aspect of the right hand.

   B. weak right finger flexors.

   C. diminished sensation over the right lateral forearm.

   D. weak right finger extensors.

13. A 45-year-old male presents with symptoms of painful dysesthesias in his dominant hand, primarily involving digits 1 to 3. Physical examination reveals diminished sensation over digits 1 to 3 and reproduction of symptoms tapping over the volar wrist. Median sensory nerve conduction testing across the symptomatic wrist recording at digit 2 is within normal limits. Likewise, the median motor nerve conduction study recording from the abductor pollicis brevis in the symptomatic hand is within normal limits. The next best step would be to

   A. perform a sympathetic skin response test recording at the palm and stimulating the median nerve at the wrist.

   B. perform a comparison study of median and ulnar sensory conduction between the wrist and ring finger.

   C. perform a median F wave study measuring minimal F wave latency and chronodispersion.

   D. conclude that the electrodiagnostic study shows no evidence of median mononeuropathy at the wrist.

14. A patient with radiculopathy can have a normal needle electromyography (EMG) examination if

   A. the radiculopathy is purely demyelinating.

   B. the EMG is performed too early in the course of an acute radiculopathy.

   C. different myotome fascicles are preferentially affected or spared.

   D. all of the above

15. Which motor nerve type consists of small, unmyelinated, preganglionic autonomic fibers?

    A. type A-δ

    B. type B

    C. type C

    D. type A-γ

16. A 49-year-old male school custodian presents with painful paresthesias and numbness involving his right wrist and thumb for 6 months. Physical examination is positive for decreased sensation to pinprick over the dorsal and thenar surfaces of the right thumb. The electrodiagnostic study data tables are listed below:

Nerve Conduction Studies

Motor Nerve	Distal Latency (ms)	Amplitude (mV)	Conduction Velocity (m/s)
R. median motor (abductor pollicis brevis)	Wrist: 5.1 (norm <4.7) Elbow: 10.6	S1: 5.6 (norm >4.2) S2: 4.9	S1-S2: 51 (norm >47)
R. ulnar motor (abductor digiti minimi)	Wrist: 3.5 (norm <3.9) Below elbow: 7.3 Above elbow: 9.8	S1: 9.9 (norm >7.8) S2: 9.4 S3: 8.9	S1-S2: 58 (norm >52) S2-S3: 56 (norm >43)

Abbreviations: R., right; S1, wrist; S2, elbow; S3, above elbow.

Sensory Nerve	Recording Site	Stimulation Site	Peak Latency (ms)	Amplitude (µV)
R. radial	Base of thumb	Forearm: 10 cm	2.0 (norm <2.9)	23.6 (norm >11.0)
R. median comparison	Thumb	Wrist: 10 cm	4.9 (norm <3.1)	25.4 (norm >11.0)
R. radial comparison	Thumb	Forearm: 10 cm	2.2 (norm <3.0) Med − Rad = 2.7 (norm <0.5)	23.7 (norm >3.0)

Abbreviation: R., right.
All *left* side comparison nerve conduction studies were within normal limits.

Electromyography

Muscle	Insertion at Rest	MUAP Morphology	Recruitment
R. abductor pollicis brevis	Normal	Normal	Normal
R. pronator teres	2+ FIB and PSW	↑ duration, 2+ poly	Decreased
R. extensor digitorum communis	Normal	Normal	Normal
R. triceps	1+ FIB and PSW	↑ duration, 1+ poly	Decreased
R. deltoid	2+ FIB and PSW	↑ duration, 2+ poly	Decreased
R. rhomboid major	Normal	Normal	Normal
R. C1-3 paraspinal muscles	Normal		
R. C4-6 paraspinal muscles	1+ PSW		
R. C7-T1 paraspinal muscles	Normal		

Abbreviations: FIB, fibrillation potential; MUAP, motor unit action potential; PSW, positive sharp wave; R., right.

The study impression is most consistent with a right

A. median mononeuropathy.

B. C6 radiculopathy.

C. radial sensory neuropathy.

D. both A and B

---

17. Which of the following is true regarding the occurrence of anodal block during routine nerve conduction studies?

A. It indicates nerve pathology.

B. It is unlikely to occur.

C. It occurs due to focal nerve compression.

D. It occurs when the active and reference electrodes are inadvertently switched.

---

18. Normal needle electromyography (EMG) insertional activity

A. lasts between 300 and 500 milliseconds.

B. has an irregular firing pattern at the endplate region.

C. represents the summated voltage of the muscle fibers from one motor unit.

D. results from mechanical muscle fiber depolarization.

19. Which of the given needle electromyography (EMG) tracings depicts a short-duration spontaneous muscle fiber depolarization with a regular firing rate?

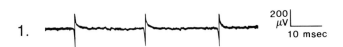

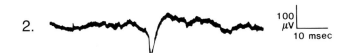

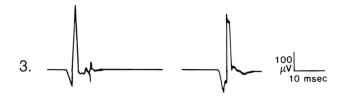

Adapted with permission from Frymoyer JW, Wiesel SW, An HS, et al, eds. *The Adult & Pediatric Spine*. 3rd ed. Philadelphia, PA: Lippincott Williams & Wilkins; 2004.

A. 1

B. 2

C. 3

D. none of the above

20. The "all-or-none" principle in nerve cell membrane action potential generation refers to

A. a period during an action potential when Na⁺ channels remain inactivated and no further action potential can be produced, regardless of strength of stimulus.

B. a stimulus reaching the activation threshold will generate an action potential with constant size and configuration.

C. a stimulus producing a local current that does not reach the activation threshold will not generate an action potential.

D. both B and C

21. You consult on a 65-year-old male who has been in a subacute rehabilitation facility for 9 months after being hospitalized for pneumonia. Prior to hospitalization, the patient was independent in activities of daily living. He is now confined to a wheelchair with complaints of stiffness, pain, and weakness in all four limbs. Physical examination is significant for retracted bilateral facial muscles, tongue weakness with fasciculations, severe widespread muscle atrophy, diffuse muscle weakness, and spasticity in all four limbs. Nerve conduction studies demonstrate reduced compound muscle action potential (CMAP) amplitudes in absence of conduction block and normal latencies and conduction velocities. Sensory nerve conduction studies are within normal limits. Needle electromyography (EMG) shows diffuse fibrillation potentials in proximal and distal muscles of the upper and lower limbs; the genioglossus; as well as the cervical, thoracic, and lumbar paraspinal muscles. Fasciculation potentials are also present in multiple muscles. Motor units are long duration and very large amplitude with decreased recruitment. What are the next best steps in clinical care?

A. Inform the patient that his disease is treatable, start him on steroids and intravenous immunoglobulin (IVIG), and transfer him to an acute inpatient rehabilitation facility.

B. Assemble an interdisciplinary or multidisciplinary team to coordinate care, schedule a family meeting, and perform additional neuroimaging or electrodiagnostic studies if appropriate.

C. Inform the patient that he most likely had a stroke with superimposed critical illness polyneuropathy, consult neurology, and medically clear him for transfer to acute inpatient rehabilitation.

D. Inform the patient that his condition is terminal and transfer to inpatient hospice.

22. During a peroneal motor nerve study recording at the extensor digitorum brevis (EDB) muscle, supramaximal stimulation at the ankle yields a compound muscle action potential (CMAP) with amplitude of 3.0 mV. Supramaximal stimulation below the fibular head and lateral to the popliteal fossa yields CMAPs of 8.0 mV and 7.8 mV, respectively. All latencies and conduction velocities are within normal limits. The amplitude difference between the distal and proximal sites can be explained by

A. normal temporal dispersion.

B. conduction block.

C. muscle atrophy.

D. anomalous innervation.

23. Decreased temperature affects the nerve action potential by

A. decreasing the action potential duration.

B. increasing time to reach peak depolarization.

C. increasing nerve conduction velocity.

D. decreasing action potential amplitude.

24. Which of the following muscles would be spared in a brachial panplexopathy involving the upper, middle, and lower trunks?

A. deltoid

B. rhomboid major

C. latissimus dorsi

D. pectoralis major

25. The following are the nerve conduction study test results for a 53-year-old left-handed female with a past medical history of left carpal tunnel release surgery 2 years ago presenting with a 3-month history of pain in her left thumb.

Before Carpal Tunnel Surgery

Motor Nerve	Distal Latency (ms)	Amplitude (mV)	Conduction Velocity (m/s)
L. median motor (abductor pollicis brevis)	Wrist: 5.5 (norm <4.4) Elbow: 11.3	5.3 (norm >4.2) 5.0	Wrist-elbow: 35 (norm >51)
Sensory Nerve	**Stimulation Site**	**Peak Latency (ms)**	**Amplitude (μV)**
L. median (record digit 2)	Wrist: 14 cm	5.8 (norm <4.0)	21.5 (norm >19.0)

Abbreviation: L., left.

Two Years After Carpal Tunnel Surgery

Motor Nerve	Distal Latency (ms)	Amplitude (mV)	Conduction Velocity (m/s)
L. median motor (abductor pollicis brevis)	Wrist: 4.2 (norm <4.4) Elbow: 9.0	5.5 (norm >4.2) 5.3	Wrist-elbow: 44 (norm >51)
Sensory Nerve	**Stimulation Site**	**Peak Latency (ms)**	**Amplitude (μV)**
L. median (record digit 2)	Wrist: 14 cm	3.5 (norm <4.0)	24.0 (norm >19.0)

Abbreviation: L., left.

What can be determined from the given information?

A. The prior carpal tunnel release surgery was unsuccessful.

B. The abnormal nerve conduction study findings have improved since the initial study.

C. The carpal tunnel syndrome has recurred in this patient.

D. The abnormal nerve conduction study findings have worsened since the initial study.

---

26. All of the following electromyography (EMG) needle electrodes have unidirectional recording properties, EXCEPT

A. bipolar concentric.

B. standard concentric.

C. monopolar.

D. single-fiber.

---

27. When performing surface nerve stimulation using standard bipolar surface electrodes:

A. Nerve hyperpolarization typically occurs under the cathode.

B. Nerve depolarization typically occurs under the anode.

C. Nerve depolarization typically occurs under the cathode.

D. both A and B

---

28. During a nerve conduction study, the stimulus intensity is increased until it is first noted that there is no further increase in the evoked potential's amplitude. The magnitude of the stimulus described above is at

A. maximal stimulus.

B. subthreshold stimulus.

C. supramaximal stimulus.

D. threshold stimulus.

29. A patient with shoulder weakness in abduction and external rotation is scheduled for needle electromyography (EMG). Which of the following statements is true in distinguishing among C5 radiculopathy, suprascapular neuropathy, and upper brachial plexopathy in a hypothetical scenario where there is no fascicular sparing or anomalous innervation?

A. In an isolated C5 radiculopathy, the infraspinatus muscle would be expected to test normal.

B. In an isolated suprascapular neuropathy, the teres minor muscle would be expected to test normal.

C. In an isolated upper trunk brachial plexopathy, the rhomboid major muscle would be expected to test abnormal.

D. In both a C5 radiculopathy and a suprascapular neuropathy, the latissimus dorsi muscle would be expected to test abnormal.

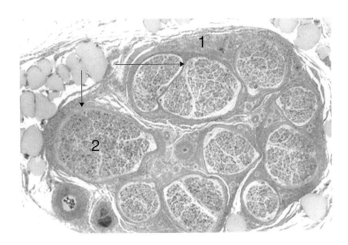

Adapted with permission from Mills SE. *Histology for Pathologists*. 3rd ed. Philadelphia, PA: Lippincott Williams & Wilkins; 2007.

30. The microscopic image above represents a cross-sectional view of the sural nerve. The black arrows point to which connective tissue structure surrounding the nerve bundles?

A. endoneurium

B. epineurium

C. perineurium

D. sarcolemma

31. Which anatomic structure remains intact in axonotmesis and Sunderland types 2 to 4 nerve injuries?

A. axon

B. endoneurium

C. epineurium

D. perineurium

32. A 32-year-old male presents with left forearm pain radiating to his hand with associated weakness flexing the left thumb, index, and middle fingers. Needle electromyography (EMG) demonstrates denervation and reduced recruitment in the following muscles: flexor pollicis longus, pronator quadratus, and the flexor digitorum profundus to digits 2 and 3. The lesion most likely involves which nerve?

A. ulnar

B. radial

C. posterior interosseous

D. anterior interosseous

33. Which electrodiagnostic motor unit action potential (MUAP) parameter is the most sensitive indicator of myopathy?

A. decreased duration

B. decreased amplitude

C. increased jitter

D. increased number of phases

34. When could a notch filter be utilized during electrodiagnostic testing?

A. attenuating the effects of electrode impedance

B. extracting a time-locked action potential from background noise over successive averaged stimulations

C. amplifying a biologic signal before noise from the leads and cables are introduced

D. minimizing the effects of electrical power line noise

35. A 35-year-old patient presents with a 1-day history of nontraumatic acute flaccid paralysis of his right shoulder girdle muscles preceded by 2 days of intense burning periscapular pain. Review of systems was positive for a recent viral illness. Physical examination reveals 1/5 strength in the right deltoid, supraspinatus, infraspinatus, and biceps muscles as well as decreased sensation in the right lateral upper arm. STAT magnetic resonance imaging (MRI) of the cervical spine and shoulder shows no evidence of mass lesion, disc herniation, spinal cord abnormality, nerve root compression, or stenosis. There is high signal intensity on T2 weighted imaging in the right deltoid, supraspinatus, infraspinatus, and biceps muscles. This patient's suspected condition

   A. statistically has a poor prognosis for recovery.

   B. results from arterial or venous occlusion.

   C. more commonly affects males.

   D. can be confirmed immediately with electrodiagnostic testing.

36. Myopathic motor unit action potential (MUAP) recruitment results from

   A. initiation of inactive motor units and more rapid firing of already active units as the force of muscle contraction is gradually increased.

   B. loss of active motor units offset by an increased firing rate of the first motor unit to generate the required muscle contractile force.

   C. multiple rapid firing motor units generating minimal contractile force to compensate for a reduced number of muscle fibers per motor unit.

   D. central nervous system dysfunction leading to an inability to increase the firing rate to maintain the force required for maximal voluntary muscle contraction.

37. The impulses that generate somatosensory evoked potentials (SSEPs) are widely believed to primarily travel to the cerebral cortex via which central nervous system pathway(s)/tract(s)?

   A. corticospinal

   B. dorsal column

   C. anterior spinocerebellar

   D. spinothalamic

38. Which of the following electrodiagnostic study findings should be present in order to properly identify the affected nerve root level when diagnosing a radiculopathy?

   A. prolonged sensory nerve action potential (SNAP) peak latency of a peripheral nerve corresponding to a nerve root level

   B. needle electromyography (EMG) abnormalities in two or more muscles innervated by the same nerve root but different peripheral nerves

   C. needle EMG abnormalities in the paraspinal muscles

   D. reduced motor compound muscle action potential (CMAP) amplitudes of a peripheral nerve corresponding to a nerve root level

39. Which hand digit could be studied to test ulnar nerve cutaneous sensory fibers?

   A. digit 1

   B. digit 3

   C. digit 5

   D. none of the above

40. Which muscle receives innervation from all the nerve roots and trunks of the brachial plexus?

   A. pectoralis major

   B. serratus anterior

   C. teres minor

   D. teres major

41. A 30-year-old female developed postoperative right foot drop and presents for electrodiagnostic testing 6 weeks later. Data tables from the study are listed below.

Motor Nerve	Distal Latency (ms)	Amplitude (mV)	Conduction Velocity (m/s)
R. tibial motor (abductor hallucis)	Ankle: 6.0 (norm <6.1) Knee: 12.2	5.4 (norm >5.8) 5.0	Ankle-knee: 62 (norm >42)
R. peroneal motor (extensor digitorum brevis)	Ankle: 6.4 (norm <6.5) Below fibula: 11.2 Popliteal fossa: 12.9	1.0 (norm >2.6) 0.8 0.7	Ankle-below fibula: 64 (norm >43) Below fibula-popliteal fossa: 59 (norm >49)

Abbreviation: R., right.

Sensory Nerve	Stimulation Site	Peak Latency (ms)	Amplitude (µV)
R. sural (behind lateral malleolus)	Calf: 14 cm	4.4 (norm <4.5)	3.7 (norm >4)
R. superficial peroneal (dorsum of foot)	Leg: 14 cm	4.3 (norm <4.2)	1.9 (norm >5)

All *left* side comparison nerve conduction studies were within normal limits. Abbreviation: R., right.

Electromyography

Muscle	Insertion at Rest	MUAP Morphology	Recruitment
R. vastus medialis	Normal	Normal	Normal
R. tibialis anterior	3+ FIB and PSW	Normal	Reduced
R. peroneus longus	2+ FIB and PSW	Normal	Reduced
R. tibialis posterior	1+ FIB and PSW	Normal	Normal
R. gastrocnemius	1+ FIB and PSW	Normal	Normal
R. biceps femoris (short head)	2+ FIB and PSW	Normal	Reduced
R. tensor fasciae latae	Normal	Normal	Normal
R. posterior primary rami (L1-S1)	Normal		

Abbreviations: FIB, fibrillation potential; MUAP, motor unit action potential; PSW, positive sharp wave; R., right.

The electrodiagnostic test findings are most consistent with

A. peroneal neuropathy.

B. sciatic neuropathy.

C. L5 radiculopathy.

D. lumbosacral plexopathy.

42. A fasciculation potential differs from a recruited motor unit action potential (MUAP) in that it

   A. is under voluntary control.

   B. always denotes pathology.

   C. fires in a semirhythmic pattern.

   D. is able to fire at a rate less than 2 Hz.

43. Bilateral blink reflex study findings: Stimulation of the right supraorbital nerve shows prolonged latencies of the right R1 and R2 (ipsilateral) responses and a normal left R2 (contralateral). Stimulation of the left supraorbital nerve shows normal left R1 and R2 responses and prolonged latency of the right R2 (contralateral) response. These findings are most consistent with a partial lesion of the right

   A. trigeminal nerve.

   B. facial nerve.

   C. mid pons.

   D. medulla.

44. During a routine median motor nerve conduction study, you notice that the amplitude of the compound muscle action potential (CMAP) obtained with distal stimulation (10 mV) is considerably higher than the proximal CMAP at the elbow (5 mV). One reason to explain this could be a

   A. Martin-Gruber anastomosis.

   B. costimulation of adjacent nerves at the wrist.

   C. submaximal stimulation at the wrist.

   D. mononeuropathy at the wrist.

45. In a motor neuron, where are most voltage-gated calcium channels found?

   A. axon terminals

   B. synaptic clefts

   C. nodes of Ranvier

   D. internode regions

46. All of the following can cause radiculopathy, EXCEPT

A. gene mutation at chromosome 17.

B. Lyme disease.

C. diabetes mellitus.

D. neurofibroma.

---

47. A 69-year-old female who recently lost 100 lb after bariatric surgery developed left foot drop and presents for electrodiagnostic testing. Data tables from the study are listed below.

Motor Nerve	Distal Latency (ms)	Amplitude (mV)	Conduction Velocity (m/s)
R. tibial motor (abductor hallucis)	Ankle: 4.2 (norm <6.1) Knee: 10.6	8.0 (norm >5.8) 7.3	Ankle-knee: 64 (norm >42)
R. peroneal motor (extensor digitorum brevis)	Ankle: 6.0 (norm <6.5) Below fibula: 12.2 Popliteal fossa: 14.9	6.0 (norm >2.6) 5.8 1.5	Ankle-below fibula: 50 (norm >43) Below fibula-popliteal fossa: 37 (norm >49)

Abbreviation: R., right.

Sensory Nerve	Stimulation Site	Peak Latency (ms)	Amplitude (µV)
L. sural (behind lateral malleolus)	Calf: 14 cm	3.2 (norm <4.5)	5.6 (norm >4)
L. superficial peroneal (dorsum of foot)	Leg: 14 cm	4.0 (norm <4.2)	4.8 (norm >5)

Abbreviation: L., left.
All *right* side comparison nerve conduction studies were within normal limits.

Electromyography

Muscle	Insertion at Rest	MUAP Morphology	Recruitment
L. vastus medialis	Normal	Normal	Normal
L. tibialis anterior	1+ FIB and PSW	Normal	Reduced
L. peroneus longus	1+ FIB and PSW	Normal	Reduced
L. tibialis posterior	Normal	Normal	Normal
L. gastrocnemius	Normal	Normal	Normal
L. biceps femoris (short head)	Normal	Normal	Normal
L. tensor fasciae latae	Normal	Normal	Normal
L. posterior primary rami (L1-S1)	Normal		

Abbreviations: FIB, fibrillation potential; L., left; MUAP, motor unit action potential; PSW, positive sharp wave.

The electrodiagnostic test findings localize the lesion to the

A. superficial peroneal nerve.

B. deep peroneal nerve.

C. common peroneal nerve.

D. peroneal division of the sciatic nerve.

---

48. Which myopathic condition can demonstrate both clinical myotonia and myotonic discharges on needle electromyography (EMG)?

A. hypokalemic periodic paralysis

B. hyperkalemic periodic paralysis

C. inclusion body myositis (IBM)

D. Duchenne muscular dystrophy (DMD)

---

49. The muscle listed below with the highest muscle fiber to motor unit innervation ratio is the

A. gastrocnemius.

B. external rectus.

C. first lumbrical.

D. brachioradialis.

---

50. Bioelectric current flow through the human body is inversely proportional to

A. conductance.

B. impedance.

C. voltage.

D. Ohm law.

51. Which of the following electrophysiologic test findings could be present in the rare case of true neurogenic thoracic outlet syndrome (TOS)?

   A. reduced median sensory nerve action potential (SNAP) amplitude on the affected side

   B. median compound muscle action potential (CMAP) amplitude that is more reduced than the ulnar CMAP amplitude on the affected side

   C. thenar muscle sparing on the affected side as evidenced by normal median motor nerve conduction studies and normal needle electromyography (EMG) of thenar muscles

   D. reduced lateral antebrachial cutaneous SNAP amplitude on the affected side

52. Slowing the electrodiagnostic instrument's sweep speed and increasing its gain can alter the visualization and interpretation of nerve action potential waveforms by

   A. decreasing the onset latency.

   B. increasing the resolution.

   C. decreasing the amplitude.

   D. both A and C

53. A 42-year-old plumber presents with a right foot "slap" during ambulation. Physical examination is significant for 4/5 strength in the right foot and ankle muscles innervated by the superficial and deep peroneal nerves. Nerve conduction studies show evidence of a partial conduction block involving the right common peroneal motor nerve at the fibular head. Needle electromyography (EMG) testing of the right tibialis anterior muscle should demonstrate

   A. normal motor unit recruitment.

   B. reduced motor unit recruitment.

   C. increased motor unit recruitment.

   D. absent motor unit recruitment.

54. Assuming the normal recruitment ratio (RR) of motor unit action potentials (MUAPs) during routine electromyography (EMG), when the first MUAP is firing at 30 Hz, how many other motor units are expected to be simultaneously firing?

   A. three

   B. four

   C. five

   D. six

55. In a transcarpal median mixed nerve study, the

   A. median nerve is stimulated at the wrist and recorded at mid-palm.

   B. muscle spindle Ia fibers are stimulated and recorded.

   C. study is antidromic for the sensory fibers and orthodromic for the motor fibers.

   D. mixed nerve conduction velocity (NCV) is typically slower than NCVs obtained in motor and sensory studies.

56. Pathology specifically involving the posterior division of the sacral plexus would affect which nerve?

   A. obturator

   B. tibial

   C. peroneal

   D. femoral

57. You perform electrodiagnostic studies on a 35-year-old female reporting a 3-month history of neck pain with left upper extremity pain and numbness. The nerve conduction studies are within normal limits. Needle electromyography (EMG) of the left triceps, flexor carpi radialis (FCR), and extensor digitorum communis (EDC) muscles shows 2+ positive sharp waves, 1+ fibrillation potentials, and reduced motor unit action potential recruitment. There is a mild degree of spontaneous muscle fiber activity in the left cervical paraspinal muscles at rest. The remaining muscles studied are within normal limits, including the deltoid and first dorsal interosseous (FDI). Physical examination findings correlating with the nerve root level of pathology could include

   A. weakness of left supinator muscle.

   B. diminished left biceps deep tendon reflex.

   C. weakness of left brachioradialis muscle.

   D. decreased sensation over the left middle finger.

58. Which of the following nerve conduction study findings would support a diagnosis of tarsal tunnel syndrome?

    A. decreased sural sensory nerve action potential amplitude on the affected side

    B. drop in the tibial compound muscle action potential amplitude of greater than 60% from the ankle to popliteal fossa stimulation sites on the affected side

    C. prolonged or absent tibial H reflex on the affected side

    D. prolonged medial and lateral plantar latencies on the affected side

59. A patient with facioscapulohumeral dystrophy would be expected to have substantial weakness and atrophy in all of the following muscles, EXCEPT

    A. biceps.

    B. orbicularis oculi.

    C. tibialis anterior.

    D. flexor carpi radialis.

60. The compound muscle action potential (CMAP) onset latency is composed of all of the following, EXCEPT

    A. terminal latency.

    B. latency of activation.

    C. nerve conduction.

    D. neuromuscular junction (synaptic) transmission.

61. Which needle electromyography (EMG) stable potentials arise from terminal axon suprathreshold muscle fiber depolarization provoked by needle insertion, fire irregularly, and are usually biphasic with an initial negative deflection?

    A. miniature endplate potentials (MEPPs)

    B. endplate potentials (EPPs)

    C. fibrillation potentials (FIBs)

    D. positive sharp waves (PSWs)

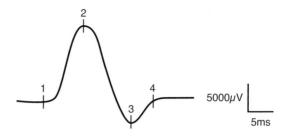

62. The recorded compound muscle action potential (CMAP) depicted above is labeled 1 through 4. The interval 1 to 2 represents

   A. peak-to-peak amplitude.

   B. rise time.

   C. baseline-to-peak amplitude.

   D. both B and C

63. You are performing a standard ulnar motor nerve conduction study as part of an evaluation for suspected neuropathy at the elbow. Comparing the data parameters obtained from below and above the elbow stimulation sites, partial conduction block can distinguished from focal slowing (i.e., abnormal temporal dispersion [ATD]) by all of the following, EXCEPT

   A. amplitude.

   B. area.

   C. duration.

   D. conduction velocity.

64. After axonal injury, regenerated nerve fibers possess

   A. thicker myelin sheaths.

   B. shorter internodal distances.

   C. increased diameters.

   D. increased conduction velocities distal to the injury site.

65. A 21-year-old female lost control driving an all-terrain vehicle (ATV) and fell down a steep embankment sustaining head/neck trauma and multiple fractures, including a right clavicle fracture. She is admitted from a level 1 trauma center to acute inpatient rehabilitation 6 weeks postinjury with a flail, insensate right arm and ipsilateral ptosis. The trauma center faxes you the results of electrodiagnostic studies performed 4 weeks postinjury:

Nerve Conduction Studies

Motor Nerve	
R. median motor (abductor pollicis brevis)	Wrist: no response Elbow: no response
R. ulnar motor (abductor digiti minimi)	Wrist: no response Below elbow: no response Above elbow: no response

Abbreviation: R., right.

Sensory Nerve	Stimulation Site	Peak Latency (ms)	Amplitude (μV)
R. median (record digit 2)	Wrist: 14 cm	2.9 (norm <4.0)	21.0 (norm >19.0)
R. ulnar (record digit 5)	Wrist: 14 cm	3.2 (norm <4.0)	19.5 (norm >13.0)
R. radial (record base of thumb)	Forearm: 10 cm	2.3 (norm <2.8)	24.0 (norm >11.0)
R. medial antebrachial cutaneous (record medial forearm)	Elbow: 12 cm	1.9 (norm <2.6)	14.5 (norm >3.0)
R. lateral antebrachial cutaneous (record lateral forearm)	Elbow: 12 cm	2.0 (norm <2.3)	16.0 (norm >6.0)

Abbreviation: R., right.
All *left* side comparison nerve conduction studies were within normal limits. No sensory nerve action potential (SNAP) side-to-side differences.

Electromyography

Muscle	Insertion at Rest	MUAP Morphology	Recruitment
R. abductor digiti minimi	3+ FIB and PSW	No MUAPs	Absent
R. abductor pollicis brevis	3+ FIB and PSW	No MUAPs	Absent
R. flexor pollicis longus	3+ FIB and PSW	No MUAPs	Absent
R. extensor indicis	3+ FIB and PSW	No MUAPs	Absent
R. triceps	3+ FIB and PSW	No MUAPs	Absent
R. biceps	3+ FIB and PSW	No MUAPs	Absent
R. deltoid	3+ FIB and PSW	No MUAPs	Absent
R. rhomboids	3+ FIB and PSW	No MUAPs	Absent
R. C1-4 paraspinals	Normal		
R. C5-T1 paraspinals	3+ FIB and PSW		

Abbreviations: FIB, fibrillation potential; MUAP, motor unit action potential; PSW, positive sharp wave; R., right.

Based on the given information, this patient's injury is best described as

A. preganglionic.

B. postganglionic.

C. retroclavicular.

D. infraclavicular.

66. Which muscle disorder is characterized by autosomal dominant inheritance with genetic anticipation, wasting of the facial and temporal muscles, prominent distal muscle weakness, dysphagia, ptosis, and multiple systemic abnormalities?

A. Welander distal myopathy

B. myotonia congenita (Thomsen disease)

C. myotonic dystrophy

D. limb-girdle muscular dystrophy

67. Which of the following is true regarding electrical safety in nerve conduction studies?

A. The neutral input lead from a wall power outlet dissipates leakage current.

B. Using an extension cord decreases stray current leakage from the power source.

C. Nerve conduction studies are safe to perform in patients with external pacemakers.

D. Intensive care unit (ICU) patients are at higher risk of electrical injury than outpatients.

68. A 52-year-old male with diabetes presents with burning, numbness, and tingling in both feet. The physical examination reveals decreased warm and cold thermal perception in both feet as well as hyperalgesia. The skin in both feet appears dry and cracked with loss of distal leg hair. Vibration, light touch, pressure, proprioception, and motor strength are all intact in both the lower and upper extremities. Based solely on the findings, routine motor and sensory nerve conduction studies in both lower extremities would be expected to

  A. test normal.

  B. show a mixed sensorimotor peripheral neuropathy.

  C. demonstrate segmental demyelination involving both the motor and sensory nerves.

  D. exhibit a pattern of diffuse axon loss involving the motor and sensory nerves.

69. In newborns, nerve conduction velocities are typically

  A. 2 times greater than adult values.

  B. 50% of adult values.

  C. equivalent to adult values.

  D. 80% of adult values.

70. The femoral nerve originates from the

  A. anterior division of lumbar plexus.

  B. anterior division of the sacral plexus.

  C. posterior division of the lumbar plexus.

  D. posterior division of the sacral plexus.

71. You consult on a 60-year-old male intensive care unit (ICU) patient for weakness that presumably developed during the 18 days he has been hospitalized for streptococcal sepsis with multisystem organ failure. He is intubated but awake and able to follow commands. On physical examination, there is (distal greater than proximal) muscle weakness with atrophy, decreased sensation to touch, and diminished to absent reflexes in all four limbs. Cerebrospinal fluid (CSF) cell count and protein levels are within normal limits. Lab studies show normal creatine phosphokinase (CPK) levels and the absence of antiganglioside antibodies. Standard nerve conduction studies show severely decreased amplitudes of both the motor and sensory responses. Motor and sensory distal latencies and conduction velocities are in the normal to mildly abnormal range. The repetitive nerve stimulation study is normal. The needle electromyography (EMG) shows abnormal spontaneous muscle fiber activity in the distal limb muscles with reduced motor unit action potential recruitment. Motor unit morphology is normal. The most likely diagnosis is

A. critical illness polyneuropathy.

B. critical illness myopathy.

C. neuromuscular junction block.

D. axonal variant of Guillain-Barré syndrome (GBS).

72. Motor unit action potentials (MUAPs) with long duration, large amplitude, and polyphasic morphologies are characteristic of

A. acute axon loss.

B. chronic axon loss.

C. acute muscle fiber loss.

D. chronic demyelination.

73. Averaging sensory nerve conduction stimulations improves the

A. resolution of the biologic signal.

B. signal-to-noise ratio.

C. vertical magnification of the signal's waveform.

D. bandwidth corresponding to the signal.

74. A 53-year-old male with Hodgkin lymphoma presented with a 3-month history of progressive symmetric weakness, numbness, and tingling in his arms and legs. Physical examination showed diminished motor strength in multiple proximal and distal muscles, including the neck flexors. Sensation to light touch and deep tendon reflexes are diminished in all four limbs. Nerve conduction studies are consistent with demyelination of both sensory and motor nerves with motor partial conduction block in more than one nerve. The diagnosis can be further established by

A. visual evoked potentials.

B. magnetic resonance imaging (MRI) of the brain with and without contrast.

C. cerebral spinal fluid analysis.

D. cervical myelogram.

75. Electrophysiologic findings that could be present in cobalamin deficiency include

A. reduced SNAP amplitudes and prolonged late responses.

B. fibrillation potentials and positive sharp waves in distal lower limb muscles.

C. prolongation in central conduction time during somatosensory evoked potentials.

D. all of the above

76. Which of the following occurs during a nerve action potential when the conductance of K^+ (gK) exceeds that of Na+ (gNa)?

A. depolarization

B. repolarization

C. local current flow

D. resting membrane potential

77. Calculate the tibial nerve conduction velocity from the knee to the ankle.
Distal tibial latency = 6.0 milliseconds
Proximal tibial latency = 12.0 milliseconds
Distance from proximal to distal tibial nerve stimulation sites = 360 mm

A. 20 m/s

B. 36 m/s

C. 50 m/s

D. 60 m/s

78. A 42-year-old male presents with a 2-month history of low back pain radiating down the lateral aspect of his right lower extremity with associated numbness on the top of the right foot. Physical examination is significant for a positive straight leg raise test on the right, mildly diminished right medial hamstring reflex, diminished sensation to pinprick over the dorsum of the right foot, and 4/5 strength in the right extensor hallucis longus muscle. Lumbosacral magnetic resonance imaging (MRI) shows a right paracentral disc extrusion at L4-5 impinging on the traversing nerve root in the right lateral recess. Given the clinically suspected pathology, the needle electromyography (EMG) study could demonstrate

A. reduced motor unit recruitment in the right vastus medialis muscle.

B. polyphasic motor unit action potentials in the right soleus muscle.

C. positive sharp waves in the right upper lumbar paraspinal muscles.

D. fibrillation potentials in the right tibialis posterior muscle.

79. Which subtype of Guillain-Barré syndrome (GBS) is characterized by ophthalmoplegia, ataxia, and areflexia?

A. acute inflammatory demyelinating polyradiculoneuropathy

B. Miller Fisher

C. acute motor and sensory axonal neuropathy

D. pharyngeal-cervical-brachial

80. Which type of sensory nerve fiber innervates the Golgi tendon organ?

   A. Ia (A-α)

   B. Ib (A-α)

   C. II (A-β)

   D. III (A-γ)

81. Findings suggestive of a Martin-Gruber anastomosis include

   A. median compound muscle action potential (CMAP) lower in amplitude upon stimulation at the elbow than at the wrist.

   B. ulnar CMAP higher in amplitude upon stimulation below the elbow than at the wrist.

   C. a recorded CMAP upon stimulation of the median nerve at the elbow and recording at the first distal interosseous (FDI) muscle.

   D. an initial positive deflection in the distal median CMAP when there is superimposed carpal tunnel syndrome (CTS).

82. You are performing a needle electromyography (EMG) study on a 27-year-old male who presents with a chief complaint of left wrist and hand weakness upon returning from his honeymoon 4 weeks ago. You suspect a radial nerve lesion at the spiral groove based on your history and thorough physical examination. Which muscle would be expected to test normal?

   A. triceps

   B. brachioradialis

   C. extensor carpi radialis

   D. supinator

83. The fastest conducting neurons have which of the following properties?

   A. small diameter, myelinated

   B. small diameter, unmyelinated

   C. large diameter, myelinated

   D. large diameter, unmyelinated

84. You are testing a patient for a possible diagnosis of myasthenia gravis, recording at the adductor digiti minimi muscle. Initial compound muscle action potential (CMAP) amplitude is within normal limits with supramaximal stimulus. There is a 5% maximum decrement during initial baseline 3 Hz stimulation at rest. What is the next best step in evaluation?

    A. Test a more proximal muscle.

    B. Conclude that the test is normal.

    C. Exercise the muscle.

    D. Cool the limb.

85. Which needle electromyography (EMG) potentials are absent after complete denervation?

    A. miniature endplate potentials

    B. endplate potentials

    C. fibrillation potentials

    D. both A and B

86. Paramyotonia congenita electrophysiologic findings can include

    A. short-duration, small amplitude motor unit action potentials (MUAPs) with an early recruitment pattern.

    B. compound muscle action potential (CMAP) increment after a short period of exercise with a rapid recovery to baseline.

    C. sustained runs of myotonic discharges elicited by muscle warming.

    D. electrical silence after extreme muscle cooling.

87. Which is NOT true regarding the physiology at the neuromuscular junction?

    A. Binding of two acetylcholine (ACh) molecules to a postsynaptic receptor initiates the opening of cation channels.

    B. A miniature endplate potential (MEPP) is equal to the release of a one quantum of ACh.

    C. An endplate potential (EPP) is formed by an "all-or-none" response.

    D. More than one MEPP can summate to create a local EPP.

88. A 67-year-old female admitted to acute inpatient rehabilitation in a wheel-chair 3 weeks status post-left total hip arthroplasty is found to have diffuse pain, numbness, and weakness in the left lower extremity. Physical examination reveals diffusely diminished left lower extremity reflexes, decreased sensation with sparing of the left medial thigh, and 2/5 strength in the left lower extremity muscles with the exception of hip adduction at 4+/5. The electrodiagnostic test findings are provided below:

Nerve Conduction Studies
Left peroneal and tibial motor nerves showed mild prolongation of distal latencies, severely reduced compound muscle action potential (CMAP) amplitudes at all stimulation sites, and mild diffuse conduction velocity slowing. Patient could not tolerate left femoral motor nerve testing. Left superficial peroneal, sural, and saphenous sensory nerve action potentials (SNAPs) were absent. All right side comparison nerve conduction studies were within normal limits.

Needle Electromyography
Needle evaluation of the left vastus medialis, anterior tibialis, peroneus longus, gastrocnemius, posterior tibialis, biceps femoris short head, and gluteus medius muscles showed increased insertional activity, 3+ positive sharp waves, 3+ fibrillation potentials, and severely diminished recruitment. The left adductor longus and gracilis muscles were unremarkable. The bilateral upper, middle, and lower lumbar paraspinal muscles were unremarkable. All right side lower limb muscles were within normal limits.

Based on the findings, the impression is most consistent with an acute left

A. multifocal motor neuropathy.

B. L5 radiculopathy.

C. sciatic neuropathy.

D. lumbosacral plexopathy.

---

89. Which of the following can be the earliest electrophysiologic abnormality in a patient with Guillain-Barré syndrome (GBS)?

A. prolonged or absent sural sensory response

B. positive sharp waves and fibrillations in the paraspinal muscles

C. prolonged or absent minimum F wave latency

D. reduced motor amplitudes at distal stimulation sites

90. Which type of nerve injury has the worst recovery prognosis?

    A. axonotmesis

    B. neurotmesis

    C. neurapraxia

    D. axonopraxia

91. Placing the recording electrodes less than 4 cm apart during a sensory nerve conduction study can affect which sensory nerve action potential (SNAP) parameter?

    A. onset latency

    B. conduction velocity

    C. amplitude

    D. stability

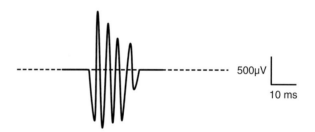

92. The motor unit action potential (MUAP) pictured above contains

    A. eight phases.

    B. nine phases.

    C. four turns/serrations.

    D. eight turns/serrations.

93. A patient with a suspected metabolic myopathy is undergoing needle electromyography during a typical attack of muscle cramping. The needle electrode is inserted into the symptomatic muscle, and the motor unit action potential interference pattern is observed to decline until complete electrical silence occurs. The muscle remains contracted despite electrical silence on electromyography (EMG). This finding is characteristic of

A. acid maltase deficiency (Pompe disease).

B. carnitine deficiency myopathy.

C. myophosphorylase deficiency myopathy (McArdle disease).

D. mitochondrial myopathies.

94. Which of the following is NOT an example of a far field potential?

A. compound muscle action potential (CMAP) negative spike

B. stimulus artifact

C. premotor potential

D. P14 upper limb somatosensory evoked potential (SSEP) (recorded at channel 3: CPi-EPc)

95. A 51-year-old right-handed female presents a 3-month history of numbness and painful tingling sensations in all fingers of the right hand. There is no history of injury, and the physical examination is normal. The following are the nerve conduction study data tables.

Motor Nerve	Distal Latency (ms)	Amplitude (mV)	Conduction Velocity (m/s)
R. median motor (abductor pollicis brevis)	Wrist: 6.5 (norm <4.4) Elbow: 12.3	5.3 (norm >4.2) 5.0	Wrist-elbow: 36 (norm >51)
R. ulnar motor (abductor digiti minimi)	Wrist: 2.7 (norm <3.7) Below elbow: 5.8 Above elbow: 7.9	8.5 (norm >7.9) 8.4 8.0	Wrist-below elbow: 58 (norm >52) Wrist-above elbow: 57(norm >43)

Abbreviation: R., right.

Sensory Nerve	Stimulation Site	Distal Latency (ms)	Amplitude (μV)
R. median (record digit 2)	Wrist: 14 cm Palm: 7 cm	4.8 (norm <3.5) 1.8 (norm <1.9)	24.0 (norm >13)
R. dorsal ulnar cutaneous (dorsum hand)	Forearm: 10 cm	2.0 (norm <2.4)	15.0 (norm >5)
R. ulnar (record digit 5)	Wrist: 14 cm	1.8 (norm <3.2)	22.0 (norm >10)

Abbreviation: R., right.

The nerve entrapment site can be localized to the

A. median nerve at the wrist.

B. median nerve in the forearm.

C. ulnar nerve at the elbow.

D. ulnar nerve at the wrist.

---

96. Which type of neuron is part of a motor unit innervating only extrafusal muscle fibers?

A. alpha

B. beta

C. gamma

D. delta

---

97. Which HIV medication can cause a myopathy with appearance of "ragged red" fibers on muscle biopsy histochemical analysis?

A. didanosine (ddI)

B. lamivudine (3TC)

C. zalcitabine (ddC)

D. zidovudine (AZT)

---

98. Which autonomic test measures both parasympathetic and sympathetic function?

A. heart rate (HR) variability with deep breathing

B. sympathetic skin response

C. HR change in standing (30:15 ratio)

D. quantitative Valsalva maneuver

---

99. Which of the following is NOT a potential proximal median nerve entrapment site?

A. arcade of Frohse

B. ligament of Struthers

C. lacertus fibrosus

D. pronator teres

100. Findings indicative of a neuropathic pattern of motor unit action potential (MUAP) recruitment include

   A. increased recruitment interval.

   B. decreased recruitment ratio.

   C. increased recruitment frequency.

   D. all of the above

101. The physical examination findings of spasticity, hyperreflexia, and extensor (upgoing) plantar response can be present in all of the following diseases, EXCEPT

   A. primary lateral sclerosis (PLS).

   B. spinal muscular atrophy (SMA).

   C. amyotrophic lateral sclerosis (ALS).

   D. middle cerebral artery stroke.

102. Which of the following electrodiagnostic test findings is most suggestive of an ulnar nerve lesion proximal to the wrist?

   A. reduced ulnar sensory nerve action potential (SNAP) amplitude obtained by recording at digit 5 and stimulating (14 cm) proximally at the wrist

   B. same-side latency difference of greater than 2.0 milliseconds between the abductor digiti minimi (ADM) and first dorsal interosseous (FDI) compound muscle action potentials (CMAPs) at the wrist stimulation site

   C. absent or abnormal dorsal ulnar cutaneous (DUC) SNAP

   D. a normal needle electromyography (EMG) examination of the flexor carpi ulnaris (FCU) muscle

103. The amplitude of a needle electromyography (EMG) motor unit action potential (MUAP) is

   A. measured from baseline to negative peak.

   B. influenced by the number of motor units near the needle electrode.

   C. reduced by lowering the high-frequency filter.

   D. representative of total number of muscle fibers in a motor unit.

104. A 65-year-old female who has a past medical history of L5-S1 disc herniation and "sciatica" 6 years ago presents with vague bilateral posterior thigh pain of 3 months duration. She has no other associated symptoms. Spine and neurologic examinations are normal. Last month, she had electrodiagnostic testing of the bilateral lower limbs at an outside facility showing absent bilateral tibial H reflex responses. The remainder of the sensorimotor nerve conduction and motor F wave studies were within normal limits. Needle electromyography studies of the bilateral lower limbs, hips, and lumbosacral paraspinal muscles were within normal limits. These electrodiagnostic study findings are consistent with

   A. recurrent bilateral S1 radiculopathies.

   B. acute bilateral sciatic neuropathies.

   C. early polyneuropathy.

   D. none of the above

105. The characteristic single-fiber electromyography (SFEMG) findings in patients with amyotrophic lateral sclerosis (ALS) are

   A. decreased jitter and increased fiber density.

   B. decreased jitter and decreased fiber density.

   C. increased jitter and decreased fiber density.

   D. increased jitter and increased fiber density.

106. Which peripheral nervous system structure contains both motor and sensory nerve fibers?

   A. dorsal root ganglion

   B. dorsal root

   C. ventral root

   D. dorsal ramus

107. Mononeuritis multiplex

   A. predominantly affects the upper limbs.

   B. is associated with conduction block at uncommon nerve entrapment sites.

   C. is a common pattern of vasculitic neuropathy.

   D. is treated with intravenous immunoglobulin (IVIG).

108. All of these needle electromyography (EMG) potentials consist of motor unit action potentials (MUAPs), EXCEPT

A. cramps.

B. complex repetitive discharges.

C. fasciculation.

D. myokymic discharges.

109. During a needle electromyography (EMG) study, the patient is asked to minimally contract the affected muscle yielding only one motor unit action potential (MUAP) firing at 15 Hz. Further muscle contraction causes the MUAP to increase its firing rate to 30 Hz with the appearance of a second motor unit action potential firing at 20 Hz. Maximal contraction is achieved and yields 5 motor units: the first MUAP firing at 50 Hz and the other four firing between 20 and 30 Hz with an incomplete interference pattern. The findings are consistent with

A. neurogenic recruitment.

B. myopathic recruitment.

C. decreased activation.

D. both A and C

110. Compared with a radiation-induced brachial plexopathy, a recurrent neoplastic brachial plexopathy in a postradiation cancer survivor is more likely to

A. present with pain.

B. occur with radiation doses less than 10,000 rads.

C. involve the upper trunk.

D. demonstrate fasciculation potentials on needle electromyography (EMG).

111. In standard bipolar nerve stimulator electrodes, the positive terminal is the

A. anode.

B. cathode.

C. active electrode.

D. amplifier.

112. A doctor in another specialty refers a patient to you for "EMG/NCV to rule out postpolio syndrome." Which of the following statements is true?

   A. Postpoliomyelitis syndrome has characteristic findings on needle electromyography (EMG) that distinguish it from clinically stable previous poliomyelitis infection.

   B. Postpoliomyelitis syndrome is a clinical diagnosis, and electrodiagnostic tests exclude other conditions.

   C. Postpoliomyelitis syndrome occurs due to reactivation of latent polio virus in the spinal sensory ganglia and is detected by needle EMG paraspinal muscle examination.

   D. Postpoliomyelitis syndrome is rapidly progressive and potentially fatal if not diagnosed and treated early.

113. Calculate the median sensory nerve conduction velocity for an antidromic study recording at 2nd digit and stimulating at only one site (at the wrist 140 mm from the recording electrode). The median *onset* latency is 2.9 milliseconds.

   A. 47 m/s

   B. 48 m/s

   C. 50 m/s

   D. not enough information to calculate

114. Normal needle electromyography (EMG) insertional activity

   A. lasts between 300 and 500 milliseconds.

   B. has an irregular firing pattern at the endplate region.

   C. represents the summated voltage of the muscle fibers from one motor unit.

   D. results from mechanical muscle fiber depolarization.

115. All of the following represent electrodiagnostic features of acquired demyelinating polyneuropathy, EXCEPT

   A. conduction block of compound muscle action potentials (CMAPs).

   B. abnormal temporal dispersion.

   C. prolonged minimal F wave latency.

   D. normal to mildly slowed conduction velocities.

116. What is the most sensitive electrodiagnostic test for diagnosis of neuromuscular junction disorders?

    A. repetitive nerve stimulation

    B. single-fiber electromyography

    C. monopolar needle electromyography of the orbicularis oculi muscle

    D. motor nerve conduction study of the facial nerve

117. A repetitive nerve stimulation study finding that aids in distinguishing a presynaptic from a postsynaptic neuromuscular junction disorder is

    A. a reduced compound muscle action potential (CMAP) amplitude to initial supramaximal nerve stimulus in only postsynaptic disorders.

    B. a decremental CMAP amplitude in response to preexercise slow stimulation rates only in presynaptic disorders.

    C. an incremental CMAP amplitude in response to fast stimulation rates only in presynaptic disorders.

    D. a progressive decrement in CMAP amplitude below initial baseline levels occurring minutes after maximum activation in only presynaptic disorders.

118. What is the effect of lowering an electrodiagnostic instrument's high-frequency (low-pass) filter from 10,000 Hz to 500 Hz when recording nerve action potentials?

    A. decreasing the onset latency

    B. decreasing the duration

    C. increasing the amplitude

    D. increasing the peak latency

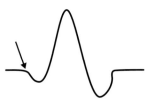

119. The arrow in the compound muscle action potential (CMAP) pictured above points to a deflection from the baseline the could be explained by all of the following, EXCEPT

    A. submaximal stimulation.

    B. tendon potential.

    C. volume conduction.

    D. recording electrode off the motor point.

120. Which pharmaceutical is known to cause toxicity, exclusively to sensory nerves?

    A. vincristine

    B. cisplatin

    C. rituximab

    D. duloxetine

121. Sensory nerve action potentials (SNAPs), specifically obtained from proximal stimulation, are difficult to interpret secondary to

    A. phase cancellation.

    B. stimulus artifact.

    C. temporal dispersion.

    D. both A and C

122. A 25-year-old male with sacrum and pelvic fractures from a high-speed motor vehicle collision is referred for electrodiagnostic testing, specifically to evaluate for nerve injury involving the S2 to S4 nerve roots. In planning your needle electromyography (EMG) study, all of the following muscles typically would represent at least one of these nerve roots, EXCEPT

  A. external anal sphincter.

  B. adductor hallucis.

  C. extensor digitorum longus.

  D. abductor digiti minimi.

123. Peripheral polyneuropathy associated with HIV infection and AIDS can present as

  A. distal sensory polyneuropathy.

  B. inflammatory demyelinating polyneuropathy.

  C. mononeuropathy multiplex.

  D. all of the above

124. Which of the following machine settings are most appropriate for a routine sensory nerve conduction study?

  A. sweep speed: 5 milliseconds; sensitivity: 5,000 μV; filters: 2 to 10,000 Hz

  B. sweep speed: 2 milliseconds; sensitivity: 20 μV; filters: 20 to 2,000 Hz

  C. sweep speed: 5 milliseconds; sensitivity: 1,000 μV; filters: 2 to 10,000 Hz

  D. sweep speed: 10 milliseconds; sensitivity: 2,000 μV; filters: 20 to 2,000 Hz

125. The most common pattern in diabetic polyneuropathy is

  A. axonal and demyelinating sensorimotor.

  B. axonal motor > sensory axonal.

  C. axonal sensorimotor.

  D. demyelinating sensorimotor.

126. Which of the following is true regarding neuromuscular junction pathophysiology?

   A. Myasthenia gravis most commonly arises from a genetic defect in the acetylcholine receptor.

   B. Lambert-Eaton syndrome arises from a reduced number of acetylcholine molecules per vesicle.

   C. Botulinum toxins inactivate the proteins required for the fusion and release of acetylcholine vesicles at the presynaptic membrane.

   D. Curare toxin depletes acetylcholinesterase in the synaptic space.

127. Which type of electromyography (EMG) needle electrode has the smallest recording surface?

   A. bipolar concentric

   B. standard concentric

   C. monopolar

   D. single-fiber

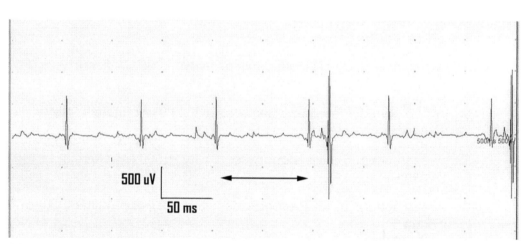

500 uV

50 ms

Adapted with permission from Pease WS, Lew HL, Johnson EW, eds. *Johnson's Practical Electromyography.* 4th ed. Philadelphia, PA: Lippincott Williams & Wilkins; 2006.

128. Which of the following statements is true regarding the motor unit action potential (MUAP) recruitment in the above needle electromyography (EMG) tracing?

   A. It depicts normal MUAP recruitment.

   B. It depicts reduced MUAP recruitment.

   C. It depicts early MUAP recruitment.

   D. It cannot be determined.

129. A disease commonly associated with axonal sensorimotor polyneuropathy is

   A. alcoholism.

   B. Friedrich ataxia.

   C. leprosy (Hansen disease).

   D. renal failure (uremia).

130. The pattern of electrophysiologic findings typical of hereditary motor sensory neuropathy (Charcot-Marie-Tooth disease) type I would show

   A. abnormal temporal dispersion.

   B. motor nerve conduction block.

   C. focal nerve conduction velocity slowing at common nerve entrapment sites.

   D. uniform slowing of nerve conduction velocity involving all segments.

131. The following muscles can be recorded when performing peroneal nerve motor conduction studies, EXCEPT

   A. extensor digitorum brevis.

   B. tibialis anterior.

   C. peroneus longus.

   D. abductor hallucis.

132. Which of the following technical factors could falsely decrease the onset latency measurement of a recorded nerve or muscle action potential?

   A. increasing the stimulus intensity above supramaximal

   B. increasing the stimulus duration

   C. lowering the high-frequency filter

   D. lowering the gain

133. The F wave late response can be described as

A. obtained by a submaximal stimulus.

B. a monosynaptic reflex.

C. produced by motor neuron backfiring.

D. resulting from activated afferent muscle spindle fibers.

134. A 45-year-old right-handed female who has a past medical history of breast cancer presents with a 3-month history of pain and numbness involving the right medial forearm and last two fingers of her right hand. Physical examination reveals weakness in both the thenar and hypothenar muscles of the right hand as well as diminished sensation in the last two digits of the right hand and medial forearm. The electrodiagnostic study data tables are listed below:

Nerve Conduction Studies

Motor Nerve	Distal Latency (ms)	Amplitude (mV)	Conduction Velocity (m/s)
R. median motor (abductor pollicis brevis)	S1: 2.9 (norm <4.4) S2: 6.3	S1: 2.2 (norm >4.2) S2: 2.1	S1-S2: 58 (norm >51)
R. ulnar motor (abductor digiti minimi)	S1: 2.8 (norm <3.7) S2: 6.1 S3: 7.7	S1: 1.9 (norm >7.9) S2: 1.8 S3: 1.8	S1-S2: 60 (norm >52) S2-S3: 62 (norm >43)

Abbreviation: R., right; S1, wrist; S2, elbow; S3, above elbow.

Sensory Nerve	Stimulation Site	Peak Latency (ms)	Amplitude (μV)
R. median (record digit 2)	Wrist: 14 cm	3.0 (norm <4.0)	24.0 (norm >19.0)
R. ulnar (record digit 5)	Wrist: 14 cm	2.8 (norm <4.0)	2.1 (norm >8.0)
R. radial (record base of thumb)	Forearm: 10 cm	1.8 (norm <2.8)	22.0 (norm >11.0)
R. medial antebrachial cutaneous (record medial forearm)	Elbow: 12 cm	2.1 (norm <2.6)	1.3 (norm >3.0)
R. lateral antebrachial cutaneous (record lateral forearm)	Elbow: 12 cm	2.0 (norm <2.5)	18.0 (norm >6.0)

Abbreviation: R., right.
All *left* side comparison nerve conduction studies were within normal limits.

Electromyography

Muscle	Insertion at Rest	MUAP Morphology	Recruitment
R. abductor digiti minimi	3+ FIB and PSW	↑ duration, 2+ poly	Decreased
R. abductor pollicis brevis	3+ FIB and PSW	↑ duration, 2+ poly	Decreased
R. flexor pollicis longus	3+ FIB and PSW	↑ duration, 2+ poly	Decreased
R. extensor indicis	1+ FIB and PSW	↑ duration, 1+ poly	Decreased
R. flexor digitorum profundus	3+ FIB and PSW	↑ duration, 2+ poly	Decreased
R. flexor digitorum superficialis	1+ FIB and PSW	↑ duration, 1+ poly	Decreased
R. flexor carpi radialis	Normal	Normal	Normal
R. triceps	Normal	Normal	Normal
R. deltoid	Normal	Normal	Normal
R. C1-T2 paraspinal muscles	Normal		

Abbreviations: FIB, fibrillation potential; MUAP, motor unit action potential; PSW, positive sharp wave; R., right.

All *left* side comparison muscles were within normal limits.

Based on the findings, the impression is most consistent with right

A. C8-T1 radiculopathies.

B. lower trunk brachial plexopathy.

C. median and ulnar mononeuropathies.

D. both A and C

---

135. Repetitive nerve stimulation is performed on a subject immediately after 10 seconds of maximal muscle contraction. The tracing shows progressively larger compound muscle action potential (CMAP) amplitudes from the baseline with repeated stimulation well as a decrease in the duration of each successive waveform. Negative peak area is found to be unchanged. These findings are most likely the result of a

A. movement artifact from inadequate limb immobilization.

B. postsynaptic disorder of neuromuscular transmission.

C. limb temperature below 34° C.

D. normal synchronization of muscle fiber action potentials.

136. Stimulus artifact during surface nerve excitation

   A. is recorded and preamplified before the biologic signal.

   B. can be counteracted by rotating the stimulator's cathode about the anode.

   C. represents impedance at the skin–electrode interface.

   D. occurs due to ambient noise.

137. A severe form of which hereditary motor sensory neuropathy (HMSN) represents a congenital hypomyelination neuropathy that clinically manifests as generalized weakness and hypotonia at birth?

   A. HMSN type I

   B. HMSN type II

   C. HMSN type III

   D. HMSN type IV

138. In electrodiagnostic instrumentation, the amplifier should possess which of the following characteristics?

   A. low amplifier input impedance and high common mode gain

   B. high differential gain and low common mode gain

   C. low common mode rejection ratio and low differential gain

   D. high common mode gain and low differential gain

139. You are testing a patient with a suspected diagnosis of myasthenia gravis, recording at the abductor pollicis brevis muscle. Initial compound muscle action potential (CMAP) amplitude is within normal limits with supramaximal stimulus. There is a 30% decrement between the first and fourth responses during 3 Hz stimulation. You would expect to observe all of the following additional findings, EXCEPT

   A. 200% increment in CMAP amplitude immediately following 10 seconds of exercise.

   B. 50% decrement between the first and second responses during preexercise low-rate stimulation.

   C. 60% decrement in CMAP amplitude recorded 2 minutes after exercise.

   D. 40% decrement in CMAP amplitude recorded 6 minutes after exercise.

140. Which type of study or technique could be used in order to accurately isolate the proximal median nerve compound muscle action potential (CMAP) elicited by stimulation at the axilla?

A. collision

B. F wave

C. A wave

D. H reflex

141. Neurapraxia injury is characterized by

A. conduction block.

B. Wallerian degeneration.

C. axon discontinuity.

D. small unmyelinated nerve fibers being most susceptible to injury.

142. Which needle electromyography (EMG) spontaneous discharges are associated with radiation-induced plexopathy?

A. neuromyotonic

B. myotonic

C. myokymic

D. cramp

143. All of the following muscles could be tested for a facial nerve (CN VII) motor study, EXCEPT

A. nasalis.

B. orbicularis oculi.

C. masseter.

D. orbicularis oris.

144. A patient is referred to you for electrodiagnostic testing of the "right upper extremity to rule out right cervical radiculopathy." Nerve conduction studies (NCS) of the right upper extremity show mildly prolonged median and ulnar compound muscle action potential (CMAP) distal latencies with moderately reduced amplitudes and normal conduction velocities. Right median, ulnar, and radial sensory nerve action potential (SNAP) responses are normal. Needle electromyography (EMG) study shows small amplitude positive sharp waves and fibrillation potentials, increased motor unit action potential amplitudes and durations, increased polyphasic potentials, and diminished recruitment in all muscles tested (representing myotomes C5-T1). The right cervical C5-T1 paraspinal muscles also show spontaneous muscle fiber activity at rest. What is the next best step in evaluation?

A. Perform a single-fiber EMG study of the right upper extremity.

B. Obtain somatosensory evoked potentials recording the right median and ulnar nerves.

C. Arrange for EMG and NCS testing of the contralateral limb.

D. Document a right upper extremity polyradiculopathy in your impression and recommend the referring physician obtain a cervical spine magnetic resonance imaging (MRI) study.

145. Which needle electromyography (EMG) discharge potentials would persist after a neuromuscular junction blockade?

A. neuromyotonic

B. myotonic

C. multiplet

D. tremor

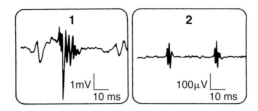

Adapted with permission from Stovitz SD, Swiontkowski MF, eds. *Manual of Orthopaedics*. 6th ed. Philadelphia, PA: Lippincott Williams & Wilkins; 2005.

146. The graphics above (labeled 1 and 2) depict two types of motor unit action potentials (MUAPs) seen in motor unit reinnervation. Which of the following statements is true regarding these graphics?

A. Graphic 1 can occur after complete denervation.

B. Graphic 2 signifies direct axon regrowth from injury site.

C. Both graphics 1 and 2 are found only in myopathies.

D. Both graphics 1 and 2 represent collateral sprouting from adjacent motor units.

147. Features of hereditary motor sensory neuropathy (HMSN) (Charcot-Marie-Tooth disease) type II include

A. axonal atrophy and degeneration.

B. onion bulb formation on histopathology.

C. elevated serum phytanic acid levels.

D. hypertrophy of peripheral nerves.

148. Which needle electromyography (EMG) grouped discharge potentials arise from a single muscle fiber, represent spread of depolarization to adjacent fibers, fire consecutively over recurrent cycles, possess a regular rhythm and stable morphology, and are time-linked together?

A. myokymic discharges

B. myotonic discharges

C. neuromyotonic discharges

D. complex repetitive discharges

149.   Which concept refers to the difference between the magnitude of the end-plate potential generated at the neuromuscular junction and the threshold potential required for initiating an action potential?

    A. safety factor

    B. rundown phenomenon

    C. potentiation

    D. facilitation

150.   Increasing an electrodiagnostic instrument's low-frequency (high-pass) filter affects the nerve action potential waveform by

    A. increasing the onset latency.

    B. increasing the amplitude.

    C. decreasing the duration.

    D. decreasing the number of phases.

ANSWER KEY WITH EXPLANATIONS

1. The correct answer is B.

The spinal cord ventral (anterior) horn cell bodies give rise to efferent neurons (transmit signals from the central nervous system to the peripheral nervous system) whose myelinated axons form the ventral root and provide motor innervation to skeletal muscle. Conversely, afferent (sensory) neurons transmit signals from peripheral receptors back to the central nervous system. The nerve cell bodies of sensory neurons are located outside of the central nervous system within the dorsal root ganglia. Unmyelinated neurons can be found in the central nervous system gray matter and in peripheral C fiber (type IV) sensory nerves.

2. The correct answer is B.

Orthodromic refers to nerve impulse conduction in the direction of normal physiologic function. A motor nerve is stimulated proximally while recording at a distal muscle innervated by that nerve. The generated action potential travels in the direction efferent motor nerve impulses normally travel in order to activate their corresponding muscle fibers (i.e., proximal to distal). Conversely, antidromic conduction is in the opposite direction of normal physiologic function. Sensory nerve conduction studies can be performed either antidromically or orthodromically. Sensory afferent nerve impulses travel distal to proximal; therefore, a sensory study recording proximally and stimulating distally would be considered orthodromic.

3. The correct answer is A.

If you are choosing additional L4 innervated muscles to test, the iliopsoas muscle would not be appropriate as it receives L2 and L3 innervation. The gracilis muscle receives L2, L3, and L4 innervation. The tensor fasciae latae and gluteus minimus muscles receive L4, L5, and S1 innervation.

4. The correct answer is B.

Steroid myopathy affects type II muscle fibers causing atrophy. There would be normal recruitment observed during needle EMG because type I fibers are initially recruited with mild to moderate muscle contraction. No spontaneous muscle fiber activity would be seen because the pathogenesis of steroid myopathy does not involve necrosis, inflammation, or other conditions that break down the muscle fiber connection to the neuromuscular junction. The other answer choices listed affect type I muscle fibers and would be expected to show needle EMG abnormalities.

5. The correct answer is C.

Arsenic toxicity causes painful paresthesias in the hands and feet as well as progressive weakness. With high-dose exposure, the weakness may progress to involve the respiratory and cranial muscles, which mimics Guillain-Barré syndrome.

6. The correct answer is C.
According to the Henneman size principle, small alpha motor units (type I) are recruited first during voluntary muscle contraction as they generate low force at a low threshold of excitation for low-intensity activity and are more fatigue-resistant than type II fibers. Type I (slow-twitch) motor units also have a smaller innervation ratios, nerve cell bodies, and axon diameters than type II (fast-twitch) motor units. When greater muscle contractile force is needed, type II (A and B) motor units are next recruited as they are larger in size and innervate a larger number of muscle fibers to generate high force at a high threshold of excitation for high-intensity activity.

7. The correct answer is C.
The median nerve is formed from both the medial and lateral cords of the brachial plexus and contains both sensory and motor fibers. The lateral cord (derived from the anterior divisions of the upper and middle trunks) supplies median sensory fibers to digits 1 to 3 and motor fibers to the proximal median innervated forearm muscles. The medial cord (derived from anterior division of the lower trunk) supplies median sensory fibers to the lateral half of digit 4 and motor fibers to the median innervated distal forearm and hand muscles.

8. The correct answer is D.
The Na^+-K^+-ATP pump maintains the nerve cell membrane potential by using ATP as an energy source to actively transport two potassium ions into the cell for every three sodium ions it exports. This counteracts the natural tendency for K^+ to passively diffuse out of the cell and Na^+ into the cell via leak channels, which if not counteracted, would eventually dissipate the membrane potential. Voltage-gated ion channels are activated during action potential generation and remain closed when the cell is at resting membrane potential.

9. The correct answer is A.
The H reflex is a true monosynaptic reflex obtained by submaximal stimulation with a stable latency from one stimulus to the next. Unlike the H reflex, the A wave is not a true reflex; it arises from antidromic motor stimulation of a collateral sprout in a reinnervated axon with orthodromic backfiring. Like the H reflex, the A wave is elicited by a submaximal stimulus with a stable latency from one stimulus to the next. The A wave is visualized between the M response and the F wave.

10. The correct answer is B.
The absent CMAP response above the elbow on initial testing suggests failure of nerve action potentials to propagate past the site of injury. This could represent either a complete conduction block or a complete axonal injury at the elbow. At 3 weeks postinjury, the additional absent CMAP responses at the wrist and below elbow stimulation sites indicate that distal denervation has occurred, which is consistent with a complete axonal injury. Conduction block injuries are focal and reversible with normal CMAP responses distal to the site of injury on repeat testing. Partial conduction block would initially present with a reduced CMAP amplitude and area above the elbow. Needle electromyography test results 3 weeks postinjury were not included in this case but also can distinguish between conduction block and axonal injury.

11. The correct answer is D.

Decreased reflexes, fasciculations, and a normal sensory examination are characteristics of both MMN and motor neuron disease. MMN is distinct because the pattern of weakness is in a peripheral nerve distribution, which is often asymmetric and in the distal arm muscles. MMN shows characteristic multifocal conduction block on nerve conduction studies. A pattern of weakness in a myotomal distribution is characteristic of motor neuron disease.

12. The correct answer is C.

The lateral antebrachial cutaneous nerve is derived from the upper trunk of the brachial plexus and supplies sensation to the lateral forearm. Hence, an upper trunk brachial plexopathy can present with diminished sensation over the right lateral forearm. The sensation over the medial aspect of the hand is supplied by the lower trunk of the brachial plexus. The finger flexors and extensors receive innervation from the middle and lower trunks of the brachial plexus.

13. The correct answer is B.

A more sensitive test would be more likely to detect the presence of median mononeuropathy at the wrist. The test sensitivity for median sensory nerve conduction between the wrist and digit is about 65%. The sensitivity of a comparison median-to-ulnar study between the wrist and ring finger is about 85%. The American Association of Electrodiagnostic Medicine (AAEM) practice parameter for electrodiagnostic studies in carpal tunnel syndrome recommends additional testing in this scenario (see summary statement article in *Muscle Nerve* 2002;25:918-922). Sympathetic and F wave tests are not as sensitive.

14. The correct answer is D.

All of the statements are correct. Additionally, if only the sensory nerve root is affected, the study also would be normal.

15. The correct answer is B.

Type B motor fibers are small, unmyelinated, preganglionic autonomic fibers. Type A-δ fibers are sensory only and consist of small, myelinated touch, pain, and temperature fibers. Type C fibers consist of small, unmyelinated motor and sensory fibers; the C motor fibers are postganglionic autonomics. Type A-γ fibers are small, myelinated motor neurons to intrafusal muscle fibers.

16. The correct answer is D.

The evaluation of "numb thumb" is a favorite topic for clinical case studies. This study is just one example of many ways clinicians can tailor their electromyography (EMG)/nerve conduction study (NCS) examination to the differential diagnoses. The right median sensory and motor latencies are prolonged at the wrist, suggestive of a median mononeuropathy. The remaining nerves tested are within normal limits, excluding polyneuropathy. The right radial sensory latency and amplitude are normal, excluding radial sensory neuropathy. Normal median and radial sensory nerve action potentials (SNAPs) make an upper/middle trunk or posterior/lateral cord brachial plexopathy unlikely. The EMG shows abnormalities in three separate limb muscles supplied by different peripheral nerves with right C6 nerve root innervation in common. Paraspinal abnormalities further serve to confirm the lesion as a radiculopathy. In this case, the impression was both a right median mononeuropathy and C6 radiculopathy. Clinically, the sensation disturbance over the thenar eminence would indicate a more proximal lesion because that area would be spared in an isolated median mononeuropathy at the wrist.

17. The correct answer is B.

Anodal block is a theoretical nonpathologic phenomenon that is unlikely to occur during routine nerve conduction studies. The action potential beneath the cathode travels bidirectionally; in theory, hyperpolarization beneath the anode could block propagation in this direction. However, this has not been proven to occur in humans as inadvertently switching the position of the anode and cathode during surface nerve stimulation still generates an action potential waveform of similar magnitude. Switching the polarity of the stimulating electrode does affect latency and conduction velocity measurements. Focal nerve compression can cause conduction block, which is a separate pathologic phenomenon. When the active and reference electrodes are switched, the recorded waveform is inverted in appearance.

18. The correct answer is D.

Normal insertional activity is less than 300 milliseconds in duration and results from the mechanical depolarization of individual muscle fibers by the needle electrode. There is the brief appearance of individual spike waveforms but no sustained firing pattern.

19. The correct answer is A.

All three tracings depict types of spontaneous activity. Tracing 1 depicts a train of fibrillation potentials, which are believed to be secondary to spontaneous muscle fiber depolarization. Fibrillation potentials are typically short duration (1 to 5 milliseconds), biphasic with initial positive deflection, and fire at a regular rate (as depicted in tracing 1). Tracing 2 depicts a single positive sharp wave, which is also a spontaneous muscle fiber depolarization. Tracing 3 depicts two separate fasciculation potentials of different morphologies representing the spontaneous discharge of single motor units.

20. The correct answer is D.

The "all-or-none" principle refers to the constant magnitude of the nerve cell action potential once the threshold stimulus is reached; a stimulus intensity greater than that needed to reach the threshold will not produce a larger action potential, and a subthreshold stimulus will not produce an action potential at all. The absolute refractory period is a period during an action potential when Na^+ channels remain inactivated and no further action potential can be produced, regardless of strength of stimulus.

21. The correct answer is B.

You might encounter a similar scenario in your own practice. This patient appears to have an undiagnosed progressive neurologic illness. In this case, his clinical features most closely resemble amyotrophic lateral sclerosis (ALS). The El Escorial World Federation of Neurology Criteria clearly establishes the clinical criteria in the absence of pathologic evidence or neuroimaging evidence of other diseases that might explain the observed clinical and electrophysiologic signs. Thus, other testing is appropriate to exclude other conditions that could cause upper and lower motor neuron signs. Scientific studies support the use of multidisciplinary teams in improving survival and quality of life in patients with ALS. The American Academy of Neurology position statement on ALS care places a high priority on patient autonomy in decision making. Thus, deciding on your own to send the patient to hospice is not appropriate, as the patient himself or another family member should be involved in that decision.

22. The correct answer is D.

The most common anomalous innervation in the lower extremity is the accessory peroneal nerve (APN). The APN is derived from the superficial peroneal nerve, travels posterior to the lateral malleolus, and innervates the lateral portion of the EDB. The fibers of the APN are excited by proximal stimulation at and above the fibular head, yielding larger peroneal CMAP amplitudes proximally than distally. Temporal dispersion would cause a slight decrease in proximal CMAP amplitudes compared to distally. A conduction block would cause a decrease in CMAP amplitude above the injury site. Muscle atrophy of the EDB is common but would result in uniformly decreased CMAP amplitudes at all stimulation sites.

23. The correct answer is B.

Decreasing a nerve's temperature increases the opening time and delays the inactivation of voltage-gated sodium channels during action potential generation. The depolarizing current flows for a longer period of time; thus, the time to reach peak depolarization increases. The prolonged current flow increases the action potential amplitude and duration. Decreasing temperature also prolongs inactivation of sodium channels and increases the refractory periods; thus, action potential propagation slows and the nerve's conduction velocity decreases.

24. The correct answer is B.

Assuming typical plexus anatomy, the dorsal scapular nerve is formed directly off of the C5 nerve root, innervates the rhomboid muscles, and contributes to the innervation of the levator scapulae muscle. Because this nerve originates at the nerve root level, the muscles it innervates would be typically spared in a panplexopathy distal to the roots. The serratus anterior (not an answer choice) would also be spared as it is innervated by the long thoracic nerve formed by the fifth through seventh cervical nerve roots. The latissimus dorsi and pectoralis major muscles receive innervation from all trunks of the brachial plexus. The deltoid receives innervation from the upper trunk of the brachial plexus.

25. The correct answer is B.

Indeed, the data tables show that the abnormal values in the presurgery study have either improved or normalized in the postsurgery study. Be aware that it is common to see persistent conduction velocity slowing even after undergoing carpal tunnel release surgery. After nerve decompression, some remyelinated areas do not regrow as thick of a myelin sheath as before, and there is increased internode distance. From the data tables alone, one cannot conclude that this was a failed surgery or recurrent carpal tunnel syndrome. This is where the clinical history, physical examination, and differential diagnosis become integral in making the determination of what is causing the thumb pain.

26. The correct answer is C.

The monopolar needle electrode has a spherical, multidirectional surface area that records motor unit action potentials (MUAPs) with higher amplitudes and more polyphasic potentials than unidirectional needle electrodes. The other listed needle electrodes have a beveled design that only allows unidirectional recording within a limited hemispheric area. The monopolar needle electrode is less painful and less expensive than the standard concentric needle electrode but is less durable and more prone to electrical interference.

27. The correct answer is C.

When a standard bipolar surface stimulator probe applies an electrical impulse to the skin overlying the nerve being studied, large numbers of intracellular positive charges are attracted to the area beneath the cathode due to the high negative extracellular voltage at that terminal. This causes nerve depolarization typically to occur first beneath the cathode. Conversely, large numbers of intracellular negative charges are attracted to the area beneath the anode causing nerve hyperpolarization in this region. In atypical circumstances, the area beneath the anode could be depolarized if excessive stimulus current were applied to the nerve.

28. The correct answer is A.

Maximal stimulus is the intensity at which there is no further increase in the evoked potential. Supramaximal stimulus is 20% to 30% above maximal stimulus and is used in most nerve conduction studies because it ensures all axons of the nerve have been stimulated (both large and small nerve fibers). Threshold stimulus is only of sufficient strength to produce a detectable evoked potential. Subthreshold stimulus will not produce a detectable response.

29. The correct answer is B.

In an isolated suprascapular neuropathy, the teres minor muscle (innervated by the axillary nerve) would test normal. In an isolated C5 radiculopathy, the C5-6 innervated infraspinatus muscle would test abnormal. In an isolated upper trunk brachial plexopathy, the rhomboid major (dorsal scapular nerve via direct branch of C5 nerve root) would test normal. In both a C5 radiculopathy and a suprascapular neuropathy, the latissimus dorsi (thoracodorsal nerve C6-8) muscle would be expected to test normal.

30. The correct answer is C.

The black arrows point to the perineurium, which is composed of connective tissue that surrounds nerve bundles (fascicles/funiculi) containing both myelinated and unmyelinated fibers. The endoneurium (located in the image region labeled 2) surrounds individual axons within the fascicle. The epineurium (located in the image region labeled 1) surrounds the entire nerve and binds the fascicles together. The sarcolemma is the plasma membrane of a muscle fiber and is not related to microscopic nerve anatomy.

31. The correct answer is C.

Axonotmesis (Seddon classification) and types 2 to 4 (Sunderland classification) nerve injuries are characterized by disruption of the axon with an intact epineurium. Type 2 nerve injury involves damage to the axon with all connective tissue structures intact.

Type 3 nerve injury involves damage to the axon and endoneurium. Type 4 nerve injury involves damage to the axon, endoneurium, and perineurium. Neurotmesis and type 5 nerve injuries involve damage to the axon and all connective tissue structures, including the epineurium.

32. The correct answer is D.

The anterior interosseous nerve innervates the flexor pollicis longus, pronator quadratus, and the flexor digitorum profundus muscle to digits 2 and 3. Weakness on physical examination and needle EMG abnormalities suggest neuropathy.

33. The correct answer is A.

The most consistent measured parameter supporting the diagnosis of myopathy is decreased MUAP duration, as it represents all fibers of a motor unit. MUAP duration is best measured via quantitative electromyography (EMG). Amplitude is variable depending on the distance of the needle electrode to the motor unit. Polyphasic MUAPs can be found in both neurogenic and myogenic disease due to various physiologic processes. Performing single-fiber EMG does not add significant information beyond that obtained with needle or quantitative EMG as increased jitter also can be found in other diseases.

34. The correct answer is D.

A notch filter is used to eliminate a specific frequency from the composite waveform. The 50- or 60-Hz notch filters are commonly used in electromyography to minimize the effects of electrical power line noise. High amplifier impedance attenuates the effect of electrode impedance in circuit by preserving the electrical voltage of the biologic signal. Averaging extracts a time-locked action potential from background noise. The preamplifier amplifies the signal before lead/cable noise is introduced.

35. The correct answer is C.

The rapid onset of unilateral right shoulder paresis preceded by a brief period of severe pain and recent illness is the classic presentation of neuralgic amyotrophy (also known as acute idiopathic brachial plexitis/neuritis or Parsonage-Turner syndrome). The incidence is 1.64/100,000 patients with a male predominance (2.4:1 male-to-female ratio). A clear etiology has not been established. The prognosis for functional recovery is generally good, although it could take as long as 3 years. If electromyography (EMG)/nerve conduction study (NCS) are performed immediately in this patient, it would likely not provide useful information to support the diagnosis or localize the lesion as it takes at least 7 to 21 days from the initial nerve injury/insult for the characteristic EMG/NCS findings of axonal loss to appear. The MRI findings are often nonspecific and include muscle edema.

36. The correct answer is C.

Myopathic conditions are characterized by loss of active muscle fibers and less muscle fibers per motor unit. In order to generate minimal muscle contractile force, multiple rapid firing motor units are recruited early (i.e., increased recruitment). Answer choice A describes normal recruitment. Answer choice B describes neurogenic (i.e., reduced) recruitment. Answer choice D describes decreased activation.

37. The correct answer is B.

SSEPs are widely believed to primarily travel to the cortex via the dorsal (posterior) column-medial lemniscus central nervous system tract, which carries myelinated afferent fibers mediating vibration, pressure, muscle stretch, and proprioception. The first-order neurons synapse in either the nucleus gracilis or nucleus cuneatus of the medulla. The second-order neurons cross over to the contralateral side forming the medial lemniscus and subsequently synapse in the ventral posterior lateral nucleus of the thalamus. The third-order neurons terminate in the somatosensory cortex. There has also been a proposed second fiber route from the lower limbs via the posterior (dorsal) spinocerebellar tract.

38. The correct answer is B.

Most published experts in the field of electrodiagnostic medicine agree that a radiculopathy is diagnosed when needle EMG abnormalities are found in two or more muscles innervated by the same nerve root but different peripheral nerves. The muscles innervated by adjacent nerve roots should be normal if no other superimposed pathology is present. Ideally, needle EMG abnormalities also should be present in the corresponding paraspinal muscles to confirm that the lesion is proximal to the dorsal root ganglion. The exact level of radiculopathy cannot be determined reliably by paraspinal EMG alone as polysegmental innervation can exist in some cases. SNAP latencies should be normal in an isolated radiculopathy. CMAP amplitudes can be reduced in some severe radiculopathies, but this alone is insufficient in distinguishing a radiculopathy from a peripheral neuropathy.

39. The correct answer is C.

The ulnar sensory nerve fibers innervate digit 5 and the medial half of digit 4 in normal (i.e., nonanomalous) individuals. Digits 1 and 3 are in the cutaneous distributions of the median and radial nerves.

40. The correct answer is A.

The pectoralis major muscle is innervated by both the medial and lateral pectoral nerves. The lateral pectoral nerve is derived from C5 and C6 nerve roots and the upper trunk of the brachial plexus. The medial pectoral nerve is derived from the C7, C8, and T1 nerve roots as well as the middle and lower trunks of the brachial plexus. The serratus anterior is innervated by the C5, C6, and C7 nerve roots. The teres minor is innervated by the axillary nerve, which is derived from C5 and C6 nerve roots and the upper trunk of the brachial plexus. The teres major is innervated by the lower subscapular nerve, which is derived from C5 and C6 nerve roots and the upper trunk of the brachial plexus.

41. The correct answer is B.

The differential diagnosis for this patient includes all of the answer choices. L5 radiculopathy is less likely given a normal paraspinal needle electromyography (EMG) examination and the presence of abnormal sensory studies. Plexopathy is less likely given a normal tensor fasciae latae (TFL) muscle on needle EMG. Peroneal neuropathy would be a likely choice, except the short head of the biceps femoris muscle tested abnormal, indicating a lesion above the peroneal nerve. The lesion involves the peroneal division of the sciatic nerve, which is more often injured than the tibial division due to the arrangement of the nerve fibers.

42. The correct answer is D.

Unlike a recruited MUAP, a fasciculation potential is not under voluntary control. A fasciculation potential can fire irregularly at rates as slow as 0.1 Hz. MUAPs under voluntary control start firing at 2 to 3 Hz and typically reach a semirhythmic firing pattern at 4 to 5 Hz. Thus, a MUAP under voluntary control is unable to fire at a rate of less than 2 Hz. Fasciculation potentials are not always pathologic and can be found in normal individuals.

43. The correct answer is B.

A partial right facial nerve lesion would present as delayed right R1 and R2 responses with normal left R1 and R2 responses. A partial right trigeminal nerve lesion would present as a delay in all responses obtained with right-sided stimulation and all normal responses obtained with left sided stimulation. A partial right mid pons lesion would present as a delayed right R1 with all other responses normal. A partial right medullary lesion would present as a delayed right R2 with both right- and left-sided stimulation. *The author recommends reviewing the anatomic pathways and components of the blink reflex for a deeper understanding of the various patterns of abnormalities.*

44. The correct answer is B.

Costimulation of the adjacent median and ulnar nerves at the wrist leads to a falsely high distal median CMAP amplitude. A Martin-Gruber anastomosis causes increased median CMAP amplitude proximally. Submaximal stimulation of the median nerve at the wrist yields a CMAP with a lower distal than proximal amplitude. Mononeuropathy at the wrist can lower both the distal and proximal CMAP amplitudes if axon loss is present.

45. The correct answer is A.

Voltage-gated calcium channels play an important role at the axon terminal in mediating neuromuscular conduction. Opening of voltage-gated channels causes influx of calcium ions into the axon terminal, facilitating the fusion of acetylcholine vesicles to the presynaptic membrane. The synaptic clefts contain acetylcholinesterase and comprise the space between the axon terminal and the postsynaptic membrane of the motor endplate. Nodes of Ranvier contain voltage-gated sodium channels and allow saltatory conduction in myelinated nerves. Internode regions are myelinated segments between nodes of Ranvier, and their underlying axon membranes contain some potassium channels.

46. The correct answer is A.

A gene mutation at chromosome 17 actually is implicated in the hereditary form of neuralgic amyotrophy. This question illustrates that there are other (albeit less common) causes of radiculopathy aside from disc herniation and spondylosis. Infectious, metabolic, and inflammatory causes as well as tumor should be considered in the differential diagnosis of radiculopathy.

47. The correct answer is C.

The vignette illustrates that those who undergo rapid weight loss can be vulnerable to developing neuropathies at common compression sites. This unfortunate patient developed a common peroneal neuropathy at the fibular head as evidenced by the conduction block at the popliteal stimulation site, the conduction velocity slowing across the fibular head segment, and a mild degree of axon injury detected in common peroneal innervated muscles on needle electromyography (EMG).

48. The correct answer is B.

Hyperkalemic periodic paralysis can manifest with both clinical and electrical myotonia; one way to memorize this is to think of it as "HYPER[active] with myotonia." Contrast this to hypokalemic periodic paralysis, where myotonia is not a prevalent clinical feature, and no electrical myotonia is found on EMG. There is no clinical or electrical myotonia in acquired IBM. There is no clinical myotonia in DMD, and electrical myotonia is rare.

49. The correct answer is A.

The innervation ratio is defined as the total number of fibers in a particular muscle divided by the number of motor units innervating that muscle. Large muscles involved in gross movements that do not require dexterity have high innervation ratios (i.e., a large number of muscle fibers innervated by each motor unit). Gastrocnemius is the largest muscle out of the answer choices and has the highest innervation ratio (1,934 fibers per motor unit in the Feinstein et al. 1955 study). Small muscles associated with fine movements that require high dexterity have low innervation ratios (e.g., the external rectus ocular muscle with a ratio of 9 fibers per motor unit).

50. The correct answer is B.

Impedance is a measure of opposition to current flow in an alternating current circuit that takes into account properties of resistors, capacitors, and inductors. The human body is analogous to a circuit made up of resistive and capacitive elements (i.e., tissues and membranes). Bioelectric current flow in the human body occurs via ion movements facilitated by voltage differences (bioelectric potentials) across these elements. Ohm law [I (current) = E (voltage) / R (resistance)] can be applied to biologic systems [I = E / Z], where the bioelectric current flow (I) is inversely proportional to the impedance (Z). Conductance (g) is the inverse of resistance (R = 1 / g). According to Ohm law, current flow is directly proportional to the applied voltage (E = IR).

51. The correct answer is B.

The incidence of true neurogenic TOS is approximately one in a million. A fibrous band extending from the C7 transverse process to an anomalous cervical rib is thought to compress and injure the lower trunk of the brachial plexus. It is hypothesized that the T1 fibers innervating the thenar muscles are disproportionally more affected, providing an explanation for the classic finding of the median motor amplitude recording at the abductor pollicis brevis (APB) more reduced than the ulnar motor amplitude recording at the abductor digiti minimi (ADM) on the affected side. Otherwise, the electrophysiologic test findings in neurogenic TOS are those found in a lower trunk brachial plexopathy. The remaining answer choices are not consistent with a lower trunk brachial plexopathy.

52. The correct answer is A.

Slowing (increasing the numerical value of) the sweep speed and increasing the gain/sensitivity both alter the display of the action potential waveform and result in a perceived decrease in the onset latency. It is important to recognize this as a potential pitfall in interpreting nerve conduction studies. Sweep speed refers to the horizontal axis of the instrument's display screen and is measured in milliseconds per division. Gain (sensitivity) refers to the vertical axis and is measured in microvolts or millivolts per division. Slowing (increasing the numerical value of) the sweep speed compresses the waveform, shifts it to the left of the screen, and decreases its resolution. The compressed waveform with decreased resolution appears to have a faster departure from the baseline (decreased onset latency). Similarly, increasing the gain magnifies the waveform, and its departure from the baseline also appears faster. Amplitude is unchanged by increasing both settings. It is recommended that an instrument's settings replicate the reference laboratory's settings for a given set of normative data values.

53. The correct answer is B.

Partial conduction block should demonstrate reduced motor unit recruitment on needle EMG testing due to its pathophysiology of motor unit dropout. Motor unit recruitment is normal in demyelinating injury not due to conduction block because there is slowing but no loss of viable motor units. Increased recruitment is found in myopathy. Absent recruitment would occur in the case of a complete conduction block.

54. The correct answer is D.

The RR is the ratio of the firing rate of the first MUAP to the number of active MUAPs on the screen during EMG voluntary activation. Normal RR is 5:1. Thus, when the first MUAP is firing at 30 Hz, there should be six total active firing motor units: 30:6 = 5:1. Alternately, 30 / 5 = 6.

55. The correct answer is B.

Mixed nerve studies stimulate and record the sensory afferent (Ia) muscle spindle fibers. In a transcarpal median mixed nerve study, the median nerve is recorded at the wrist and stimulated at mid-palm. The study is orthodromic for sensory fibers and antidromic for motor fibers. The mixed NCV is typically faster than that of motor and sensory studies because the Ia fibers are the fastest conducting population of nerve fibers.

56. The correct answer is C.

The sacral plexus derived from the lumbosacral trunk (branch of L4 ventral ramus that joins the L5 ventral ramus) and the ventral rami of S1, S2, S3, and part of S4. The upper cord that forms the sciatic nerve consists of the anterior and posterior divisions of the sacral plexus. The posterior division contains the fibers that will become peroneal nerve. The anterior division contains the fibers that will become the tibial nerve. The obturator and femoral nerves are formed by the divisions of the lumbar plexus.

57. The correct answer is D.

The electrodiagnostic studies in this case show evidence most consistent with a C7 radiculopathy. Although the triceps and FCR muscles receive both C6 and C7 innervation, the deltoid muscle (C5 and C6) is normal. Although the triceps and EDC muscles receive both C7 and C8 innervation, the FDI (C8 and T1) is normal. Correlating physical examination findings could include decreased sensation over the middle finger (C7 dermatome distribution), diminished triceps reflex, and weakness in C7 innervated muscles. The supinator and brachialis muscles both receive innervation from the C5-6 nerve roots and would test normal in a C7 radiculopathy. The biceps reflex represents C5.

58. The correct answer is D.

Electrophysiologic tests to support a diagnosis of tarsal tunnel syndrome include medial and lateral plantar mixed nerve or sensory studies and motor studies recording at the abductor hallucis (AH) or abductor digiti minimi (ADM) muscles. Evidence to support a diagnosis of tarsal tunnel syndrome can include prolonged latencies or reduced amplitudes, especially when compared to the unaffected side. The H reflex is recorded proximal to the tarsal tunnel. A drop in tibial compound muscle action potential (CMAP) amplitude at the popliteal fossa stimulation site could indicate a neuropathy proximal to the tarsal tunnel.

59. The correct answer is D.

In a patient with facioscapulohumeral dystrophy, the deltoid and forearm muscles are relatively spared in comparison to the other muscles affected. The spared muscles give the characteristic appearance of a "Popeye" arm. The flexor carpi radialis is a forearm muscle. Facial muscles, such as orbicularis oculi, will be affected early in course of disease along with the scapular muscles. The biceps and triceps will also be affected. The tibialis anterior is the first lower limb muscle to be affected, resulting in foot drop.

60. The correct answer is A.

The CMAP onset latency is composed of the latency of activation (time between nerve stimulation and depolarization, typically 0.1 millisecond), nerve conduction (propagation of the nerve action potential to the neuromuscular junction, of variable time), and synaptic transmission (electrochemical generation of muscle action potential, typically 1.0 milliseconds). The onset latency represents the arrival time of the fastest conducting nerve fibers and is represented by the initial departure of the negative spike from the baseline. Terminal latency refers to the time at which the positive spike of the waveform intersects the baseline and represents the termination of the CMAP. The total CMAP duration occurs between the onset and terminal latencies.

61. The correct answer is B.

EPPs are propagating suprathreshold muscle fiber depolarizations in the endplate region provoked by needle insertion. They are usually biphasic with an initial negative deflection when originating under the tip of the needle electrode but sometimes appear triphasic with an initial positive deflection. Although EPPs can appear to have similar morphology to FIBs, EPPs can be distinguished from FIBs by their irregular firing rate. EPPs and MEPPs represent normal spontaneous activity at the endplate. MEPPs represent the release of spontaneous quanta of acetylcholine at the endplate. Spontaneous muscle fiber potentials outside the endplate region (FIBs and PSWs) are considered abnormal and due to active denervation.

62. The correct answer is D.

The CMAP is a summated waveform representing the depolarization of muscle fibers from multiple motor units. By convention, negative spikes are depicted as upward deflections from the baseline and positive spikes are downward deflections from the baseline. The interval labeled 1 to 2 represents both the rise time of the waveform's negative spike (measured via horizontal x axis) and the baseline to peak (negative spike) amplitude (measured via vertical y axis). Baseline to peak is the most commonly used amplitude measurement in motor studies as it depicts the summated voltage of the depolarized muscle fibers recorded over the motor endplate. The CMAP's peak-to-peak amplitude is represented on the vertical axis by interval 2 to 3 (measured from the maximum negative peak to the maximum positive peak); it is less commonly measured as it can be influenced by phase cancellation and far field potentials.

63. The correct answer is D.

Conduction block (CB) can be distinguished from abnormal temporal dispersion (ATD) by comparing the compound muscle action potential (CMAP) amplitude, area, and duration at the distal and proximal stimulation sites. Nerve conduction velocity (NCV) is not helpful in distinguishing between CB and focal slowing as variable degrees of NCV slowing across the injured segment can occur in both CB and ATD but for different reasons. Numeric percentage values to determine CB show variation in the literature by the site and nerve studied. In general, amplitude drops of greater than 50% strongly favor CB over ATD; however, area and duration parameters must also be analyzed. The American Association of Neuromuscular & Electrodiagnostic Medicine (AANEM) published their proposed consensus criteria in 1999 (available at aanem.org).

64. The correct answer is B.

After axonal injury, regenerated nerve fibers possess thinner myelin sheaths, shorter intermodal distances, decreased diameters, and decreased conduction velocities distal to the injury site.

65. The correct answer is A.

The nerve roots from C5 to T1 were found to be completely avulsed from the spinal cord in this unfortunate patient. Nerve root avulsions are preganglionic and supraclavicular brachial plexus injuries as they occur proximal to the dorsal root ganglion. The T1 avulsion damaged the preganglionic sympathetic fibers causing an ipsilateral Horner syndrome. The normal sensory nerve action potential (SNAP) studies and abnormal needle electromyography (EMG) examination of the cervicothoracic paraspinal muscles suggest a lesion proximal to the dorsal root ganglion. Postganglionic injuries are distal to the dorsal root ganglion. Retroclavicular injuries are uncommon and involve the divisions of the brachial plexus. Infraclavicular injuries involve the cords and branches of the brachial plexus.

66. The correct answer is C.

All of the answer choice options are myopathies that affect the limb muscles and can be inherited in an autosomal dominant pattern. However, myotonic dystrophy is the only answer choice that demonstrates genetic anticipation (the phenotypic symptoms are more severe in each successive generation due to unstable nucleotide repeats). Multiple systemic abnormalities also distinguish myotonic dystrophy from the other answer choices.

67. The correct answer is D.

ICU patients are more vulnerable to electrical injury than outpatients because the skin's protective barrier against the flow of electrical current is breeched secondary to peripheral and central lines, fluid leakage around catheters, and wounds. ICU patients are connected to various machines which all have the potential for current leakage. The most dangerous situation occurs when a patient has an external pacemaker; this provides a direct pathway for stray electrical currents to reach the heart. Thus, nerve conduction studies absolutely are contraindicated in externally paced patients. The neutral input lead actually can be a source of leakage current. The ground lead dissipates leakage current. Using an extension cord can actually increase current leakage and is not advised.

68. The correct answer is A.

An important limitation of routine motor and sensory nerve conduction studies is the fact that these studies only test large nerve fibers. Physical examination findings suggestive of large fiber peripheral neuropathy include diminished proprioception, vibration, light touch, pressure, and motor strength. Physical examination findings suggestive of small fiber neuropathy include decreased temperature perception, allodynia, hyperalgesia, and symptoms of autonomic dysfunction. Based on the symptoms and examination alone, routine nerve conduction studies would be expected to appear normal in this particular case.

69. The correct answer is B.

Nerve conduction velocities are 50% of adult values in newborns, reach 80% of adult values by the first year, and are equivalent to adult values by 3 to 5 years of age.

70. The correct answer is C.
The lumbar plexus is derived from ventral rami of L1, L2, L3, and part of L4. The posterior division of the lumbar plexus forms the femoral nerve and the lateral femoral cutaneous nerve. The anterior division of the lumbar plexus forms the obturator nerve. The sacral plexus forms the sciatic nerve and its divisions, pudendal nerve, superior gluteal nerve, inferior gluteal nerve, and branches to innervate buttock muscles.

71. The correct answer is A.
The factors making critical illness neuropathy that most likely diagnosis include sepsis with organ failure, difficulty weaning from ventilator, primary distal muscle involvement, decreased amplitudes on all nerve conduction studies, denervation potentials on EMG, and normal creatine kinase (CK) level. The largely elevated CK level, short-duration/low-amplitude motor units, and normal sensory studies often found in critical illness myopathy were not present. Repetitive nerve stimulation tests are normal making a transient neuromuscular blockade by pharmacologic agents less likely. Normal CSF and the absence of antiganglioside antibodies make the axonal variant of GBS less likely.

72. The correct answer is B.
In chronic neuropathic conditions, axon loss and denervation is followed by reinnervation by direct axonal regrowth or collateral sprouting. Reinnervation increases the number of muscle fibers per motor unit, spatial summation of electrical activity, and temporal dispersion of action potentials. This produces polyphasic, large amplitude, and long-duration MUAPs. These MUAP morphology changes take weeks to months to manifest. In acute axon loss, the MUAP morphology initially appears normal because Wallerian degeneration and reinnervation have not yet occurred. Acute muscle fiber loss decreases both the number of muscle fibers per motor unit and the firing synchronicity—resulting in short-duration, small-amplitude, and polyphasic MUAPs. The MUAP morphology remains normal in chronic demyelination.

73. The correct answer is B.
Averaging extracts a time-locked sensory nerve action potential from background noise over successive stimulations, thus improving the signal-to-noise ratio by a factor of the square root of the total number of averaged stimulations. The resolution of the biologic signal is determined by the analog to digital convertor and the computer display settings. The vertical magnification of the signal's waveform can be improved by increasing the sensitivity (gain) setting. The bandwidth corresponding to the signal is determined by the low- and high-frequency filter settings.

74. The correct answer is C.
Chronic inflammatory demyelinating polyneuropathy (CIDP) can be associated with Hodgkin lymphoma. CIDP is an acquired demyelinating polyneuropathy typically demonstrating partial conduction block of more than one motor nerve, reduced conduction velocities and prolonged distal latencies of two or more nerves, and absent F waves. The diagnosis is supported by analyzing cerebrospinal fluid, which characteristically shows elevated protein levels greater than 45 mg/dL without pleocytosis and a white cell count of less than 10 cells/mm^3. A nerve biopsy can also be performed.

75. The correct answer is D.

All of the following electrodiagnostic test findings can be found in vitamin B_{12} deficiency neuropathy. This is usually consistent with a sensory or sensorimotor axonal polyneuropathy. In addition to peripheral nervous system damage, it can cause central nervous system and psychiatric disturbances.

76. The correct answer is B.

Conductance (g) refers to the ability of electrical charge to move easily through the nerve cell membrane. During nerve action potential generation, changes in ionic conductance occur due to opening of voltage-gated ion channels. When a voltage-gated ion channel opens, the permeability and electrical conductance to that respective ion increases and alters the membrane potential. During depolarization, the influx of Na^+ into the cell causes gNa to rise and exceed that of gK (gK lags behind gNa, initially, due to the delayed opening of K^+ channels). During repolarization, Na^+ channels are inactivated and gK exceeds gNa due to the efflux of K^+. Both local transmembrane current flow and the steady state resting membrane potential do not involve changes in ionic conductance due to an action potential.

77. The correct answer is D.

The nerve conduction velocity (distance over time in units of meters per second) between two stimulation points can easily be calculated by dividing the distance between the two points (360 mm) by the latency difference between the two points (12.0 − 6.0 milliseconds = 6.0 milliseconds): 360 mm ÷ 6 milliseconds = 60 mm/ms (millimeters cancel out to 60 m/s).

　　Alternately: 0.36 m ÷ 0.006 second = 60 m/s.

78. The correct answer is D.

The clinical history, physical examination, and MRI imaging strongly suggest a right L5 radiculopathy. The needle EMG study is useful for confirming the presence of a radiculopathy if abnormalities are found in two or more muscles with L5 innervation but different peripheral nerves. The tibialis posterior muscle receives both L5 and S1 innervation; therefore, this muscle could test abnormal on needle EMG in the case of an L5 radiculopathy. The vastus medialis muscle receives innervation from L2 to L4. The right soleus muscle receives innervation from S1 to S2. Abnormalities in the upper lumbar paraspinal muscles would not confirm an L5 radiculopathy.

79. The correct answer is B.

The Miller Fisher variant of GBS classically presents with ophthalmoplegia, ataxia, and areflexia. The other subtypes listed in the answer choices have their own distinguishing characteristics.

80. The correct answer is B.

The Lloyd and Hunt classification (I to IV) is used to describe sensory nerve fibers. Types I to III fibers are myelinated, and type IV fibers are unmyelinated. The nerve fiber diameter decreases with increasing number (e.g., I = largest, IV = smallest). The Golgi tendon organ is innervated by Ib nerve fibers, which are A-α fibers. Ia fibers are also A-α fibers, but they innervate the muscle spindles. Type II fibers innervate the muscle spindles and carry touch, pain, and vibration. Type III fibers carry touch, pain, and temperature.

81. The correct answer is C.

A Martin-Gruber anastomosis (a median-to-ulnar motor nerve fiber crossover) in the forearm could be detected by recording at the ulnar-innervated FDI muscle while stimulating the median nerve in the antecubital fossa—yielding a CMAP with a negative deflection. Other findings include proximal median CMAP *higher* in amplitude than the distal CMAP, ulnar CMAP *lower* in amplitude below the elbow than at the wrist, and an initial positive deflection in the *proximal* median CMAP when there is superimposed CTS.

82. The correct answer is A.

This is the classic case vignette for "honeymoon palsy" (radial nerve compression neuropathy). The radial nerve innervates the triceps before it wraps around the spiral groove; therefore, it is expected to test normal in the case of a lesion at the spiral groove. The brachioradialis is expected to be normal in all lesions distal to spiral groove. The extensor carpi radialis is expected to be normal in a lesion of the posterior interosseous nerve. The supinator is expected to test normal in a lesion at or below the arcade of Frohse.

83. The correct answer is C.

The fastest conducting neurons are large diameter and myelinated (i.e., A-α motor and sensory fibers and 1a sensory fibers). Increasing axon cross-sectional diameter decreases the internal resistance to current flow and increases the conduction velocity. The internode segments of myelinated neurons are insulated from transmembrane current, allowing action potential current to propagate from node (of Ranvier) to node via saltatory conduction, thus increasing the nerve conduction velocity. Unmyelinated neurons are the slowest conducting, as they rely on a stepwise depolarization of the entire axon membrane.

84. The correct answer is C.

The standard slow-rate repetitive nerve stimulation (RNS) protocol for evaluating suspected myasthenia gravis (MG) is to obtain a baseline train of repetitive stimulations at rest, exercise the muscle, and then perform postexercise RNS at regular intervals for up to 4 to 5 minutes. In this particular case, the baseline tracing did not show the expected reproducible decrement of 10% or more. Therefore, the muscle should be exercised to look for postexercise exhaustion. In mild cases of MG, an abnormal decrement can sometimes only be seen postexercise. If there is still no decrement after exercise, a more proximal muscle can then be studied. There are many other muscles that can be tested before concluding that the study is normal. Cooling the limb will mask any decrement and is not a good idea in RNS. On the contrary, warming the limb could be useful in enhancing decrements.

85. The correct answer is D.

All potentials arising at the motor endplate are absent after denervation due to Wallerian and neuromuscular junction degeneration. Fibrillation potentials arise from denervated muscle fibers.

86. The correct answer is D.

Periodic paralysis disorders, such as paramyotonia congenita, display a characteristic finding of electromyography (EMG) electrical silence after cold exposure. Cooling causes sustained muscle cell membrane depolarization due to a defect in the sodium channel. This will appear on EMG initially as myotonic bursts of fibrillation potentials followed by electrical silence. Clinically, this would cause muscle flaccid paralysis due to cell membrane inexcitability.

87. The correct answer is C.

Unlike a muscle fiber or nerve action potential, an EPP is a local endplate depolarization formed by a "graded" response; the magnitude is determined by the quantity of ACh molecules released from the nerve axon terminal and the sensitivity of the postsynaptic receptors to ACh. The postsynaptic binding of two ACh molecules initiates the opening of Na^+ channels and endplate depolarization. EPPs are able to initiate an "all or none" muscle action potential if enough ACh is released or if two or more EPPs summate and exceed the membrane threshold value. Each MEPP represents a small endplate depolarization equal to the spontaneous release of one quantum of ACh. More than one MEPP can summate to create a local EPP.

88. The correct answer is D.

Lumbosacral plexopathy can occur from a traction injury during hip arthroplasty. This particular patient had a panplexopathy with sparing of the anterior division of the lumbar plexus. The absent SNAP responses suggest an axonal sensory lesion distal to the dorsal root ganglion, excluding both L5 radiculopathy and multifocal motor neuropathy (as it is a pure motor disorder). The vastus medialis (femoral nerve) and gluteus medius (superior gluteal nerve) muscles were abnormal on needle electromyography (EMG), excluding a sciatic neuropathy.

89. The correct answer is C.

F waves are most useful for testing the proximal nerve segments in patients with demyelinating neuropathies, such as GBS. The proximal nerve roots are the earliest affected segments in GBS. There is a noted phenomenon of sparing of the sural nerve (i.e., normal response) that can be found in GBS. Spontaneous muscle fiber activity in the paraspinal muscles is an early finding in motor neuron disease but not in GBS.

90. The correct answer is B.

Neurotmesis (Seddon classification) describes a nerve transection injury where there is damage to axons and supporting connective tissue structures of the peripheral nerve to varying degrees. The loss of continuity in the axons, the deformed connective tissue elements, and scar tissue formation make nerve regrowth difficult. Thus, it has the worst recovery prognosis. Axonotmesis involves loss of axon continuity but intact and aligned connective tissue structures, allowing a path for nerve regrowth to occur. Neurapraxia involves reversible conduction block with preservation of axon and connective tissue continuity and has the best prognosis. There is no such thing as "axonopraxia."

91. The correct answer is C.
An interelectrode distance of less than 4 cm results in a truncated SNAP amplitude. The closely spaced recording electrodes do not allow enough separation for optimal differential amplification, and there is common mode rejection of SNAP waveform components. This technical issue also decreases the SNAP peak latency, duration, rise time, and area. The remaining parameters are unaffected.

92. The correct answer is B.
The pictured MUAP is polyphasic in configuration (five or more baseline crossings). A phase is a portion of the MUAP between a departure from and return to the baseline. The number of MUAP phases is calculated by counting the number of baseline crossings and adding 1. There are 8 baseline crossings + 1 = 9 phases. Turns or serrations describe changes in the direction of the MUAP that *do not cross the baseline*. In this particular MUAP waveform, there are no turns, as all changes in direction cross the baseline.

93. The correct answer is C.
McArdle disease is a metabolic myopathy known for the EMG finding of electrical silence during attacks of muscle cramping/contracture.

94. The correct answer is A.
The CMAP negative spike is a near field potential; its parameters are measured during routine nerve conduction studies using a standard bipolar montage where the recording electrodes are in proximity to one another. The near field refers to the close distance to the electrical field generated at the site of nerve depolarization with action potential propagation resulting in current flow and variable distribution of electrical charge. The far field refers to a distance away from the site of nerve depolarization where the electrical field remains relatively invariable. Stimulus artifact, premotor potentials, and SSEPs recorded with a referential (noncephalic) montage are examples of far field potentials.

95. The correct answer is A.
This is most consistent with a median mononeuropathy at the wrist. The nerve conduction study data table demonstrates a prolonged median motor distal latency with abnormal slowing of the conduction velocity between the wrist and elbow segments. Additionally, there is a prolonged median sensory distal latency at the wrist segment. The median motor amplitudes show no significant drop between the wrist and elbow, so a forearm neuropathy is unlikely. The ulnar nerve response data is within normal range.

96. The correct answer is A.
Alpha motor neurons innervate only extrafusal fibers (i.e., skeletal muscle). *Beta* motor neurons innervate *both* intrafusal (i.e., muscle spindle) and extrafusal fibers. Gamma motor neurons innervate only intrafusal fibers. Delta neurons are classified only as sensory neurons. Alpha, beta, gamma, and delta neurons all belong to the "A group" of peripheral nerves, which consist of large diameter, myelinated nerve fibers.

97. The correct answer is D.

Mitochondrial myopathy is a known side effect of azidothymidine (AZT) use but is difficult to clinically distinguish from other myopathies associated with HIV infection. The finding of ragged red fibers on muscle specimen staining is suggestive of mitochondrial myopathy, which is the proposed pathogenesis of AZT myopathy as AZT inhibits mitochondrial DNA polymerase. The number of ragged red fibers on muscle biopsy correlates with the cumulative dose of AZT received by the patient.

98. The correct answer is D.

Quantitative Valsalva testing involves open glottis exhalation into a mouthpiece maintaining 40 to 50 mm Hg for 15 seconds while recording HR and blood pressure (BP) changes. Exhalation lowers cardiac input/output and BP. The normal baroreflex response is parasympathetic (vagal) mediated reflex tachycardia and sympathetic mediated peripheral vasoconstriction. The vasomotor response elevates BP with an overshoot, followed by transient reflex bradycardia. The Valsalva ratio (ratio of the longest R-R interval after the maneuver divided by the shortest R-R interval during the test) and beat-to-beat BP changes are measured; together, these measures reflect parasympathetic and sympathetic function. HR variability with deep breathing and HR change in standing both measure parasympathetic activity only. Sympathetic skin response measures only sympathetic sudomotor nerve activity.

99. The correct answer is A.

The ligament of Struthers, lacertus fibrosus, pronator teres, and sublimis bridge are all potential sites where the median nerve can become entrapped. The arcade of Frohse is a potential site of radial nerve entrapment.

100. The correct answer is C.

Neurogenic recruitment is characterized by loss of active motor units compensated by an increased firing rate of the first motor unit to generate the required muscle contractile force until additional motor units can be recruited. The recruitment frequency is the firing rate of the first MUAP when the second MUAP starts to fire and increases in neuropathic recruitment. The recruitment interval is measured as the interspike interval between two discharges of the first MUAP when the second MUAP begins to fire and decreases in neuropathic recruitment. The recruitment ratio is the ratio of the firing rate of the first MUAP to the number of active MUAPs on the screen and increases in neurogenic recruitment.

101. The correct answer is B.

SMA is a lower motor neuron disease of the spinal cord and therefore would not show the described clinical signs of upper motor neuron disease. PLS is an upper motor neuron disease with the expected physical examination signs. ALS would demonstrate both upper motor neuron and lower motor neuron signs on examination. Spasticity, hyperreflexia, and extensor (upgoing) plantar response can be present in the setting of stroke as well.

102. The correct answer is C.

The finding of an abnormal or absent DUC nerve is useful in diagnosing ulnar neuropathy proximal to the wrist. The DUC branches off from the ulnar nerve proximal to the wrist; therefore, an abnormal DUC response in addition to other abnormal ulnar findings can help to localize the lesion above the wrist. Decreased ulnar SNAP amplitude at the wrist alone does not localize the lesion. Abnormal needle EMG findings in the FCU muscle suggest a proximal lesion, but a normal FCU is not useful. Latency differences between ADM and FDI localize the lesion to the wrist.

103. The correct answer is C.

The MUAP amplitude consists of high-frequency waveform components; therefore, lowering the high-frequency filter will reduce the amplitude of a recorded MUAP. The MUAP amplitude is measured from peak to peak; it is influenced by the number of *muscle fibers* near the needle electrode and decreases with increasing recording distance from the motor unit. MUAP amplitude is not an accurate measure of the muscle fibers in a motor unit; the MUAP duration best represents the total number of muscle fibers in a motor unit.

104. The correct answer is D.

The findings are not consistent with any of the listed answer choices. The isolated finding of absent bilateral tibial H reflexes in an otherwise normal electrodiagnostic study cannot localize a lesion or determine its chronicity. The findings do suggest blocked signal transmission through the S1 reflex arc bilaterally. A lesion to any portion of this reflex arc, including the peripheral nerves (sciatic and tibial) and S1 nerve roots, can cause absent H reflexes. Once the reflex arc has been damaged, the H reflex will remain delayed or absent indefinitely. Tibial H reflex abnormalities can support diagnoses of peripheral neuropathy or S1 radiculopathy along with corresponding clinical history, physical examination, nerve conduction, F wave, and/or needle EMG findings. The tibial H reflex can be absent bilaterally in some healthy individuals; however, a study by Falco et al. found the tibial H reflex to be present bilaterally in 92% of elderly subjects.

105. The correct answer is D.

Both increased jitter and increased fiber density are SFEMG findings in ALS due to ongoing denervation and reinnervation. Nevertheless, these findings are NOT specific for ALS as they can be found in other motor neuron, neurogenic, and myopathic disorders.

106. The correct answer is D.

The dorsal (afferent sensory) and ventral (efferent motor) nerve roots join to form a spinal nerve (mixed fibers); the spinal nerve divides into both dorsal and ventral rami, each containing motor and sensory fibers. The dorsal ramus innervates the deep muscles of the trunk and supplies skin sensation to the dermatome corresponding to a specific axial segment. The dorsal root ganglion contains the unipolar cell bodies of the afferent sensory neurons.

107. The correct answer is C.

Mononeuritis multiplex is a common pattern of vasculitic neuropathy characterized by an asymmetric pattern of nerve involvement involving the lower and upper limbs. It is treated with corticosteroids and cyclophosphamide. Conduction block at uncommon nerve entrapment sites describes the pattern of acquired demyelinating neuropathy.

108. The correct answer is B.

Complex repetitive discharges (CRDs) consist of a group of muscle fibers firing regularly, consecutively, and repetitively. Cramps, fasciculation, and myokymic discharges all consist of MUAPs not under voluntary control. Cramps are actually multiple MUAPs firing synchronously at high frequencies causing painful involuntary muscle contractions. Fasciculations consist of individual MUAPs firing spontaneously and irregularly at slow rates. Myokymic discharges are groups of MUAPs firing repetitively and semiregularly in bursts with a variable number of MUAPs.

109. The correct answer is A.

Neurogenic conditions are characterized by loss of active motor units compensated for by increasing the firing rate of the first motor unit to generate the required muscle contractile force until additional motor units can be recruited. The recruitment ratio (RR) is the ratio of the firing rate of the first MUAP to the number of active MUAPs on the screen during EMG voluntary activation. Normal RR is 5:1. The RR increases in neurogenic conditions as there are less active motor units (i.e., reduced recruitment). When the first MUAP is firing at 50 Hz, there normally should be 10 active MUAPs. In this case, there are only 5 (RR of 10:1). Myopathic recruitment would yield a low RR and a full interference pattern with minimal contraction. Decreased activation would manifest as an inability to increase the firing rate of the first MUAP.

110. The correct answer is A.

Recurrent neoplastic brachial plexopathies are more likely to present with pain, involve the lower trunk, and occur with radiation doses less than 6,000 rads within 1 year of radiation. Radiation-induced brachial plexopathies are more likely to involve the upper trunk, demonstrate fasciculation potentials on needle EMG, and occur with radiation doses of greater than 6,000 rads within 1 year of radiation. If the plexopathy develops after more than 1 year has elapsed after radiation treatment, the radiation dose is no longer a significant factor in determining etiology.

111. The correct answer is A.

The anode (designated as +) is the positive current terminal and attracts negative ions (anions). The cathode (designated as −) is the negative current terminal and attracts positive ions (cations). The active (E1) electrode records electrical potentials directly over the site of interest, whether a muscle or nerve segment. The amplifier is part of the electrophysiologic instrumentation and magnifies the biologic signal recorded at the active electrode while reducing common noise recorded at both the active and reference electrodes.

112. The correct answer is B.

Postpolio syndrome is a clinical diagnosis. Electrodiagnostic studies often show non-specific chronic neurogenic changes indicating prior denervation and reinnervation. No active denervation (i.e., no spontaneous muscle fiber activity) would be expected in the needle EMG study. The presence of active denervation would indicate another overlapping nerve or muscle disorder.

113. The correct answer is C.

Unlike motor nerve conduction velocities, sensory nerve conduction velocities can be calculated from one distal stimulation site as there is no neuromuscular junction transmission time to consider. Nevertheless, the latency of activation (0.1 milliseconds) should be subtracted from the *onset* latency. *The above does NOT apply to peak latencies.* The nerve conduction velocity (distance over time in units of m/s): 140 mm ÷ (2.9 − 0.1 milliseconds) = 140 mm ÷ 2.8 milliseconds = 50 mm/ms (millimeters cancel out to 50 m/s). Alternately: 0.14 m ÷ 0.0028 second = 50 m/s.

114. The correct answer is D.

Normal insertional activity is less than 300 milliseconds in duration and results from the mechanical depolarization of individual muscle fibers by the needle electrode. There is the brief appearance of individual spike waveforms but no sustained firing pattern.

115. The correct answer is D.

CMAP conduction block, abnormal temporal dispersion, and prolonged minimal F wave latency are found in acquired demyelinating neuropathies. There is more than one criteria for acquired demyelination as some conduction velocity (CV) and latency thresholds are dependent on CMAP amplitude. In general, CV less than 70% of the lower limit of normal is in the demyelinating range and cannot be attributed to axon loss alone.

116. The correct answer is B.

Single-fiber electromyography is the most sensitive electrodiagnostic test for neuromuscular junction disorders. The characteristic finding is increased jitter and/or blocking without increased fiber density. Fiber density is unchanged because the pathophysiology does not involve reinnervation.

117. The correct answer is C.

The presynaptic neuromuscular junction disorders (i.e., Lambert-Eaton syndrome and botulism) demonstrate a CMAP amplitude increment in response to fast stimulation rates. Presynaptic disorders demonstrate reduced CMAP amplitude to initial supramaximal nerve stimulus. Both pre- and postsynaptic disorders can show decremental CMAP amplitudes in response to preexercise slow stimulation rates. A progressive decrement in CMAP amplitude below initial baseline levels occurring minutes after maximum activation occurs in postsynaptic disorders.

118. The correct answer is D.

Lowering the high-frequency (low-pass) filter eliminates more high-frequency signals above the cutoff value, reducing the high-frequency components of the composite action potential waveform. The high-frequency components represent the fast changing parts of the waveform (i.e., rise time of negative spike and the latencies) and contribute to the amplitude. Sequential lowering of the high-frequency filter results in increases in both onset and peak latencies, increased duration, and decreased amplitude.

119. The correct answer is A.

An initial positive deflection in the CMAP waveform can arise secondary to a tendon potential from an electrically active region under the reference electrode, volume conduction from nearby muscles, or by the recording electrode being off the motor point. It can also represent evidence of an anomalous innervation (i.e., proximal median CMAP appearance with Martin-Gruber anastomosis and concurrent carpal tunnel syndrome [CTS]). Submaximal stimulation results in a CMAP with a falsely low amplitude and prolonged latency as not all of the motor fibers are being depolarized.

120. The correct answer is B.

Cisplatin affects only sensory nerves in a pattern of a length dependent "dying back" axonal neuropathy or neuronopathy. Vincristine affects both sensory and motor nerves (sensory nerves are more affected than motor nerves). Rituximab and duloxetine are used as treatment for chemotherapy-induced peripheral neuropathy.

121. The correct answer is D.

Proximal SNAPs are affected by normal temporal dispersion and phase cancellation; hence, they are not widely utilized. Increasing the distance between the recording and stimulation sites accentuates the difference in the depolarization times between the fast and slow conducting sensory nerve fibers. This temporal dispersion of individual nerve fiber conduction times increases the duration and decreases the amplitude of the SNAP. Additionally, the trailing positive waveforms of the fast conducting fibers overlap with the leading negative waveforms of the slow conducting fibers. This produces a phase cancellation which decreases the area of the SNAP. Stimulus artifact can nonspecifically interfere with SNAP recording any at site, whether distal or proximal.

122. The correct answer is C.

It is important to appropriately tailor your needle EMG examination to the referring provider's request and to your history and physical examination. The adductor hallucis and abductor digiti minimi muscles receive innervation from the S1-3 nerve roots. The external anal sphincter receives innervation from the S2-4 nerve roots. The extensor digitorum longus receives innervation from the L5-S1 nerve roots.

123. The correct answer is D.

The most common HIV-associated neuropathies (HIV-N) are distal sensory polyneuropathy (a predominantly axonal neuropathy which develops late in the disease) and antiretroviral toxic neuropathies. Other forms of HIV-N include acute or chronic inflammatory polyneuropathies, which are less common and occur mostly during seroconversion or early stages of HIV infection. Opportunistic infections in AIDS can lead to mononeuritis multiplex or radiculopathies.

124. The correct answer is B.

Settings of sweep speed (2 milliseconds), sensitivity (20 µV), and filters (20 to 2,000 Hz) are suitable for a sensory nerve conduction study. Sensory responses require increased horizontal resolution to measure latency (i.e., faster [lower numerical] sweep speeds) and increased vertical resolution (i.e., increased [lower numerical] sensitivity/gain) to measure sensory amplitudes typically ranging from 1 to 50 µV. Sensory responses are composed of frequencies up to 2,000 to 3,000 Hz (high-frequency filter set at 2,000 Hz). They are susceptible to the effects of 0 to 20 Hz baseline noise, which is filtered out (low-frequency filter set at 20 Hz). Answer choices A and C are examples of settings that could be used for a motor nerve conduction study. Answer choice D is a distractor.

125. The correct answer is A.

The most common pattern in diabetic polyneuropathy is an axonal and demyelinating (mixed) sensorimotor polyneuropathy.

126. The correct answer is C.

The statement regarding botulinum toxins is true. Myasthenia gravis most commonly arises from autoantibodies against the acetylcholine receptor. Lambert-Eaton syndrome arises from a reduced number of calcium channels. Curare toxin blocks the acetylcholine receptor.

127. The correct answer is D.

The single-fiber needle electrode has the smallest recording surface (approximately 25 µm in diameter) with the active wire (E1) located in a side port proximal to and on the opposite side of the needle cannula reference electrode (E2). The bipolar concentric electrode has the second smallest recording surface and consists of a cannula with two separate ports for the active (E1) and reference (E2) electrodes. The standard concentric needle contains a port for E1 with E2 located within the cannula. The monopolar needle has the largest recording surface (approximately 0.17 mm^2) and requires a separate surface electrode for E2; E1 is contained in the bare metal at the conical needle tip.

128. The correct answer is A.

The 0.5-second tracing shows two distinct firing motor units. The recruitment interval (RI) is measured as the interspike interval between two discharges of the first MUAP when the second MUAP begins to fire. The double arrowheads depict this interval, which is slightly less than 100 milliseconds (90 milliseconds to be exact). Normal RI is at or around 100 milliseconds. The recruitment frequency (RF) is the firing rate of the first MUAP when the second MUAP starts to fire. The RF is the reciprocal of the RI: 1/90 = 11.1 Hz (to be exact) or 1/100 = 10 Hz (rough estimate). Normal RF is 10 to 20 Hz. The recruitment ratio (RR) is the RF divided by the number of different firing MUAPs on the screen. In this case, 10:2 = 5:1. Normal RR is 5:1. All these parameters indicate that the tracing depicts normal MUAP recruitment.

129. The correct answer is A.

Heavy alcohol use for a prolonged period of time can produce an axonal sensorimotor polyneuropathy. Friedrich ataxia can produce a sensory axonal polyneuropathy. Leprosy can produce a sensorimotor demyelinating polyneuropathy. Renal disease (uremia) can produce an axonal and demyelinating sensorimotor polyneuropathy.

130. The correct answer is D.
Uniform slowing of nerve conduction velocity involving all segments is characteristic of hereditary demyelinating peripheral polyneuropathies. Abnormal temporal dispersion, motor nerve conduction block, and focal nerve conduction velocity slowing at common nerve entrapment sites are characteristics of acquired demyelinating peripheral polyneuropathies.

131. The correct answer is D.
The abductor hallucis is innervated by the medial plantar branch of the tibial nerve. The common peroneal motor nerve divides into superficial and deep branches below the knee. The deep peroneal innervates the tibialis anterior and extensor digitorum brevis among other muscles. The superficial peroneal innervates the peroneus longus among other muscles.

132. The correct answer is A.
Stimulus intensities above supramaximal can falsely decrease the recorded potential's onset latency; the site of nerve depolarization spreads distal to the cathode via volume conduction, analogous to the cathode being moved closer to the recording site. There is also spread of the current to nearby nerves causing coactivation. Increasing the stimulus duration, lowering the high-frequency filter, and lowering the gain can all result in an increase in the recorded latency.

133. The correct answer is C.
The F wave is produced by supramaximal motor antidromic stimulation of anterior horn cells with orthodromic backfiring and is not a true reflex. In contrast, the H reflex is a monosynaptic reflex resulting from submaximal stimulation of afferent muscle spindle fibers which synapse in the spinal cord with a resultant efferent motor response.

134. The correct answer is B.
This patient was found to have a metastatic lymph node compressing the lower trunk of the brachial plexus. The reduced median and ulnar compound muscle action potential (CMAP) amplitudes suggest a lesion affecting the C8-T1 nerve roots, lower brachial plexus, or both the median and ulnar nerves. The reduced sensory nerve action potential (SNAP) amplitudes and the normal cervicothoracic paraspinal muscle examination further localize the lesion distal to the dorsal root ganglion, excluding C8-T1 radiculopathies. Median mononeuropathy is unlikely given that the digit 2 sensory study and the flexor carpi radialis muscle (both representing the lateral cord, upper and middle trunks of the brachial plexus) are both normal. The abnormal ulnar and medial antebrachial cutaneous nerve responses as well as the abnormal muscles on the needle electromyography (EMG) study all are derived from the lower trunk of the brachial plexus.

135. The correct answer is D.
This vignette describes the characteristic findings of pseudofacilitation, which is a normal physiologic finding on repetitive nerve stimulation that should not be mistaken for pathology. Movement artifact from inadequate limb immobilization can cause a false decremental response. A cold limb can hide an abnormal decremental response and cause false-negative findings in patients with neuromuscular disorders.

136. The correct answer is A.
Stimulus artifact is a volume-conducted, low-frequency signal arising from the nerve stimulator that is rapidly recorded and preamplified before the actual biologic signal. It appears at the beginning of the cathode ray tube tracing and can obscure the onset of the nerve action potential's waveform. One of the strategies to counteract stimulus artifact is to rotate the *anode* about the cathode. Impedance mismatch between the active and reference electrode can lead to further magnification of stimulus artifact; however, stimulus artifact is a distinct phenomenon from skin–electrode impedance. Ambient noise is also a separate problem that can be counteracted by various components of the electrodiagnostic equipment/instrumentation.

137. The correct answer is C.
The answer choices include the HMSN and their Charcot-Marie-Tooth subtypes. HMSN III includes a severe form of Dejerine-Sottas disease, which is a rapidly fatal congenital hypomyelination neuropathy with hypotonia and significant respiratory distress at birth. Less severe forms of this disorder manifest as delayed motor milestones.

138. The correct answer is B.
The amplifier used in electrodiagnostic studies should possess a high differential gain and low common mode gain; this is represented by the common mode rejection ratio (CMRR = differential gain / common mode gain). Most instruments have a high CMRR of at least 10,000 to 1. Differential gain is the biologic signal's output after amplification divided by the input of the potential difference between the active and reference electrodes. Common mode gain is the output of signal (i.e., noise) common to the active and reference electrodes divided by input of these common signals. Both the amplifier and the electrodes are sources of impedance in the transmission of the biologic signal. High amplifier impedance actually preserves the signal's electrical potential by counteracting the diminutive effect of electrode impedance.

139. The correct answer is A.
Answer choices B through D describe the typical repetitive nerve stimulation findings in a patient with myasthenia gravis. Answer choice A describes a characteristic finding in a patient with Lambert-Eaton syndrome.

140. The correct answer is A.
It is difficult to isolate the proximal median CMAP with stimulation at the axilla because the ulnar nerve is often costimulated due to the close proximity of the two nerves in this region. The collision technique is designed to temporally separate the median response by delivering two simultaneous stimulations—one to the ulnar nerve at the wrist and the other to the median nerve in the axilla. Any ulnar nerve impulse traveling distally from the axilla will be negated by collision with a proximal impulse traveling from the wrist. The F wave, A wave, and H reflex are late responses recorded by special nerve conduction studies that allow study of proximal nerve segments.

141. The correct answer is A.

Conduction block is the hallmark characteristic of neurapraxia (Seddon classification of nerve injury). It most commonly occurs due to transient focal compression resulting in failure of the nerve to conduct an impulse across the affected segment, but conduction proximal and distal to the segment is preserved. Conduction block is reversible if the offending cause of injury is removed. Neurapraxia involves demyelination of the affected segment, but the axon remains intact; thus, Wallerian degeneration does not occur. Large myelinated motor fibers are more susceptible to injury than small myelinated or unmyelinated fibers in neurapraxia; this is manifested clinically by weakness or loss of motor control.

142. The correct answer is C.

Myokymic discharges are a type of spontaneous activity consisting of grouped motor unit action potentials firing repetitively and semiregularly in bursts. In a needle EMG study where findings are consistent with plexopathy, the presence of myokymic discharges aids in establishing an etiology of radiation-induced plexopathy.

143. The correct answer is C.

The trigeminal nerve (mandibular division) innervates the masseter muscle. The facial nerve innervates the nasalis, orbicularis oculi, and the orbicularis oris muscles. Any of these muscles could be recorded in a facial nerve conduction study, but the nasalis is the most commonly tested muscle. Stimulation could be performed anterior or posterior to the ear. Anterior stimulation can yield a volume-conducted potential from the trigeminal-innervated masseter muscle that can be erroneously mistaken for a facial nerve response.

144. The correct answer is C.

This clinical case brings up important concepts: (1) The findings alone cannot distinguish polyradiculopathy from motor neuron disease, neuromuscular disease, or superimposed polyneuropathy. (2) EMG/NCS of at least the contralateral limb is the next step in evaluation. (3) EMG ideally should not be used as a blanket "screening test" for radiculopathy as it is more specific than sensitive in establishing a diagnosis. (4) The testing clinician ideally should perform a detailed history and physical examination in order to establish a working/provisional or differential diagnosis prior to EMG/NCS.

Single-fiber EMG of the right limb could be considered later, but contralateral limb testing is the next best step. Somatosensory evoked potentials would be of little value in this case where motor axon loss is the primary pathology. Polyradiculopathy diagnosis is premature for reasons stated previously, but cervical MRI could be considered.

145. The correct answer is B.

Theoretically or experimentally blocking transmission at the neuromuscular junction would prohibit the firing of potentials generated by motor units. Neuromyotonic, multiplet, and tremor discharges are all generated by motor units, resulting in secondary muscle contraction. Myotonic discharges are generated by muscle fibers and would persist after a neuromuscular junction blockade.

146. The correct answer is B.

Graphic 1 depicts a long-duration polyphasic MUAP, and graphic 2 depicts a nascent MUAP. Long-duration polyphasic MUAPs represent collateral sprouting from adjacent motor units; they are absent in complete denervation as there are no adjacent intact motor units to form collateral sprouts. Nascent potentials represent early direct axon regrowth from the injury site and can occur after complete denervation; they are short duration, small amplitude, and polyphasic. Both types of MUAPs are found in neuropathic conditions and represent reinnervation. Long-duration polyphasic MUAPs can also be found in some chronic myopathies.

147. The correct answer is A.

HMSN/Charcot-Marie-Tooth type II is an axonal polyneuropathy; this feature distinguishes it from the other hereditary motor sensory neuropathy subtypes, which are demyelinating. Onion bulb formation is a histopathologic finding in demyelinating disorders due to demyelination and remyelination. Elevated serum phytanic acid levels are found in HMSN IV Refsum disease. Hypertrophy of peripheral nerves can be found in HMSN/Charcot-Marie-Tooth type I.

148. The correct answer is D.

Complex repetitive discharges (CRDs) arise from a single muscle fiber that acts as a pacemaker with ephaptic spread of depolarization to adjacent fibers in a closed loop circuit. These grouped potentials have the same stable appearance with each firing cycle, possess a regular rhythm, and start and stop abruptly. Myotonic discharges also arise from single muscle fibers, but their morphology and firing rate vary with a characteristic waxing and waning rhythm. Myokymic and neuromyotonic discharges both arise from motor unit action potentials (MUAPs). *The author recommends making a study table to compare and contrast the characteristics of abnormal EMG potentials.*

149. The correct answer is A.

The concept of the safety factor is often difficult to explain but important to understand in terms of neuromuscular junction pathology. In order to reliably and continually generate postsynaptic muscle membrane action potentials, there is normally a high safety factor where an endplate potential magnitude greatly exceeds what is required to generate an action potential. This guarantees an action potential even when there are reduced numbers of acetylcholine quanta immediately available for release (as can occur during normal repetitive physiologic activity, such as exercise). Neuromuscular junction disorders cause a decrease in the safety factor. In the case of a low safety factor, the endplate potential magnitude will fall below the threshold needed to generate a muscle action potential.

150. The correct answer is C.

Increasing the low-frequency (high-pass) filter eliminates more low-frequency signals below the cutoff value, reducing the low-frequency components of the composite action potential waveform and making the high-frequency components more predominant. The waveform duration, peak latency, and amplitude consist of low-frequency components. Less low frequencies in the waveform result in a shorter (decreased) duration; more low frequencies result in a longer (increased) duration. Increasing the low-frequency filter also will decrease the peak latency, decrease the amplitude, and increase the number of phases in the composite waveform. The onset latency is unchanged as it is composed solely of high-frequency signals.

Board Review Points ("Pearls") for Electrodiagnostic Medicine

Anatomy and Neurophysiology

- Type I motor units are recruited first during voluntary muscle contraction as they generate low force at a low threshold of excitation for low-intensity activity and are more fatigue-resistant than type II fibers. Type I (slow-twitch) motor units also have a smaller innervation ratios, nerve cell bodies, and axon diameters than type II (fast-twitch) motor units.
- The Na$^+$-K$^+$-ATP pump maintains the nerve cell membrane potential by using ATP as an energy source to actively transport two potassium ions into the cell for every three sodium ions it exports.
- The H reflex is a true monosynaptic reflex obtained by submaximal stimulation with a stable latency from one stimulus to the next.
- The most common anomalous innervation in the lower extremity is the APN, which is derived from the superficial peroneal nerve, travels posterior to the lateral malleolus, and innervates the lateral portion of the EDB.
- Decreasing a nerve's temperature increases the time to reach peak depolarization, increases the action potential amplitude and duration, increases the refractory period, and decreases the conduction velocity.
- The latissimus dorsi and pectoralis major muscles receive innervation from all trunks of the brachial plexus.
- The anterior interosseous nerve innervates the flexor pollicis longus, pronator quadratus, and the flexor digitorum profundus muscle to digits 2 and 3.
- Large muscles involved in gross movements that do not require dexterity have high innervation ratios. Small muscles associated with fine movements that require high dexterity have low innervation ratios.
- Bioelectric current flow (I) is inversely proportional to the impedance (Z).
- After axonal injury, regenerated nerve fibers possess thinner myelin sheaths, shorter intermodal distances, decreased diameters, and decreased conduction velocities distal to the injury site.

- The posterior division of the lumbar plexus forms the femoral nerve and the lateral femoral cutaneous nerve. The anterior division of the lumbar plexus forms the obturator nerve.
- The fastest conducting neurons are large diameter and myelinated (i.e., A-α motor and sensory fibers and 1a sensory fibers).
- Each miniature endplate potential represents a small endplate depolarization equal to the spontaneous release of one quantum of acetylcholine.
- Neurapraxia involves reversible conduction block with preservation of axon and connective tissue continuity.

Nerve Conduction Studies and Electromyography Basics

- Sensory afferent nerve impulses travel distal to proximal; therefore, a sensory study recording proximally and stimulating distally would be considered orthodromic.
- The monopolar needle electrode has a spherical, multidirectional surface area that records MUAPs with higher amplitudes and more polyphasic potentials than unidirectional needle electrodes.
- Nerve depolarization typically occurs first beneath the cathode.
- Supramaximal stimulus is 20% to 30% above maximal stimulus and is used in most nerve conduction studies because it ensures all axons of the nerve have been stimulated (both large and small nerve fibers).
- Averaging extracts a time-locked action potential from background noise.
- Unlike a recruited MUAP, a fasciculation potential is not under voluntary control. Fasciculation potentials are not always pathologic and can be found in normal individuals.
- Slowing the sweep speed and increasing the gain results in a perceived decrease in the onset latency. Increasing the gain magnifies the waveform, and its departure from the baseline also appears faster. Amplitude is unchanged by increasing both settings.
- Mixed nerve studies stimulate and record the sensory afferent (Ia) muscle spindle fibers.
- EPPs can be distinguished from FIBs by their irregular firing rate.
- Nerve conduction studies absolutely are contraindicated in patients with *external* cardiac pacing.
- An important limitation of routine motor and sensory nerve conduction studies is the fact that these studies only test large nerve fibers.
- Nerve conduction velocities are 50% of adult values in newborns, reach 80% of adult values by the first year, and are equivalent to adult values by 3 to 5 years of age.
- Reinnervation produces polyphasic, large amplitude, and long-duration MUAPs.
- An interelectrode distance of less than 4 cm results in a truncated SNAP amplitude and also decreases the SNAP peak latency, duration, rise time, and area.
- Lowering the high-frequency filter results in increases in both onset and peak latencies, increased duration, and decreased amplitude.
- Increasing the low-frequency filter increases the duration, decreases the peak latency, decreases the amplitude, and increases the number of phases in the composite waveform. The onset latency is unchanged as it is composed solely of high-frequency signals.

- CRDs consist of a group of muscle fibers firing regularly, consecutively, and repetitively.
- Cramps, fasciculation, and myokymic discharges all consist of MUAPs not under voluntary control.
- Cramps are actually multiple MUAPs firing synchronously at high frequencies causing painful involuntary muscle contractions.
- Fasciculations consist of individual MUAPs firing spontaneously and irregularly at slow rates.
- Myokymic discharges are groups of MUAPs firing repetitively and semiregularly in bursts with a variable number of MUAPs.
- The RR increases in neurogenic conditions. Myopathic recruitment would yield a low RR.
- The F wave is produced by supramaximal motor antidromic stimulation of anterior horn cells with orthodromic backfiring and is not a true reflex.
- One of the strategies to counteract stimulus artifact is to rotate the *anode* about the cathode.
- Anterior ear stimulation can yield a volume-conducted potential from the trigeminal-innervated masseter muscle that can be erroneously mistaken for a facial nerve response.
- Neuromyotonic, multiplet, and tremor discharges are all generated by motor units, resulting in secondary muscle contraction.

Radiculopathy and Plexopathy

- The rapid onset of unilateral right shoulder paresis preceded by a brief period of severe pain and recent illness is the classic presentation of neuralgic amyotrophy (also known as acute idiopathic brachial plexitis/neuritis or Parsonage-Turner syndrome). A gene mutation at chromosome 17 is implicated in the hereditary form of neuralgic amyotrophy.
- The electrophysiologic test findings in neurogenic thoracic outlet syndrome are those found in a lower trunk brachial plexopathy. There is also a classic finding of the median motor amplitude recording at the APB more reduced than the ulnar motor amplitude recording at the ADM on the affected side.
- Recurrent neoplastic brachial plexopathies are more likely to present with pain, involve the lower trunk, and occur with radiation doses less than 6,000 rads within 1 year of radiation. Radiation-induced brachial plexopathies are more likely to involve the upper trunk, demonstrate fasciculation potentials on needle EMG, and occur with radiation doses of greater than 6,000 rads within 1 year of radiation. In a needle EMG study where findings are consistent with plexopathy, the presence of myokymic discharges aids in establishing an etiology of radiation-induced plexopathy.
- SNAP latencies should be normal in an isolated radiculopathy.

Mononeuropathy and Polyneuropathy

- CMAP conduction block, abnormal temporal dispersion, and prolonged minimal F wave latency are found in acquired demyelinating neuropathies.

- MMN shows characteristic multifocal conduction block on nerve conduction studies; peripheral nerve involvement is often asymmetric and in the distal arm muscles.
- It is common to see persistent conduction velocity slowing even after undergoing carpal tunnel release surgery. After nerve decompression, there is increased internode distance.
- The most consistent measured parameter supporting the diagnosis of myopathy is decreased MUAP duration.
- In sciatic neuropathy, the peroneal division is more often injured than the tibial division due to the arrangement of the nerve fibers.
- The author recommends reviewing the anatomic pathways and components of the blink reflex for a deeper understanding of the various patterns of abnormalities.
- Motor unit recruitment is normal in demyelinating injury (not due to conduction block) because there is slowing but no loss of viable motor units.
- CIDP can be associated with Hodgkin lymphoma.
- The Miller Fisher variant of GBS classically presents with ophthalmoplegia, ataxia, and areflexia.
- A Martin-Gruber anastomosis (a median-to-ulnar motor nerve fiber crossover) in the forearm could be detected by recording at the ulnar-innervated FDI muscle while stimulating the median nerve in the antecubital fossa—yielding a CMAP with a negative deflection. Other findings include proximal median CMAP *higher* in amplitude than the distal CMAP, ulnar CMAP *lower* in amplitude below the elbow than at the wrist, and an initial positive deflection in the *proximal* median CMAP when there is superimposed CTS.
- F wave abnormalities can be the earliest findings in GBS.
- Mononeuritis multiplex is a common pattern of vasculitic neuropathy characterized by an asymmetric pattern of nerve involvement involving the lower and upper limbs.
- Cisplatin neuropathy affects only sensory nerves in an axonal pattern.
- Vincristine affects both sensory and motor nerves (sensory nerves are more affected than motor nerves).
- The most common pattern in diabetic polyneuropathy is an axonal and demyelinating (mixed) sensorimotor polyneuropathy.
- Uniform slowing of nerve conduction velocity involving all segments is characteristic of hereditary demyelinating peripheral polyneuropathies.
- HMSN/Charcot-Marie-Tooth type II is an axonal polyneuropathy.

Myopathy and Neuromuscular Disorders

- Steroid myopathy affects type II muscle fibers causing atrophy with typically normal EMG findings.
- Myopathic conditions are characterized early (increased) recruitment on needle EMG.
- Hyperkalemic periodic paralysis can manifest with both clinical and electrical myotonia; one way to memorize this is to think of it as "HYPER[active] with myotonia." Contrast this to hypokalemic periodic paralysis, where myotonia is not a prevalent clinical feature, and no electrical myotonia is found on EMG.

- In a patient with facioscapulohumeral dystrophy, the deltoid and forearm muscles are relatively spared in comparison to the other muscles affected.
- Myotonic dystrophy demonstrates genetic anticipation (the phenotypic symptoms are more severe in each successive generation due to unstable nucleotide repeats).
- Periodic paralysis disorders, such as paramyotonia congenita, display a characteristic finding of EMG electrical silence after cold exposure.
- McArdle disease is a metabolic myopathy known for the EMG finding of electrical silence during attacks of muscle cramping/contracture.
- Mitochondrial myopathy is a known side effect of AZT with the finding of ragged red fibers on muscle specimen staining.
- SMA is a lower motor neuron disease. PLS is an upper motor neuron disease. ALS involves both upper and lower motor neurons.
- Single-fiber electromyography is the most sensitive electrodiagnostic test for neuromuscular junction disorders.
- The presynaptic neuromuscular junction disorders (i.e., Lambert-Eaton syndrome and botulism) demonstrate a CMAP amplitude increment in response to fast stimulation rates and a reduced CMAP amplitude to initial supramaximal nerve stimulus.
- A progressive decrement in CMAP amplitude below initial baseline levels occurring minutes after maximum activation occurs in postsynaptic disorders.

REFERENCES & SUGGESTED READINGS

American Association of Electrodiagnostic Medicine, American Academy of Neurology, American Academy of Physical Medicine and Rehabilitation. Practice parameter for electrodiagnostic studies in carpal tunnel syndrome: summary statement. *Muscle Nerve*. 1993;16(12):1390-1391.

Barohn RJ, Saperstein DS. Guillain-Barré syndrome and chronic inflammatory demyelinating polyneuropathy. *Semin Neurol*. 1998;18(1):49-61.

Carter GT, England JD, Hecht TW, Han JJ, Weydt P, Chance PF. Electrodiagnostic evaluation of hereditary motor and sensory neuropathies. *Phys Med Rehabil Clin N Am*. 2003;14(2):347-363.

Cuccurullo S. *Physical Medicine and Rehabilitation Board Review*. 3rd ed. New York, NY: Demos Publishing; 2014.

Dreyer SJ, Dumitru D, King JC. Anodal block V anodal stimulation. Fact or fiction. *Am J Phys Med Rehabil*. 1993;72(1):10-18.

Dumitru D, Amato A, Zwartz M, eds. *Electrodiagnostic Medicine*. 2nd ed. Philadelphia, PA: Hanley & Belfus; 2001.

Feinberg J. EMG: myths and facts. *HHS J*. 2006;2(1):19-21.

Hehir MK, Logigian EL. Electrodiagnosis of myotonic disorders. *Phys Med Rehabil Clin N Am*. 2013;24(1):209-220. doi:10.1016/j.pmr.2012.08.015.

Kimura J. *Electrodiagnosis in Diseases of Nerve and Muscle: Principles and Practice*. 4th ed. New York, NY: Oxford University Press; 2013.

Krarup-Hansen A, Helweg-Larsen S, Schmalbruch H, Rørth M, Krarup C. Neuronal involvement in cisplatin neuropathy: prospective clinical and neurophysiological studies. *Brain*. 2007;130(pt 4):1076-1088.

Lateva ZC, McGill KC. Satellite potentials of motor unit action potentials in normal muscles: a new hypothesis for their origin. *Clin Neurophysiol*. 1999;110(9):1625-1633.

Lee HJ, DeLisa JA. *Manual of Nerve Conduction Study and Surface Anatomy for Needle Electromyography*. 4th ed. Philadelphia, PA: Lippincott Williams & Wilkins; 2004.

Leis AA, Trapani VC. *Atlas of Electromyography*. New York, NY: Oxford University Press; 2000.

Miller RG, Jackson CE, Kasarskis EJ, et al; Quality Standards Subcommittee of the American Academy of Neurology. Practice parameter update: the care of the patient with amyotrophic lateral sclerosis: multidisciplinary care, symptom management, and cognitive/behavioral impairment (an evidence-based review): report of the Quality Standards Subcommittee of the American Academy of Neurology. *Neurology*. 2009;73(15):1227-1233. doi:10.1212/WNL.0b013e3181bc01a4.

Olney RK. Guidelines in electrodiagnostic medicine. Consensus criteria for the diagnosis of partial conduction block. *Muscle Nerve Suppl*. 1999;8:S225-S229.

Pease WS, Lew HL, Johnson EW, eds. *Johnson's Practical Electromyography*. 4th ed. Philadelphia, PA: Lippincott Williams & Wilkins; 2006.

Prahlow ND, Buschbacher ND. *Manual of Nerve Conduction Studies*. New York, NY: Demos Medical; 2005.

Tan FC. *EMG Secrets: Questions and Answers Reveal the Art & Science of Electromyography*. Philadelphia, PA: Hanley & Belfus; 2003.

Visser LH. Critical illness polyneuropathy and myopathy: clinical features, risk factors and prognosis. *Eur J Neurol*. 2006;13(11):1203-1212.

Wulff EA, Wang AK, Simpson DM. HIV-associated peripheral neuropathy: epidemiology, pathophysiology and treatment. *Drugs*. 2000;59(6);1251-1260.

Spine Trauma and Spinal Cord Injury Medicine

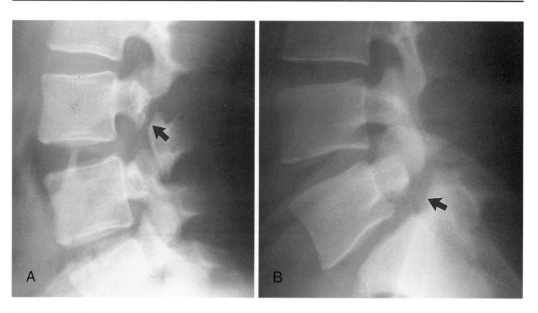

From Yochum TR, Rowe LJ. *Yochum and Rowe's Essentials of Skeletal Radiology*. 3rd ed. Philadelphia, PA: Lippincott Williams & Wilkins; 2004.

1. In the above radiographs, the black arrows depict

    A. a normal superior articular process.

    B. a normal facet (zygapophyseal) joint.

    C. an abnormal pars interarticularis.

    D. an abnormal facet (zygapophyseal) joint.

2. Features of neck hyperextension injuries include

A. preservation of the anterior longitudinal ligament with posterior ligament tear.

B. neurologic dysfunction disproportionally affecting the lower extremities.

C. anterior distraction and posterior compression.

D. both A and B

3. The fracture line in a flexion/distraction (Chance) fracture injury would pass through which of the following anatomic structure(s)?

A. spinous process

B. spinous process and lamina

C. spinous process, lamina, and pedicle

D. spinous process, lamina, pedicle, and vertebral body

4. Which of these spine fractures is most likely to be associated with spine instability?

A. bilateral facet joint dislocation

B. wedge compression fracture

C. Jefferson fracture

D. odontoid process fracture

5. Which type of fracture is most likely to cause severe spinal cord injury?

A. Jefferson fracture

B. Chance fracture

C. hangman fracture

D. flexion teardrop fracture

6. A burst fracture of a thoracolumbar vertebral body would be considered most unstable if

A. the anterior longitudinal ligament is disrupted.

B. the posterior ligaments are disrupted.

C. the posterior portion of intervertebral disc is herniated.

D. the anterior one-third of the vertebral body is fractured.

7. Which of the following would be vulnerable to injury from an occlusion of the artery of Adamkiewicz?

A. the posterior one-third of the spinal cord

B. the cervical segments of the spinal cord

C. the anterior two-thirds of the spinal cord

D. the dorsal column of the spinal cord

8. Anterior cord syndrome would manifest with all the following, EXCEPT

A. loss of vibratory sensation.

B. loss of temperature sensation.

C. loss of pain sensation.

D. flaccid paraplegia.

9. The figure shows caudal spine nervous system structures labeled from A to D.
A lesion affecting which labeled structure is considered to be a sacral spinal cord injury?

A. A

B. B

C. C

D. D

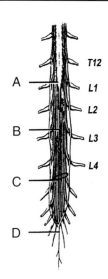

10. Central cord syndrome (CCS)

   A. is a complete spinal cord injury.

   B. occurs more commonly in younger persons.

   C. affects the lower limbs greater than the upper limbs.

   D. recovery occurs last in the intrinsic hand muscles.

11. In a classic presentation of traumatic left hemisection spinal cord injury at C6, the following feature would be present as loss of

   A. vibration sensation at the middle finger on the left side.

   B. finger flexion on the right side.

   C. pain and temperature at the lateral antecubital fossa on the right side.

   D. brachioradialis reflex on the right side.

12. A hemisection spinal cord injury (i.e., Brown-Séquard syndrome) would affect which of the following nerve tracts?

   A. dorsal column and spinocerebellar

   B. spinothalamic

   C. corticospinal

   D. all of the above

13. Traumatic spinal cord injury (SCI) statistics reveal

   A. SCI occurs with peak incidence in the month of February.

   B. diseases of the respiratory system are the leading cause of death following SCI.

   C. falls are the leading cause of SCI among all age groups.

   D. having Medicare does not predict mortality during the first year.

14. According to the International Standards for Neurological Classification of Spinal Cord Injury, sensory testing at the lateral (radial) side of the antecubital fossa slightly proximal to the elbow crease corresponds to which sensory dermatome?

A. C4

B. C5

C. C6

D. C7

15. A 29-year-old male was involved in a motor vehicle accident with a presumed spinal cord injury. The International Standards for Neurological Classification of Spinal Cord Injury were used. The motor testing data is listed below.

Motor

	R	L
C5	5	5
C6	3	4
C7	2	3
C8	0	1
T1	0	0
L1	0	0
L2	0	0
L3	0	0
L4	0	0
L5	0	0
S1	0	0

Voluntary anal contraction = no.

Based on the available information, what is the motor level for this patient?

A. C5

B. C6

C. C7

D. C8

16. A 29-year-old male was involved in a motor vehicle accident with a presumed spinal cord injury. The motor and sensory testing data is summarized below.

Sensory: right T5, left T7
Motor: right L2, left L3
Voluntary anal contraction = no
Anal sensation and deep anal pressure = yes

Based on the available information, which of the following is TRUE for this patient?

A. This represents a complete spinal cord injury because anal contraction was absent.

B. This spinal cord injury has an ASIA Impairment Scale (AIS) grade of B.

C. There should be a zone of partial preservation in this spinal cord injury.

D. The neurologic level of injury is T5.

17. A 29-year-old male was involved in a motor vehicle accident with a presumed spinal cord injury. The International Standards for Neurological Classification of Spinal Cord Injury were used. The motor and sensory testing data are listed below.

Motor

	R	L
C5	5	5
C6	5	5
C7	5	5
C8	5	4
T1	4	4
L1	4	3
L2	3	3
L3	3	1
L4	3	0
L5	2	0
S1	1	0

Voluntary anal contraction = yes.

Sensory

Light Touch	R	L	Pinprick	R	L
C2	2	2	C2	2	2
C3	2	2	C3	2	2
C4	2	2	C4	2	2
C5	2	2	C5	2	2
C6	2	2	C6	2	1
C7	2	1	C7	1	0
C8	1	1	C8	1	0
T1	1	0	T1	1	0
T2	1	0	T2	1	0
T3	1	0	T3	1	0
T4	1	0	T4	1	0
T5	1	0	T5	1	0
T6	0	0	T6	0	0
T7	0	0	T7	0	0
T8	0	0	T8	0	0
T9	0	0	T9	0	0
T10	0	0	T10	0	0
T11	0	0	T11	0	0
T12	0	0	T12	0	0
L1	1	1	L1	0	0
L2	1	0	L2	1	0
L3	0	0	L3	0	0
L4	1	0	L4	0	0
L5	0	0	L5	0	0
S1	0	0	S1	0	0
S2	0	0	S2	0	0
S3	0	0	S3	0	0
S4-5	1	1	S4-5	0	0

What is the neurologic level and ASIA Impairment Scale (AIS) for this patient?

A. C6 ASIA C

B. C6 ASIA D

C. C5 ASIA C

D. C5 ASIA D

18. The zone of partial preservation (ZPP) refers to

A. the residual sensory and motor function seen in incomplete spinal cord injuries.

B. sacral sparing at the S4-5 level.

C. innervated dermatomes and myotomes below the level of a complete spinal cord injury.

D. international standards to document remaining autonomic function after spinal cord injury.

19. While performing an admission physical on the spinal cord injury rehabilitation floor, your patient tests at 0 for all key graded muscles from C5 to S1 with absent anal contraction. The sensory level is C4. What conclusion can you reach with the given information?

A. There is no motor level for this patient.

B. The motor level is C4.

C. This patient's motor examination should be recorded as not testable (NT) because there is no motor function.

D. There is no zone of partial preservation.

20. Muscles that are OPTIONAL to include in your International Standards for Neurological Classification of Spinal Cord Injury assessment include all the following, EXCEPT

A. diaphragm.

B. deltoids.

C. finger flexors.

D. hip adductors.

21. A person with which of the following neurologic levels of spinal cord injury has the potential to be independent in transfers on level surfaces, feeding, upper body dressing, and manual wheelchair propulsion on even terrain (except curbs)?

A. C4

B. C5

C. C6

D. C7

22. A person with a neurologic level of spinal cord injury at C6 usually would be

   A. dependent with bathing.

   B. independent in manual wheelchair with coated rims on level surfaces.

   C. requiring assistance for upper body dressing.

   D. independent with lower body dressing.

23. An example of appropriate adaptive equipment to order for a patient with C5 complete tetraplegia would be a

   A. universal cuff.

   B. shoulder immobilizer.

   C. button hook.

   D. short opponens splint.

24. A tenodesis splint would be most appropriate for which neurologic level of spinal cord injury?

   A. C5

   B. C6

   C. C7

   D. C8

25. Which of the following is true about cervical spondylotic myelopathy?

   A. This condition can present with signs of hyperreflexia, lower extremity spasticity, and wasting of intrinsic hand muscles.

   B. This condition is the most common cause of gait dysfunction in persons older than 55 years.

   C. This condition is the most common cause of spinal cord dysfunction in the world.

   D. all of the above

26. Which type of spinal tumor is known for being both intradural and extra-medullary in location?

    A. schwannoma

    B. astrocytoma

    C. ependymoma

    D. hemangioblastoma

27. Which type of spinal tumor has the worst prognosis?

    A. astrocytoma

    B. ependymoma

    C. lung metastatic

    D. schwannoma

28. Which of the following statements is true regarding spinal cord injury without radiographic abnormality (SCIWORA)?

    A. Young children have a high predisposition for SCIWORA due to head to neck size and ligament elasticity.

    B. One of the major criteria for SCIWORA is the presence of a negative magnetic resonance imaging (MRI) study.

    C. The neurologic symptoms in SCIWORA characteristically appear immediately after injury.

    D. The adolescent population is most susceptible to SCIWORA through sports injuries, especially in football.

29. A 50-year-old female with past medical history of gastric bypass presents with symptoms of leg dysesthesias. Physical examination reveals loss of vibration and proprioception in the legs and a positive Romberg sign. What is the next step in assessment?

    A. Order magnetic resonance imaging (MRI) of the lumbar spine.

    B. Order spinal tap.

    C. Order serum cobalamin level.

    D. Order the Schilling test.

30. What is the primary outcome measure for functional recovery in the spinal cord injury (SCI) population?

    A. Tetraplegic and Paraplegic Functional Scale

    B. Spinal Cord Independence Measure

    C. Modified Barthel Index

    D. Quadriplegia Index of Function

31. The current recommended routine management of acute traumatic spinal cord injury (SCI) includes all of the following, EXCEPT

    A. high-dose methylprednisolone.

    B. fluid resuscitation.

    C. maintenance of mean arterial pressure (MAP) above 85 mm Hg.

    D. spine stabilization.

32. In the acute period after spinal cord injury, a characteristic finding is

    A. reflex defecation.

    B. positive Babinski sign.

    C. areflexia.

    D. spasticity.

33. Which of these answer choices lists the expected chronologic pattern of reflex recovery after spinal cord injury (SCI) (from the first reflex to recover to the latest to recover)?

    A. knee jerk → cremasteric → bulbocavernosus → delayed plantar response

    B. delayed plantar response → bulbocavernosus → cremasteric → knee jerk

    C. bulbocavernosus → knee jerk → delayed plantar response → cremasteric

    D. cremasteric → knee jerk → bulbocavernosus → delayed plantar response

34. The majority of patients with spinal cord injury will make the most functional recovery within which time frame following injury?

   A. 1 month

   B. 2 to 4 months

   C. 6 to 9 months

   D. 2 years

35. Which of the following statements typically is true regarding bowel and bladder management in the pediatric spinal cord injury population?

   A. Indwelling catheters are the treatment of choice for paraplegic children from the developmental ages 2 to 10 years.

   B. Diarrhea and/or constipation are contraindications for starting a bowel program in children younger than 2 years old unless it is causing skin breakdown.

   C. Clean intermittent catheterization should be considered starting in adolescence.

   D. Children with adequate hand function can begin self-catheterization and independent bowel program when they are developmentally 5 to 7 years old.

36. You are called to the inpatient therapy gym to evaluate a 25-year-old male 2 weeks after complete C7 spinal cord injury (SCI). He reports sudden onset of light-headedness and near syncope after being transferred from the exercise table back into his wheelchair. Vital signs are as follows: pulse = 100, supine blood pressure = 100/70 mm Hg, seated blood pressure = 80/60 mm Hg, pulse oximetry = 98% oxygen saturation (Spo_2) on room air. After reclining him in his wheelchair, his therapist comments that this is the third incident this week with these same symptoms. A combination of nonpharmacologic and pharmacologic treatment plan for this condition would be to

   A. apply functional electrical stimulation and prescribe midodrine.

   B. remove any noxious stimulus and administer clonidine.

   C. remove abdominal binder and prescribe baclofen.

   D. initiate fluid restriction and prescribe furosemide.

37. The best option for deep vein thrombosis (DVT) prophylaxis in patients with spinal cord injury (SCI) is

A. pneumatic compression stockings.

B. warfarin.

C. inferior vena cava (IVC) filter.

D. low molecular weight heparin.

38. Which of the following is TRUE regarding autonomic dysreflexia (AD) in the spinal cord injury population?

A. The pathophysiology is mainly due to unregulated and exaggerated parasympathetic activity arising from descending pathways above the lesion.

B. The characteristic symptoms are hypertension, headache, flushing, sweating, and piloerection.

C. The most common inciting event arises from a rapid change in body position to upright.

D. The condition is benign with full resolution and no further complications once the noxious stimulus is removed.

39. Which of the following would be the most appropriate respiratory management of a patient with complete tetraplegia in the acute inpatient rehabilitation setting?

A. continued secretion management, cough assist, and glossopharyngeal breathing

B. monotherapy with long-acting beta agonists to treat bronchospasm

C. phrenic nerve pacing in the acute period after injury

D. permanently discontinuing pulmonary toilet once vent weaning has commenced

40. You are making inpatient rounds on the spinal cord rehab unit with your medical students in tow and ask them: Which respiratory muscles are expected to still be functional in a patient with complete C7 tetraplegia?

   A. accessory muscles

   B. accessory muscles and diaphragm

   C. accessory muscles, diaphragm, and intercostal muscles

   D. accessory muscles, diaphragm, intercostals, and abdominal muscles

41. Which of the following parameters is the best predictor of respiratory muscle fatigue in a rehabilitation patient with acute spinal cord injury?

   A. tidal volume

   B. vital capacity

   C. residual volume

   D. arterial oxygen tension (Pao_2)

42. A 32-year-old male with 2-year history of T7 complete paraplegia returns for an outpatient clinic follow-up visit for a 6-month history urinary retention and frequent urinary tract infections. He had been reflex voiding with no difficulties prior to onset of symptoms. Prior renal diagnostic imaging showed normal anatomy of kidneys and ureters. He presents today to review the results of his cystometrogram electromyography (EMG) urodynamic study and discuss treatment options. Thus, summarized findings of the study showed elevated detrusor pressure, elevated urinary sphincter pressure, and continuous pelvic floor EMG activity with low flow during the voiding phase. Given the test findings, all of the following treatment options can be considered, EXCEPT

   A. botulinum toxin A injections to sphincter.

   B. sphincterotomy.

   C. clean intermittent catheterization (CIC) and anticholinergic medication.

   D. bethanechol.

43. Assuming all patients have normal urinary tract anatomy, choose the patient with spinal cord injury (SCI) in your inpatient rehabilitation unit who would be best suited for intermittent catheterization (IC).

A. 70-year-old female with central cord syndrome and rheumatoid arthritis

B. 18-year-old male with T5 complete paraplegia and autonomic dysreflexia

C. 35-year-old male with T9 incomplete paraplegia and hypercalcemia

D. 23-year-old female with T10 complete paraplegia and spontaneous bladder contractions

44. An example of utilizing the gastrocolic reflex in the management of neurogenic bowel would be

A. timed defecation within 1 hour after meals.

B. prescribing senna 1 to 4 tablets orally daily at noon.

C. digitally stimulating inside rectum.

D. abdominal massage.

45. Which of the following statements is true regarding sexual function in males after spinal cord injury (SCI)?

A. Most men will retain the ability to ejaculate.

B. Reflexogenic erections are uncommon.

C. Intracavernosal injection therapy can induce erections.

D. Sildenafil can induce ejaculation.

46. Regarding sexual or reproductive function in women with spinal cord injury (SCI):

A. Autonomic dysreflexia can occur with labor contractions in women with T6 or higher injury.

B. Women missing sensation in the T11-L2 dermatomes can still experience arousal and orgasm.

C. A female with T9 complete paraplegia can still feel uterine contractions.

D. SCI causes long-term infertility due to amenorrhea.

47. In a person with chronic spinal cord injury (SCI) at 2 years postinjury, the most common location for a pressure ulcer is

A. trochanter.

B. ischium.

C. heel.

D. elbow.

48. Choose the best antispasticity medication to prescribe for your patient, a 45-year-old male with paraplegia who is a heavy drinker with elevated hepatic enzymes and problems with orthostatic hypotension.

A. baclofen

B. dantrolene

C. clonidine

D. diazepam

49. A partial thickness pressure ulcer that extends through the epidermis and a portion of the dermis is considered to be

A. stage 1.

B. stage 2.

C. stage 3.

D. stage 4.

50. Which of the following treatments is NOT considered to be form of pressure ulcer debridement?

A. using a scalpel to remove necrotic tissue from wound

B. wet to dry dressings to wound

C. applying collagenase to wound bed

D. covering wound with transparent polymeric membrane dressing

51. The differential diagnosis for fever in a patient with C6 tetraplegia typically would NOT include which of the following?

   A. poikilothermia

   B. infection

   C. orthostatic hypotension

   D. heterotopic ossification

52. The most common musculoskeletal complications in people with spinal cord injury (SCI) involve

   A. the hips.

   B. the shoulders.

   C. the feet.

   D. the knees.

53. Which of the following is proper positioning of patient with spinal cord injury (SCI) to prevent contracture?

   A. shoulders in abduction and external rotation in bed

   B. posterior pelvic tilt in wheelchair

   C. place pillow under knees in bed

   D. prolonged supine in bed

54. Compared to the age-matched population without spinal cord injury (SCI), cause of death due to suicide

   A. is less for people with SCI.

   B. is higher for people with SCI.

   C. is the same for people with SCI.

   D. is inconclusive due to poor tracking data.

55. Which is an example of a colonic stimulant?

   A. docusate sodium

   B. senna

   C. psyllium

   D. metoclopramide

56. A prescription for a high back power wheelchair with tilt and recline, head-rest, modified joystick, and upper extremity support is best suited for which injury level?

A. C8

B. C5

C. C7

D. T2

57. The proper "parastance" posture for people with paraplegia is described best as standing

A. in bilateral knee ankle foot orthoses (KAFOs) with dorsiflexed ankles, extended knees, hyperextended hips, posterior lean.

B. using crutches and bilateral KAFOs while leaning forward and flexing knees.

C. with a KAFO on one leg and AFO on the other leg using exaggerated hip flexion to balance between each leg.

D. while performing alternating reciprocal weight shifts from one leg to another.

58. Which of the following is a contraindication to phrenic nerve pacing?

A. absent phrenic nerve function found on electromyography (EMG)/ nerve conduction study

B. significant lung disease

C. patient at 2 months postinjury

D. all of the above

59. Secondary complications more common in the pediatric and/or adolescent spinal cord injury (SCI) population include all of the following, EXCEPT

A. spasticity.

B. scoliosis.

C. hip dislocation.

D. hypercalcemia.

60. In the population with spinal cord injury (SCI), an expanding posttraumatic syringomyelia would

  A. most commonly present as pain in the clinical setting.

  B. communicate directly with the fourth ventricle of the brain.

  C. cause a decrease in muscle tone below the affected area.

  D. occur several levels below the injury site.

61. A 3-year-old female with L1 paraplegia from spina bifida presents with her parents evaluation for an ambulatory device. She currently uses a wheelchair. She had previously used a standing frame with success. She is very motivated and wishes to walk for exercise and short distances. She has intact upper extremity strength and normal head and neck control. Bilateral lower extremity motor strength is at maximum 2/5 in all muscle groups. She has no contractures or deformities in her lower limbs. Spasticity is not a limiting factor. Of the listed answer choices, you are most likely to prescribe

  A. parapodium.

  B. reciprocating gait orthosis (RGO).

  C. ankle foot orthoses (AFO).

  D. knee ankle foot orthoses (KAFO).

62. You are called to the acute inpatient spinal cord injury (SCI) rehab floor to see an 18-year-old male with T7 paraplegia with history of traction immobilization with symptoms of abdominal pain, fatigue, vomiting, and polyuria with physical examination showing no sign of acute abdomen. Serum ionized calcium level is 8.20 mg/dL (reference range: 4.64 to 5.28 mg/dL). What is a standard medication used to treat this condition?

  A. alendronate

  B. pamidronate

  C. prazosin

  D. piperacillin/tazobactam

63. A typical metabolic change in spinal cord injury (SCI) is

 A. a decreased testosterone.

 B. an increased basal metabolic rate.

 C. an increased rate of obesity.

 D. an increased rate of hypoglycemia.

64. Moving the wheelchair axle anteriorly,

 A. stability is increased.

 B. maneuverability is increased.

 C. both stability and maneuverability are increased.

 D. maneuverability is decreased.

65. You are doing your morning inpatient rounds on the spinal cord injury (SCI) unit and encounter on a 56-year-old male with complete T6 paraplegia 2 months postinjury. The night nurse reports patient developed a fever last night and complains of pain in his right hip. There was no reported injury. Vitals signs are stable, and he is now afebrile. Physical examination reveals soft tissue swelling involving the right hip and proximal thigh with reduced passive range of motion. STAT venous Doppler study is negative for deep vein thrombosis (DVT). STAT labs reveal normal complete blood count (CBC) with differential but elevated erythrocyte sedimentation rate (ESR) and alkaline phosphatase. What is the next best step to confirm the diagnosis?

 A. Aspirate the right hip under fluoroscopy and send the fluid to the lab for culture.

 B. Send him out to the hospital for plain radiographs of the right hip.

 C. Obtain three-phase bone scan.

 D. Order bone biopsy.

ANSWER KEY WITH EXPLANATIONS

1. The correct answer is C.
The black arrow in each of the lateral lumbar radiographs points to a defect in the pars interarticularis (spondylolysis). Radiograph A on the left demonstrates spondylolysis at L3 without a spondylolisthesis at L3-4, and the radiograph on the right demonstrates L5 spondylolysis with a grade I spondylolisthesis at L5-S1.

2. The correct answer is C.
Hyperextension cervical spine injuries are commonly found in high-velocity acceleration-deceleration motor vehicles. The mechanism is anterior distraction (often causing disruption of the anterior longitudinal ligament) and posterior compression. Clinical manifestation is traumatic central cord syndrome. The upper extremities are disproportionally affected.

3. The correct answer is D.
A flexion/distraction (Chance) fracture is a type of seat belt injury with a horizontal fracture line extending from the spinous process to the vertebral body. All anatomic structures along that path can be involved. This injury can be caused in the thoracolumbar region by wearing a lap belt type restraint (without shoulder strap) where the upper body moves forward on deceleration, whereas the lower body remains fixed with axis of rotation at the lap belt.

4. The correct answer is A.
Bilateral facet joint dislocation is an unstable injury that includes disruption of the anterior longitudinal ligament, posterior longitudinal ligament, and facet capsules. A wedge compression fracture of the anterior vertebral body is a stable fracture. Jefferson and odontoid process fractures can be stable or unstable. Unstable atlantoaxial fractures occur in the setting of transverse atlantal ligament disruption.

5. The correct answer is D.
A flexion teardrop fracture is considered to be the most severe, unstable injury of the cervical spine that results in quadriplegia with anterior cord syndrome. A severe flexion and axial compression injury (commonly diving into shallow pool) results in a fracture of the anterior inferior vertebral body (resembling a teardrop) with posterior vertebral body displacement into the spinal canal. Chance and Jefferson fractures do not commonly cause severe spinal cord injury. The hangman fracture of C2 sounds dangerous; however, it only refers to bilateral fractures through the pars interarticularis that separate the body of C2 from the posterior elements but does not compress the spinal cord.

6. The correct answer is B.
The three-column concept of spine stability in acute trauma was described by Francis Denis in his landmark 1983 paper (please review the anatomic structures of the three columns in your study notes). A burst fracture involves the anterior and middle columns. Additional disruption of the posterior (column) ligaments would indicate a three-column failure and be the most unstable. Both disruption of the anterior longitudinal ligament (ALL) and an anterior vertebral fracture imply anterior column failure only. The posterior annulus fibrosis is considered part of the middle column only.

7. The correct answer is C.
The blood supply to the anterior two-thirds of the spinal cord is from the anterior spinal artery, which arises from the vertebral arteries and travels the length of the spinal column as a single artery, receiving contributions from radicular arteries. The major anterior lumbar radicular artery, called the arteria radicularis magna (a.k.a. the artery of Adamkiewicz), joins the anterior spinal artery between the lower thoracic to upper lumbar regions and supplies the caudal two-thirds of the spinal cord. Occlusion of this artery can manifest as anterior spinal artery syndrome.

8. The correct answer is A.
The nerve tracts carrying vibratory sensation are housed in the dorsal column (posterior one-third of the spinal cord), which are supplied by the posterior spinal arteries. Anterior cord syndrome affects the anterior two-thirds of the spinal cord supplied by the anterior spinal artery. Anterior cord syndrome symptoms correspond to the anatomic spinal tracts affected and include loss of motor function below the level of the lesion (flaccid paraplegia) with loss of pain and temperature sensation.

9. The correct answer is A.
The structure labeled "A" is the conus medullaris, which is the tapered caudal end of the spinal cord. The conus medullaris contains the sacral spinal cord segments (S1-5). Answer choices B and C are below the spinal cord in the region of the lumbosacral nerve roots (i.e., cauda equina) and thus are considered to be nerve root injuries. Answer choice D is the coccygeal ligament, surrounding the filum terminale. Lesions to the lower portion of the conus medullaris and to the cauda equina would characteristically manifest with areflexic bladder and bowel. Lesions in upper conus medullaris (suprasacral lesions) would characteristically present with an upper motor neuron, including preserved bowel, bladder, and bulbocavernosus reflexes.

10. The correct answer is D.
CCS is characterized by sacral sparing (incomplete spinal cord injury). CCS occurs more often in older individuals with preexisting cervical spondylosis. The motor weakness in CCS affects the upper limbs to a much greater degree than the lower limbs. The recovery occurs earliest in the lower extremities and latest in the intrinsic hand muscles.

11. The correct answer is A.
A classic hemisection spinal cord injury (i.e., Brown-Séquard syndrome) would result in ipsilateral loss of vibration and proprioception below the lesion and thus would involve the C7 dermatome at the left middle finger. Other features of a hemisection spinal cord injury are ipsilateral motor loss at and below the level of the lesion (in this case would be on the left side), contralateral loss of pain temperature below the level of the lesion (lateral antecubital fossa is C5, so incorrect answer choice), and ipsilateral flaccid paralysis at the level of the lesion (brachioradialis reflex would be absent on left, not right).

12. The correct answer is D.
All the listed nerve tracts would be affected (please refer to your textbook illustrations to briefly review anatomy).

13. The correct answer is B.

Diseases of the respiratory system are leading cause of primary death in patients with traumatic SCI, the highest percentage due to pneumonia. Traumatic SCI occurs with peak incidence in the month of July; the month of February has the least incidence. Automobile accidents are the most common etiology of injury among all age groups, followed by falls and gunshot wounds. Falls are only the most common etiology in older adults. Medicare or Medicaid has actually been identified as a factor predicting mortality during the first year after traumatic SCI.

14. The correct answer is B.

This question describes the C5 dermatome landmark for sensory testing. Please refer back to the International Standards for Neurological Classification of Spinal Cord Injury in order to review the dermatome testing landmarks and dermatome map.

15. The correct answer is B.

The motor level for each side is the lowest (most caudal) muscle that has a testing grade of at least 3, and has intact motor innervation (muscle grade of 5) in all the levels above it. The motor level on the right is C6, and the motor level on the left is C6. Thus, the motor level is C6. If the motor levels were to differ by side of the body, a single motor level would be considered the more rostral (most cephalad level) of the two.

16. The correct answer is D.

The neurologic level of injury is determined by the lowest segment where motor and sensory function is normal on both sides. A single neurologic level would be the most rostral/cephalad of the four recorded levels. The presence of any of the following—anal sensation, deep anal pressure, or voluntary anal contraction—indicates sacral sparing. Any sacral sparing is indicative of an incomplete injury, which is defined as partial preservation of sensory and/or motor function below the neurologic level that includes the lowest sacral segments S4-5. There is not enough information provided to determine AIS classification, which require reviewing the motor and sensory data tables. This is an incomplete injury, so a zone of partial preservation is not considered.

17. The correct answer is D.

Please refer back to the International Standards for Neurological Classification of Spinal Cord Injury for detailed explanation of the classification guidelines. The right and left motor levels are T1 and C8, respectively. The sensory levels are right C6 and left C5. The single neurologic level of C5 is the lowest segment where both sensory and motor function is normal on both sides. This is an incomplete injury because there is sacral sparing. Because at least 50% of the key muscles below C5 are graded 3 or better, thus the AIS impairment grade is D.

18. The correct answer is C.

The ZPP is a term used only with complete traumatic spinal cord injuries to refer to dermatomes and myotomes caudal to the neurologic level that remain partially innervated. The most caudal segment with this partial innervation is recorded on the standard classification form as the ZPP.

19. The correct answer is B.

The International Standards for Neurological Classification of Spinal Cord Injury state that for myotomes that are not tested by the manual muscle examination (like in this case of C1-4), the motor level is presumed to be the same as the sensory level. The option of marking a muscle as not testable can be done in cases of limb immobilization, severe pain, amputation, or contracture of greater than 50% of range of motion. There is no information to reach a conclusion about a zone of partial preservation.

20. The correct answer is C.

The finger flexor muscle testing is NOT considered to be optional; it is a required part of the motor assessment for the innervation of the C8 myotome. The rest of the muscles are optional for testing; the optional muscles are helpful to determine if there is motor sparing in incomplete injuries but are not used to obtain a motor index score.

21. The correct answer is D.

A person with a C7 level of injury potentially will be independent in most activities of daily living using a wheelchair. A C7 still may require assistance for uneven surfaces and lower body dressing.

22. The correct answer is B.

A person with a C6 spinal cord injury would have shoulder abduction, elbow flexion, and wrist extension. This would allow manual wheelchair propulsion at least for short distances on level surfaces with a chair equipped with plastic coated rims. Bathing would require adaptive equipment with minimal assistance. Upper body dressing is usually independent with clothing modifications. Lower body dressing still requires some assistance.

23. The correct answer is A.

The C5 level includes shoulder motion and elbow flexion; this will allow the user to maintain objects, such as utensils, in a universal cuff. The shoulder usually would not be immobilized because our goal is to enhance function, not impede it. A button hook would require the user to have finger flexion. A short opponens splint requires wrist strength in extension and flexion because the orthosis does not control wrist movement. A long opponens splint (*not an answer choice*) would provide the appropriate wrist support a C5 level patient would need.

24. The correct answer is B.

The C6 muscle function of wrist extension will allow passive opposition of the thumb and the index finger. Conversely, wrist flexion will allow passive finger extension. Achieving a functional tenodesis grip is a primary rehabilitation goal in a patient with C6 spinal cord injury. Tenodesis splinting can aid in achieving this goal and in maintaining the proper position of the hand digits to facilitate the grip.

25. The correct answer is D.

All of the statements are true regarding cervical spondylotic myelopathy. Always look for it in your differential diagnosis in clinical practice.

26. The correct answer is A.

Nerve sheath tumors, such as schwannomas and neurofibromas, are known as intradural extramedullary spinal tumors. The remaining answer choices are types of intradural intramedullary spinal cord tumors; intramedullary tumors are far less common than extramedullary tumors.

27. The correct answer is C.

Metastatic spinal tumors have the worst prognosis of the answer choices. The majority of metastatic tumors are extradural from lung, breast, or prostate cancer. Metastatic malignant cells can proliferate within the epidural space, leading to spinal cord compression with a median survival of only 1.5 months for patients with lung cancer spine metastasis with cord compression. The most common treatment is palliative, consisting of steroids and radiotherapy. Nearly all spine astrocytomas and schwannomas are benign. Ependymomas are benign slow-growing tumors that respond well to resection.

28. The correct answer is A.

The prevalence of SCIWORA is highest in children younger than 8 years of age with predisposition for upper cervical injury due to head to neck size and ligament elasticity. Horizontal orientation of the cervical facets could also be a factor in children. It can also present after a fall in elderly people with preexisting spine degenerative changes. SCIWORA is the presence of clinical symptoms of traumatic myelopathy without any spine fracture or spine instability on radiographs or computed tomography. Persons with SCIWORA can be found to have spinal cord abnormalities on MRI studies. The neurologic symptoms can be delayed in SCIWORA for as long as 48 hours in some patients.

29. The correct answer is C.

This clinical vignette describes some characteristic neurologic symptoms arising from cobalamin vitamin B_{12} deficiency, namely, early signs of the myelopathy of subacute combined degeneration (SCD). SCD is known to predominantly involve the posterior/dorsal column of the spinal cord with possible later involvement of the anterolateral columns. The condition most severely affects the lower cervical region followed by the thoracic region. The initial test would be serum cobalamin (vitamin B_{12}), and subsequent laboratory tests would be ordered according to a diagnostic algorithm. The Schilling test is time-consuming and not a good choice for an initial test; it might be appropriate to order later in the workup if there is confirmed vitamin B_{12} deficiency.

30. The correct answer is B.

The Functional Recovery Outcome Measures Work Group 2008 paper in the *Journal of Spinal Cord Medicine* indicates that Spinal Cord Independence Measure (SCIM) is the primary functional recovery outcome measure designed specifically for the population with SCI; it has been found to be valid and reliable for SCI. The Modified Barthel Index has only minimal validity and little clinical utility in the population with SCI. The Quadriplegia Index of Function is limited to a nonambulatory tetraplegia subset of patients with minimal evidence for validity. The other answer choice (A) was made up.

31. The correct answer is A.

Current level 1 recommendations at time of publication are not in support of the routine use of methylprednisolone as part of an acute SCI management protocol. (Please see references at end of the chapter and review results of the Third National Acute Spinal Cord Injury Study [NASCIS III] for more information.) The 1997 Vale et al. study has shown that maintaining MAP at greater than 85 mm Hg has been associated with improved neurologic outcomes for cervical and upper thoracic injuries. Fluid resuscitation and spine stabilization are routine measures in acute traumatic SCI.

32. The correct answer is C.

A temporary loss in spinal reflex activity below the level of injury is a characteristic of spinal shock, an acute stage of neurologic dysfunction following spinal cord injury. The other answer choices involve increased reflex activity, which will appear in the subacute to chronic periods after injury.

33. The correct answer is B.

The studied return of reflex arc activity (see the "Suggested Readings" section for the 1999 study by Ko et al.) has shown the delayed plantar reflex to be the earliest reflex followed by the bulbocavernosus and cremasteric in the initial days after SCI. Later, deep tendon reflexes (i.e., ankle and knee jerk) return, usually within 1 to 2 weeks.

34. The correct answer is C.

The majority of functional recovery typically occurs within the first 6 to 9 months following injury with plateau occurring between 12 and 18 months and minimal recovery after that time.

35. The correct answer is D.

Children with adequate hand function can begin self-catheterization and independent bowel program when they are developmentally 5 to 7 years old. Clean intermittent catheterization typically begins at age 3 years or earlier if there are recurrent urinary infections or renal dysfunction. Diarrhea or constipation is an indication for starting a child's bowel program earlier than the recommended age of 2 to 4 years old.

36. The correct answer is A.

Orthostatic hypotension (OH) is a common complication in the initial postinjury period following complete SCI in those with neurologic level of T6 or above. A 2009 systemic review of OH management in patients with SCI showed level 2 evidence for functional electrical stimulation and for the selective alpha-adrenergic agonist, midodrine. Other nonpharmacologic treatments with some evidence of efficacy include elastic stockings, abdominal binders, fluids, and increased salt intake. Other pharmacologic treatments used for OH include fludrocortisone, ephedrine, salt tablets, ergot alkaloids, and L-dihydroxyphenylserine (L-DOPS).

37. The correct answer is D.

At time of publication, there are level 1 recommendations for use of low molecular weight heparin (LMWH) either as a stand-alone agent or in combination with other modalities for DVT prophylaxis in patients with SCI. Low-dose unfractionated heparin (UFH) as a stand-alone prophylactic measure is no longer recommended. UFH is most effective if used in combination with pneumatic compression stockings or electrical stimulation (level 1 recommendation). (*The author was considering including an answer choice option of heparin but did not want to confuse the readers for this reason. However, LMWH vs. UFH for SCI DVT prophylaxis is potential test question material on the subspecialty boards.*) IVC filters are only recommended for select patients and do not prevent DVT. Warfarin typically is not appropriate for DVT prophylaxis in this patient population.

38. The correct answer is B.

The characteristic symptoms of AD are hypertension with headache, flushing, sweating above the level of injury, and piloerection below the level of injury. The pathophysiology of AD involves unregulated sympathetic activity below the level of injury and absence of descending inhibitory pathways from supraspinal centers. The AD inciting events are below the level of injury, the most common being bladder distention, followed by bowel distention. The treatment involves both removing the noxious stimulus and paying close attention to controlling the resulting hypertension. Severe complications can arise from AD, including hemorrhage, cerebrovascular accident, myocardial infarction, seizure, and even death.

39. The correct answer is A.

Respiratory management in the acute inpatient rehabilitation setting centers on keeping the lungs expanded to prevent atelectasis and managing secretions to prevent mucus plugging. Pulmonary toilet is continued through vent weaning and even after tracheostomy capping has commenced. Bronchospasm and reactive airway are common complications and are typically managed short term with short-acting beta agonists along with inhaled corticosteroids. Monotherapy with long-acting beta agonists was linked to increased mortality. Careful screening must be undertaken to identify eligible candidates for phrenic pacing, and patients in the acute period of injury still may have further improvement in respiratory function and thus are not considered this early.

40. The correct answer is B.

The spinal accessory nerve innervates the accessory muscles of respiration and would be intact. Fibers from C3, C4, and C5 innervate the diaphragm (the primary inspiratory muscle) and would also be intact. Injuries above T1 would lose the external (inspiratory) and internal (expiratory) intercostals. Injuries above T7 would lose the abdominals (the primary expiratory and coughing muscles). You would then tell your medical students that is why patients with complete spinal cord injury (SCI) at T6 or above will have trouble with clearing secretions. Then, your students will think you are wise and awesome.

41. The correct answer is B.
It is important to monitor vital capacity in all patients with acute spinal cord injury at risk for respiratory insufficiency. Studies have found reduced forced vital capacity of 30% to 50% in the first week after injury. Experts in spinal cord medicine recommend obtaining a baseline vital capacity upon admission, comparing it to predicted normal values, and monitoring it thereafter for any changes. A decrease from baseline is the best indicator of respiratory muscle fatigue. A decrease in vital capacity of less than 15 mL/kg of ideal body weight is an ominous sign of impending respiratory failure. Vital capacity technically includes tidal volume plus the inspiratory and expiratory reserve volumes (reference one of your old human physiology textbook charts if you need to review). Residual volume is typically not affected (however, energy recovery ventilation [ERV] and functional residual capacity [FRC] can be reduced). PaO_2 is a physiologic parameter obtained by arterial blood gas that can be affected by the presence of atelectasis.

42. The correct answer is D.
The clinical symptoms and urodynamic study results suggest a diagnosis of detrusor sphincter dyssynergia, defined as impaired coordination between the detrusor and sphincter during voiding that is seen in as many as 75% patients with suprasacral spinal cord injury. This patient has continuous external urinary sphincter (EUS) contraction during bladder emptying phase and runs a high risk for developing serious urologic complications if this is left untreated. Treatment options focus on decreasing detrusor pressure and relieving the outflow obstruction due to the increased EUS activity. CIC combined with anticholinergic medication is a common treatment option. If this option does not provide relief, botulinum toxin A injections or sphincterotomy can be considered. Bethanechol is not a good option because it is a cholinergic medication that increases bladder contractions.

43. The correct answer is D.
IC is ideal for a normotensive patient with SCI with adequate hand function who can adhere to a fluid restriction of 2 L per day or 100 mL per hour (i.e., doesn't require IV fluids for a condition such as hypercalcemia). Once spontaneous uninhibited bladder contractions occur after spinal shock, this can be managed by combining IC with an anticholinergic medication to treat the bladder spasm. IC should be performed frequently enough to avoid bladder overdistention by keeping volume under 500 mL.

44. The correct answer is A.
The gastrocolic reflex is defined as "the increase in colonic activity after ingestion of a meal." It is thought to be mediated by acetylcholine and is typically preserved in patients with suprasacral spinal cord injury as long as the sacral reflex arc is intact. This reflex can be utilized in establishing a regular timed bowel regimen after meals, usually within 20 to 60 minutes. Digital stimulation of the rectum represents the rectocolic reflex.

45. The correct answer is C.

Intracavernosal injection therapy is one treatment option for erectile dysfunction and so is sildenafil (phosphodiesterase type 5 [PDE5] inhibitors), vacuum pumps, and penile prosthesis. In general, the majority of men with SCI will have dysfunction in ejaculation. Treatments for absent ejaculation include penile vibratory stimulation, electroejaculation, prostate massage, and surgical removal of sperm. Men with SCI can still have reflexogenic erections given that the sacral nerve roots S2-4 remain intact.

46. The correct answer is A.

Women with SCI are in the high-risk pregnancy category. In women with injury T6 or above, autonomic dysreflexia (AD) can occur during pregnancy, especially during labor contractions. Women with preserved T11-L2 sensation could experience psychogenic arousal, and those with preserved S2-5 sensation (or present bulbocavernosus reflex) could experience reflex genital arousal and orgasm. Injury above T10 will likely not feel uterine contraction due to loss of afferent input from the hypogastric innervation of the uterus.

47. The correct answer is B.

In patients with chronic SCI at 2 years, the most common pressure site is the ischium—thought to be due to greater time spent sitting in wheelchair than during the initial phases after injury. In the acute phase of injury through the first year, the most common site is the sacrum.

48. The correct answer is A.

Based on the side effect profile of the agents listed in the answer choices, baclofen would be the best choice. However, combining any of these antispasticity medications with alcohol is potentially dangerous because all these medications tend to cause sedation. Dantrolene can potentially cause toxic hepatitis and thus not a good choice for heavy drinker with elevated liver transaminases. Diazepam, a benzodiazepine, is also not a best choice for heavy drinker due to additive interaction with alcohol and is potentially habit forming. Clonidine is not a best choice for someone with orthostatic hypotension because that is a potential side effect.

49. The correct answer is B.

A stage 2 ulcer is partial thickness involving epidermis and/or dermis. Stage 1 is intact skin with nonblanching redness. Stage 3 is full thickness, extending through epidermis, dermis, and the subcutaneous tissue. Stage 4 is full thickness to the bone—extending through skin, subcutaneous tissue, and muscle.

50. The correct answer is D.
Covering a wound with transparent dressing is not a form of debridement; it serves to protect the wound and keeps it moist. The other answer choices are examples of debridement—surgical (by scalpel), mechanical, (by wet to dry dressing), and enzymatic (by collagenase ointment).

51. The correct answer is C.
Spinal cord injury (SCI) above T6 impairs temperature regulation, and body temperature can rise in hot environments, resulting in fever. Fever is also known as a presenting symptom in both infection and heterotopic ossification (HO). Orthostatic hypotension typically does not present with fever.

52. The correct answer is B.
The most common musculoskeletal issues in those with SCI involve the shoulder joints and are from overuse injuries.

53. The correct answer is A.
Patients with SCI are prone to shoulder internal rotation and adduction contracture; therefore, it is advised to avoid this position. Posterior pelvic tilt should also be avoided as it encourages head and neck forward lean and spine kyphosis. Prolonged supine positioning and placing pillows under the knees promotes hip and knee flexion contractures.

54. The correct answer is B.
Suicide rates have been reported to be 2 to 6 times greater in patients with SCI than an age-matched population without SCI. It is higher in younger age group and during first 5 years postinjury. Therefore, psychological support and screening for suicidal ideation is crucial for your patients with SCI.

55. The correct answer is B.
Senna is a colonic stimulant. Docusate sodium is a stool softener. Psyllium is a bulk-forming agent. Metoclopramide is a prokinetic agent.

56. The correct answer is B.
Patients with spinal cord injury (SCI) with level C5 and above typically require a high back power wheelchair with tilt and recline for pressure relief, headrest, and upper extremity support. Many with injury level at C5 use a modified joystick (nonproportional, head, or chin control). Levels C7 and below can typically propel a manual wheelchair and perform their own weight shifts without requiring tilting or reclining mechanism.

57. The correct answer is A.
The "parastance" refers to utilizes ankle dorsiflexion, knee extension, hip hyperextension, and posterior lean while standing using bilateral long leg braces. This standing position will provide anterior hip stability from the iliofemoral ligament and anterior capsule of the hip.

58. The correct answer is D.

All the answer choices are contraindications for phrenic nerve pacing. Candidates should be at least 6 to 12 months postinjury as some function could still recover after lower motor neuron injury to the diaphragm, and a pacer implantation requires some level of chest wall compliance. Serial EMG/nerve conduction studies are usually performed before making final decision. Pacing is only indicated if there is some intact lower motor neuron innervation of the diaphragm. Pacer is not indicated if there is consistent absent phrenic nerve function indicating damage of the phrenic nerve nucleus. Significant lung disease is also a contraindication.

59. The correct answer is A.

The pediatric population with SCI has less percentage of spasticity than the adult population. Scoliosis and hip dislocation are at a higher incidence in the pediatric population with SCI than the adult population as there are complications as a result of growth in children who sustained SCI prior to puberty. Hypercalcemia is most common in adolescent males within the first 3 months of injury.

60. The correct answer is A.

With symptomatic posttraumatic syringomyelia, the most common clinical presentation is pain. Unlike syrinx related to congenital Chiari malformation, posttraumatic syringomyelia is noncommunicating (confined to grey matter of spinal cord). Spasticity symptoms in patients with SCI can increase in syringomyelia. Syringomyelia occurs at the level of injury, not below.

61. The correct answer is B.

An RGO is a good choice for a motivated patient with thoracic to upper lumbar paraplegia with good upper body strength in the absence of limiting lower extremity contractures and spasticity. The device consists of bilateral hip knee ankle foot orthoses (HKAFOs) connected by cables with a pelvic band or girdle. Both orthoses are coupled to allow simultaneous hip extension on one side and hip flexion on the other side—a reciprocal gait pattern. Because the patient already had used a standing frame, a parapodium is not necessary at this point and would be too limiting. She does not possess enough hip and knee strength for either a KAFO or AFO.

62. The correct answer is B.

This vignette illustrates the SCI complication of hypercalcemia. The mainstay management consists of hydration with intravenous normal saline and intravenous pamidronate. There are other adjunctive treatments as well, such as furosemide (please reference your internal medicine resources if you are interested in more in depth information beyond the scope of a Physical Medicine and Rehabilitation [PM&R] board review book).

63. The correct answer is A.

Metabolic changes in SCI include decreased testosterone levels, decreased basal metabolic rate, decrease in muscle mass (consequently leading to weight), decrease in bone density, and impaired glucose tolerance.

64. The correct answer is B.

Anterior wheel position closer to the castors increases maneuverability but decreases stability by narrowing the base of support. Conversely, moving the wheel position posteriorly increases stability.

65. The correct answer is C.

The clinical vignette describes a common presentation of heterotopic ossification in the acute inpatient rehabilitation setting after acute SCI. Fever is described as one of the first symptoms, followed by joint pain, swelling, and loss of range of motion. Early markers include elevated alkaline phosphatase and erythrocyte sedimentation rate on lab results. The gold standard for diagnosis is three-phase bone scan, which can diagnose earlier than plain radiographs. The resolution of fever and normal CBC makes differential diagnosis of infection less likely. DVT is also in the differential diagnosis but was ruled out.

Board Review Points ("Pearls") for Spine Trauma and Spinal Cord Injury Medicine

Spine Trauma

- Hyperextension cervical spine injuries are commonly found in high-velocity acceleration-deceleration motor vehicles. The mechanism is anterior distraction (often causing disruption of the anterior longitudinal ligament) and posterior compression. Clinical manifestation is traumatic CCS. The upper extremities are disproportionally affected.
- A flexion/distraction (Chance) fracture is a type of seat belt injury with a horizontal fracture line extending from the spinous process to the vertebral body. This injury can be caused in the thoracolumbar region by wearing a lap belt type restraint (without shoulder strap) where the upper body moves forward upon deceleration while the lower body remains fixed with axis of rotation at the lap belt.
- Bilateral facet joint dislocation is an unstable injury which includes disruption of the anterior longitudinal ligament, posterior longitudinal ligament, and facet capsules.
- A severe neck flexion and axial compression injury (commonly diving into shallow pool) results in a fracture of the anterior inferior vertebral body (resembling a teardrop) with posterior vertebral body displacement into the spinal canal. This will commonly result in quadriplegia with anterior cord syndrome.
- The hangman fracture of C2 sounds dangerous; however, it only refers to bilateral fractures through the pars interarticularis that separate the body of C2 from the posterior elements but does not compress the spinal cord.
- Please review the anatomic structures of the three spine columns in your study notes. A burst fracture involves the anterior and middle columns.

Spine Anatomy and Spinal Cord Syndromes

■ The blood supply to the anterior two-thirds of the spinal cord is from the anterior spinal artery. Artery of Adamkiewicz supplies the caudal two-thirds of the spinal cord, and occlusion of this artery can manifest as anterior spinal artery syndrome.

■ The nerve tracts carrying vibratory sensation are housed in the dorsal column (posterior one-third spinal cord), which are supplied by the posterior spinal arteries.

■ Lesions to the lower portion of the conus medullaris and to the cauda equina would characteristically manifest with areflexic bladder and bowel. Lesions in upper conus medullaris (suprasacral lesions) would characteristically present with an upper motor neuron, including preserved bowel, bladder, and bulbocavernosus reflexes.

■ CCS is an incomplete SCI that occurs more often in older individuals with pre-existing cervical spondylosis. The motor weakness affects the upper limbs to a much greater degree than the lower limbs. The recovery occurs earliest in the lower extremities and latest in the intrinsic hand muscles.

■ Brown-Séquard syndrome would result in ipsilateral loss of vibration and proprioception below the lesion, ipsilateral motor loss at and below the level of the lesion, contralateral loss of pain temperature below the level of the lesion, and ipsilateral flaccid paralysis at the level of the lesion.

Spinal Cord Injury Evaluation and Treatment

■ The neurologic level of injury is determined by the lowest segment where motor and sensory function is normal on both sides.

■ The presence of any sacral sparing—anal sensation, deep anal pressure, or voluntary anal contraction—indicates incomplete SCI.

■ Review table showing functional abilities and goal for levels of quadriplegia and paraplegia.

■ SCIWORA is the presence of clinical symptoms of traumatic myelopathy without any spine fracture or spine instability on radiographs or computed tomography. Persons with SCIWORA can be found to have spinal cord abnormalities on MRI studies. The prevalence of SCIWORA is highest in children younger than 8 years of age with predisposition for upper cervical injury.

■ The studied return of reflex arc activity has shown the delayed plantar reflex to be the earliest reflex followed by the bulbocavernosus and cremasteric in the initial days after SCI. Later, deep tendon reflexes (i.e., ankle and knee jerk) return, usually within 1 to 2 weeks.

■ The majority of functional recovery typically occurs within the first 6 to 9 months following injury with plateau occurring between 12 and 18 months and minimal recovery after that time.

Spinal Cord Injury Complications

- The characteristic symptoms of AD are hypertension with headache, flushing, sweating above the level of injury, and piloerection below the level of injury.
- It is important to monitor vital capacity in all acute patients SCI at risk for respiratory insufficiency. A decrease in vital capacity of less than 15 mL/kg of ideal body weight is an ominous sign of impending respiratory failure.
- In patients with chronic SCI at 2 years, the most common pressure site is the ischium. In the acute phase of injury through the first year, the most common site is the sacrum.
- SCI above T6 impairs temperature regulation, and body temperature can rise in hot environments, resulting in fever.
- The most common musculoskeletal issues in those with SCI involve the shoulder joints.
- Patients with SCI are prone to shoulder internal rotation and adduction contracture.
- Scoliosis, hip dislocation, and hypercalcemia are at a higher incidence in the pediatric population with SCI than the adult population.
- Metabolic changes in SCI include decreased testosterone levels, decreased basal metabolic rate, decrease in muscle mass (consequently leading to weight), decrease in bone density, and impaired glucose tolerance.
- The gold standard for diagnosis of heterotopic ossification is three-phase bone scan.

REFERENCES & SUGGESTED READINGS

Anderson K, Aito S, Atkins M, et al. Functional recovery measures for spinal cord injury: an evidence-based review for clinical practice and research. *J Spinal Cord Med*. 2008;31(2):133-144.

Campagnolo DI, Kirshblum S. *Spinal Cord Medicine*. 2nd ed. Philadelphia, PA: Lippincott Williams & Wilkins; 2011.

Cuccurullo S. *Physical Medicine and Rehabilitation Board Review*. 3rd ed. New York, NY: Demos Medical; 2014.

Dhall SS, Hadley MN, Aarabi B, et al. Deep venous thrombosis and thromboembolism in patients with cervical spinal cord injuries. *Neurosurgery*. 2013;72:244-254. doi:10.1227/NEU.0b013e31827728c0.

Hurlbert RJ, Hadley MN, Walters BC, et al. Pharmacological therapy for acute spinal cord injury. Guidelines for the management of acute cervical spine and spinal cord injuries: chapter 8. *Neurosurgery*. 2015;76:S71-S83. doi:10.1227/01.neu.0000462080.04196.f7.

Kirshblum S, Waring W III. Updates for the International Standards for Neurological Classifications of Spinal Cord Injury. *Phys Med Rehabil Clin N Am*. 2014;25(3):505-517.

Ko HY, Ditunno JF Jr, Graziani V, Little JW. The pattern of reflex recovery during spinal shock. *Spinal Cord*. 1999;37(6):402-409.

Krassioukov A, Eng JJ, Warburton DE, Teasell R; and Spinal Cord Injury Rehabilitation Evidence Research Team. A systematic review of the management of orthostatic hypotension following spinal cord injury. *Arch Phys Med Rehabil*. 2009;90(5):876-885. doi:10.1016/j.apmr.2009.01.009.

Teasell RW, Mehta S, Aubut JA, et al; and Spinal Cord Injury Rehabilitation Evidence Research Team. A systematic review of pharmacologic treatments of pain after spinal cord injury. *Arch Phys Med Rehabil*. 2010;91(5):816-831. doi:10.1016/j.apmr.2010.01.022.

Vale FL, Burns J, Jackson AB, Hadley MN. Combined medical and surgical treatment after acute spinal cord injury: results of a prospective pilot study to assess the merits of aggressive medical resuscitation and blood pressure management. *J Neurosurg*. 1997;87:239-246.

Stroke Rehabilitation

1. Modifiable risk factors for stroke include

    A. age, sex, hypertension.

    B. hypertension and cigarette smoking.

    C. high cholesterol.

    D. both B and C

2. Is blood pressure often increased at the time of ischemic stroke and normally reduces by itself over the course of several days?

    A. Yes, and it does not require management.

    B. No, blood pressure is not a factor in ischemic stroke.

    C. No, blood pressure takes several months to stabilize in most patients with stroke.

    D. Yes, but it does require management.

3. Stroke occurring at or within 3 months from transient ischemic attack (TIA) is

    A. highly likely (occurring in 70% or more of patients).

    B. very unlikely (occurring in less than 1% of patients).

    C. likely to occur in about half of all patients.

    D. somewhat likely (occurring in more than 1% but less than 50% of patients).

4. Pneumonia after stroke is commonly due to

 A. aspiration.

 B. systemic effects of urinary tract infection.

 C. exposure to hospital pathogens.

 D. cold weather and barometric effects.

5. Risk of urinary tract infection (UTI) increases significantly in patients with stroke when the postvoid residual (PVR) is greater than

 A. about 5 mL.

 B. about 50 mL.

 C. about 100 mL.

 D. 25 mL for men and 75 mL for women.

6. Is subluxation of the glenohumeral joint a common occurrence poststroke and may be a significant source of pain?

 A. Yes, in about 30% of stroke survivors

 B. Yes, in up to about 80% of stroke survivors

 C. Glenohumeral joint subluxation can occur but is not common.

 D. Glenohumeral joint subluxation can occur but is not considered a significant source of pain.

7. _____ may be effective in the treatment of glenohumeral subluxation.

 A. Strapping

 B. Botulinum toxin

 C. External fixator

 D. Functional electrical stimulation and strapping

8. Consider the veracity of these two statements: The presence of diabetes is a risk factor for stroke, and there is a strong significant difference in the effect of diabetes on the occurrence of stroke based on gender.

   A. The first statement is true, and the second is false.

   B. Both statements are true.

   C. The first statement is false, and the second is true.

   D. Both statements are false.

9. Sedation is NOT significantly associated with which of the following antispasticity medications?

   A. valium

   B. tizanidine

   C. botulinum toxin

   D. baclofen

10. What is pusher syndrome?

   A. when a patient with stroke pushes people due to poor impulse control and frontal lobe disinhibition

   B. when a patient with stroke pushes himself or herself around in a wheelchair into walls or people

   C. when a patient with stroke pushes alarm buttons or pulls alarm cords inappropriately due to poor impulse control and frontal lobe disinhibition

   D. when a patient with stroke uses his or her strong limb to push toward his or her weak (paretic) limb

11. Mr. Smith, a writer, is very dismayed. Since his stroke, he cannot read because he has

   A. alexia.

   B. acalculia.

   C. agraphia.

   D. aphasia.

12. The 6-month prevalence of depression poststroke is

   A. about 5%.

   B. about 30%.

   C. about 75%.

   D. about 100%.

13. Do selective serotonin reuptake inhibitors (SSRIs) improve poststroke outcomes independently of relief of depression?

   A. No, the use of SSRIs poststroke is primarily for depression, and there is no additional benefit.

   B. No, SSRIs are not indicated for use poststroke.

   C. Yes, there are some data indicating that SSRIs are beneficial for patients poststroke due to relief of depression and improvement in motor function.

   D. Yes, there are some data indicating that SSRIs are beneficial for patients poststroke due to relief of depression and improvement in visual impairment.

14. Locked-in syndrome can be due to an infarct of the

   A. basilar artery affecting the pons.

   B. basilar artery affecting the occipital lobe.

   C. middle cerebral artery affecting the parietal lobes.

   D. anterior cerebral artery affecting the frontal lobe.

15. Which outcome measure can be used for stroke ranges from 0 to 6?

   A. Barthel Index

   B. National Institutes of Health Stroke Scale

   C. Modified Rankin Scale

   D. Glasgow Outcome Scale

16. Consider the veracity of these two statements: Poststroke speech language therapy is effective in the treatment of aphasia, and it is most effective as high-intensity treatments.

    A. Both statements are true.

    B. The first statement is true, and the second is false.

    C. The first statement is false, and the second is true.

    D. Both statements are false.

17. When speaking of stroke with hemiparesis, FDS means

    A. female deficit syndrome.

    B. foot depth system.

    C. first depth stimulator.

    D. foot drop stimulator.

18. Poststroke, foot drop simulator (FDS) systems are clearly better than traditional ankle foot orthoses (AFOs)

    A. in men.

    B. in women.

    C. in both men and women.

    D. It is not clear that FDS systems are better than traditional AFOs poststroke.

19. A common presentation of complex regional pain syndrome in patients with stroke is

    A. shoulder-hand syndrome.

    B. shoulder-foot syndrome.

    C. hip-foot syndrome.

    D. none of the above

20. The most common vessel for stroke is the

    A. middle cerebral artery (MCA).

    B. anterior cerebral artery (ACA).

    C. posterior cerebral artery (PCA).

    D. basilar artery.

ANSWER KEY WITH EXPLANATIONS

1. The correct answer is D.
A modifiable risk factor for a condition is one that can be changed. Factors such as age, race/ethnicity, and sex are thought of as nonmodifiable. Factors such as habits, behaviors, and certain medical conditions are thought of as modifiable. Modifiable risk factors can highlight possible interventions to improve a medical outcome, and nonmodifiable risk factors can highlight which groups might benefit most from an intervention. Hypertension, cigarette smoking, and high cholesterol are known modifiable risk factors for stroke.

2. The correct answer is D.
Increased blood pressure is a major risk factor for stroke, and blood pressure is often significantly increased around the time of an ischemic stroke. In most patients, blood pressure will naturally decrease over the course of several days, although not necessarily into the optimal range, and it should still be monitored and actively managed as needed.

3. The correct answer is D.
Exact rates of stroke occurring at or within 90 days of TIA are not known, but several studies indicate a range of about 2% to 20% is likely. (References: Amarenco P, Lavallée PC, Labreuche J, et al. One-year risk of stroke after transient ischemic attack or minor stroke. *N Engl J Med*. 2016;374:1533-1542; and Wu CM, McLaughlin K, Lorenzetti DL, Hill MD, Manns BJ, Ghali WA. Early risk of stroke after transient ischemic attack: a systematic review and meta-analysis. *Arch Intern Med*. 2007;167[22]:2417-2422.)

4. The correct answer is A.
Dysfunction in the swallowing mechanism is common after stroke and predisposes to pneumonia due to aspiration. Normally, patients should be kept "npo" (nil per os or nothing by mouth) until a swallowing evaluation has been performed to help prevent this complication.

5. The correct answer is C.
Urinary dysfunction poststroke is very common and may necessitate catheterization. Bladder scans to determine PVRs are taken routinely. The risk of UTI is increased with high PVRs. A 2003 study by Dromerick and Edwards published in *Archives of Physical Medicine and Rehabilitation* states that they found PVRs over 150 mL to be significantly associated with increased likelihood of UTI (meaning, an odds ratio [OR] confidence interval not crossing 1, with the point value being OR 3.25). A 2012 study by Kim et al. published in the *Annals of Rehabilitation Medicine* found that PVR over 100 was associated with a higher rate of UTI regardless of gender, with OR 4.87 and *P* value less than .05 by chi-square test. (References: Dromerick AW, Edwards DF. Relation of postvoid residual to urinary tract infection during stroke rehabilitation. *Arch Phys Med Rehabil*. 2003;84[9]:1369-1372; and Kim BR, Lim JH, Lee SA, et al. The relation between postvoid residual and occurrence of urinary tract infection after stroke in rehabilitation unit. *Ann Rehabil Med*. 2012;36[2]:248-253.)

6. The correct answer is B.

Glenohumeral joint subluxation is common poststroke,   in up to about 80% of stroke survivors. It is considered to be significant pain generator by many experts, through various mechanisms. (Reference: Paci M, Nannetti L, Rinaldi LA. Glenohumeral subluxation in hemiplegia: an overview. *J Rehabil Res Dev*. 2005;42[4]:557-568.)

7. The correct answer is D.

A 2005 systematic review of treatment of glenohumeral subluxation published in the *Journal of Rehabilitation Research and Development* found that shoulder strapping, some kinds of shoulder slings, and functional electrical stimulation were effective treatments for glenohumeral subluxation. (Reference: Paci M, Nannetti L, Rinaldi LA. Glenohumeral subluxation in hemiplegia: an overview. *J Rehabil Res Dev*. 2005;42[4]:557-568.)

8. The correct answer is A.

A 2016 article in the *American Journal of the Medical Sciences* notes that diabetes mellitus is a relatively modifiable risk factor for both all strokes and ischemic strokes. The studies evaluated in that article which reported separate measures of association for males versus females generally found the point estimate for the opposite sex to be within the confidence interval of the sex under consideration, implying that there is not a significant difference in the association between diabetes and stroke in men as compared to women. (Reference: Chen R, Ovbiagele B, Feng W. Diabetes and stroke: epidemiology, pathophysiology, pharmaceuticals and outcomes. *Am J Med Sci*. 2016;351[4]:380-386.)

9. The correct answer is C.

Sedation is NOT significantly associated with botulinum toxin (BOTOX, Dysport, MYOBLOC), as opposed to the other oral antispasticity medications listed.

10. The correct answer is D.

Pusher syndrome refers to the phenomenon in which a patient poststroke uses his or her strong limb to push toward his or her weak (paretic) limb, which can result in imbalance and falls.

11. The correct answer is A.

Poststroke problems with verbal communication, writing, and reading are common. Alexia refers to the inability to read. Acalculia refers to the inability to perform mathematical calculations. Agraphia refers to the inability to write. Aphasia refers to verbal impairment of various subtypes.

12. The correct answer is B.

Poststroke depression is common. According to a 2008 review article published in *Neuropsychiatric Disease and Treatment*, the prevalence of depression at 6 months poststroke is approximately 30%. (Reference: Paolucci S. Epidemiology and treatment of post-stroke depression. *Neuropsychiatr Dis Treat*. 2008;4[1]:145-154.)

13. The correct answer is C.

SSRIs are commonly used to treat depression poststroke. There are also some data that SSRIs may independently contribute to improvement in motor function post-stroke, although more research is needed in this area. (References: Siepmann T, Penzlin AI, Kepplinger J, et al. Selective serotonin reuptake inhibitors to improve outcome in acute ischemic stroke: possible mechanisms and clinical evidence. *Brain Behav.* 2015;5[10]:e00373; and Chollet F, Tardy J, Albucher JF, et al. Fluoxetine for motor recovery after acute ischaemic stroke [FLAME]: randomised placebo-controlled trial. *Lancet Neurol.* 2011;10[2]:P123-P130.)

14. The correct answer is A.

Locked-in syndrome can be due to an infarct of the basilar artery affecting the pons.

15. The correct answer is C.

The Modified Rankin Scale ranges from 0 to 6 and measures degree of disability: 0 is normal, and 6 is death. The National Institutes of Health Stroke Scale ranges from 0 to 42. The Barthel Index ranges from 0 to 100. The Glasgow Outcome Scale ranges from 1 to 5. (Reference: Lees KR, Bath PM, Schellinger PD, et al; for European Stroke Organization Outcomes Working Group. Contemporary outcomes measures in acute stroke research choice of primary outcome measure. *Stroke.* 2012;43:1163-1170.)

16. The correct answer is B.

A 2016 study from the *Cochrane Database of Systematic Reviews* found that poststroke speech language therapy is effective in the treatment of aphasia but that high-intensity treatments may not be best for all patients, as studies with that type of treatment had a somewhat higher rate of attrition of subjects. (Reference: Brady MC, Kelly H, Godwin J, Enderby P, Campbell P. Speech and language therapy for aphasia following stroke. *Cochrane Database Syst Rev.* 2016;[6]:CD000425. doi:10.1002/14651858 .CD000425.pub4.)

17. The correct answer is D.

Patients with lower extremity hemiparesis often have ankle dorsiflexion weakness, or foot drop. FDS stands for foot drop stimulator and refers to a type of functional electrical stimulator that a patient wears which stimulates ankle dorsiflexion. It is an alternative to a traditional ankle foot orthosis.

18. The correct answer is D.

After stroke, it is not clear that FDS systems are better than traditional AFOs. Recent studies indicate that improvements in functional outcomes are about the same, but patients generally prefer to use the FDS compared to traditional AFOs. (References: Everaert DG, Stein RB, Abrams GM, et al. Effect of a foot-drop stimulator and ankle-foot orthosis on walking performance after stroke: a multicenter randomized controlled trial. *Neurorehabil Neural Repair.* 2013;27[7]:579-591; and Kluding PM, Dunning K, O'Dell MW, et al. Foot drop stimulation versus ankle foot orthosis after stroke: 30-week outcomes. *Stroke.* 2013;44[6]:1660-1669.)

19. The correct answer is A.

A common presentation of complex regional pain syndrome in patients with stroke is called shoulder-hand syndrome, referring to pain at the shoulder and wrist/hand area, with relative sparing of the midportion of the upper limb.

20. The correct answer is A.

The most common vessel for stroke is the MCA.

Board Review Points ("Pearls") for Stroke Rehabilitation

Stroke Anatomy

- The most common vessel for stroke is the MCA.
- Locked-in syndrome can be due to an infarct of the basilar artery affecting the pons.

Stroke Epidemiology

- Hypertension, cigarette smoking, and high cholesterol are known modifiable risk factors for stroke.
- Diabetes mellitus is a relatively modifiable risk factor for all strokes and ischemic strokes.

Stroke Complications

- Dysfunction in the swallowing mechanism is common after stroke and predisposes to pneumonia due to aspiration. Normally, patients should be kept "npo" (nil per os or nothing by mouth) until a swallowing evaluation has been performed to help prevent this complication.
- Urinary dysfunction poststroke is very common and may necessitate catheterization. Bladder scans to determine PVRs are taken routinely. The risk of urinary tract infection is increased with high PVRs.
- Other common issues poststroke are musculoskeletal problems such as glenohumeral joint subluxation, depression, and impairments with verbal communication, writing, and/or reading.

Stroke Treatment

- A 2005 systematic review of treatment of glenohumeral subluxation published in the *Journal of Rehabilitation Research and Development* found that shoulder strapping, some kinds of shoulder slings, and functional electrical stimulation were effective treatments for glenohumeral subluxation. (Reference: Paci M, Nannetti L, Rinaldi LA. Glenohumeral subluxation in hemiplegia: an overview. *J Rehabil Res Dev*. 2005;42[4]:557-568.)

- SSRIs are commonly used to treat depression poststroke. There are also some data that SSRIs may independently contribute to improvement in motor function poststroke, although more research is needed in this area. (References: Siepmann T, Penzlin AI, Kepplinger J, et al. Selective serotonin reuptake inhibitors to improve outcome in acute ischemic stroke: possible mechanisms and clinical evidence. *Brain Behav*. 2015;5[10]:e00373; and Chollet F, Tardy J, Albucher JF, et al. Fluoxetine for motor recovery after acute ischaemic stroke [FLAME]: randomised placebo-controlled trial. *Lancet Neurol*. 2011;10[2]:P123-P130.)

- A 2016 study from the *Cochrane Database of Systematic Reviews* found that poststroke speech language therapy is effective in the treatment of aphasia but that high-intensity treatments may not be best for all patients, as studies with that type of treatment had a somewhat higher rate of attrition of subjects. (Reference: Brady MC, Kelly H, Godwin J, Enderby P, Campbell P. Speech and language therapy for aphasia following stroke. *Cochrane Database Syst Rev*. 2016;[6]:CD000425. doi:10.1002/14651858.CD000425.pub4.)

- After stroke, it is not clear that FDS systems are better than traditional AFOs. Recent studies indicate that improvements in functional outcomes are about the same, but patients generally prefer to use the FDS compared to traditional AFOs. (References: Everaert DG, Stein RB, Abrams GM, et al. Effect of a foot-drop stimulator and ankle-foot orthosis on walking performance after stroke: a multicenter randomized controlled trial. *Neurorehabil Neural Repair*. 2013;27[7]:579-591; and Kluding PM, Dunning K, O'Dell MW, et al. Foot drop stimulation versus ankle foot orthosis after stroke: 30-week outcomes. *Stroke*. 2013;44[6]:1660-1669.)

REFERENCES & SUGGESTED READINGS

Amarenco P, Lavallée PC, Labreuche J, et al. One-year risk of stroke after transient ischemic attack or minor stroke. *N Engl J Med*. 2016;374:1533-1542.

Bang OY, Ovbiagele B, Kim JS. Nontraditional risk factors for ischemic stroke an update. *Stroke*. 2015;46:3571-3578.

Bowry R, Navalkele DD, Gonzales NR. Blood pressure management in stroke: five new things. *Neurol Clin Pract*. 2014;4(5):419-426.

Braddom RL, Chan L, Harrast ME, et al, eds. *Physical Medicine and Rehabilitation*. 4th ed. St. Louis, MO: Saunders; 2011.

Brady MC, Kelly H, Godwin J, Enderby P, Campbell P. Speech and language therapy for aphasia following stroke. *Cochrane Database Syst Rev*. 2016;(6):CD000425. doi:10.1002/14651858 .CD000425.pub4.

Chen R, Ovbiagele B, Feng W. Diabetes and stroke: epidemiology, pathophysiology, pharmaceuticals and outcomes. *Am J Med Sci*. 2016;351(4):380-386.

Chollet F, Tardy J, Albucher JF, et al. Fluoxetine for motor recovery after acute ischaemic stroke (FLAME): randomised placebo-controlled trial. *Lancet Neurol*. 2011;10(2):P123-P130.

Dromerick AW, Edwards DF. Relation of postvoid residual to urinary tract infection during stroke rehabilitation. *Arch Phys Med Rehabil*. 2003;84(9):1369-1372.

Everaert DG, Stein RB, Abrams GM, et al. Effect of a foot-drop stimulator and ankle-foot orthosis on walking performance after stroke: a multicenter randomized controlled trial. *Neurorehabil Neural Repair*. 2013;27(7):579-591.

Francisco GE, McGuire JR. Poststroke spasticity management. *Stroke*. 2012;43:3132-3136.

Hannawi Y, Hannawi B, Rao CP, Suarez JI, Bershad EM. Stroke-associated pneumonia: major advances and obstacles. *Cerebrovasc Dis*. 2013;35:430-443.

Kim BR, Lim JH, Lee SA, et al. The relation between postvoid residual and occurrence of urinary tract infection after stroke in rehabilitation unit. *Ann Rehabil Med*. 2012;36(2):248-253.

Kim YW, Kim Y, Kim JM, Hong JS, Lim HS, Kim HS. Is poststroke complex regional pain syndrome the combination of shoulder pain and soft tissue injury of the wrist? A prospective observational study: STROBE of ultrasonographic findings in complex regional pain syndrome. *Medicine (Baltimore)*. 2016;95(31):e4388.

Kluding PM, Dunning K, O'Dell MW, et al. Foot drop stimulation versus ankle foot orthosis after stroke: 30-week outcomes. *Stroke*. 2013;44(6):1660-1669.

Lees KR, Bath PM, Schellinger PD, et al; for European Stroke Organization Outcomes Working Group. Contemporary outcomes measures in acute stroke research choice of primary outcome measure. *Stroke*. 2012;43:1163-1170.

McManus M, Liebeskind DS. Blood pressure in acute ischemic stroke. *J Clin Neurology*. 2016;12(2):137-146.

Paci M, Nannetti L, Rinaldi LA. Glenohumeral subluxation in hemiplegia: an overview. *J Rehabil Res Dev*. 2005;42(4):557-568.

Paolucci S. Epidemiology and treatment of post-stroke depression. *Neuropsychiatr Dis Treat*. 2008;4(1):145-154.

Siepmann T, Penzlin AI, Kepplinger J, et al. Selective serotonin reuptake inhibitors to improve outcome in acute ischemic stroke: possible mechanisms and clinical evidence. *Brain Behav*. 2015;5(10):e00373.

Wu CM, McLaughlin K, Lorenzetti DL, Hill MD, Manns BJ, Ghali WA. Early risk of stroke after transient ischemic attack: a systematic review and meta-analysis. *Arch Intern Med*. 2007;167(22):2417-2422.

Amputee Rehabilitation, Prosthetics, and Orthotics

1. A wart-like condition at the distal end of a residual limb is

   A. verrucous hyperplasia.

   B. edema.

   C. skin breakdown.

   D. pressure ulcer.

2. Depression in patients with new amputation

   A. may be an important factor that should be considered.

   B. rarely is a factor in treatment.

   C. should not be considered in treatment.

   D. is always present.

3. Hyperhidrosis is

   A. a common skin condition affecting patients with amputation.

   B. very rare in patients with amputation.

   C. not a known condition.

   D. a topic whose discussion should be avoided in patients with amputation.

4. Firm, round nodules that may be found in the popliteal fossa of transtibial amputees are

    A. ganglion cysts.

    B. epidermoid cysts.

    C. verrucose hyperplasia.

    D. hyperhidrosis.

5. When do epidermoid cysts occur?

    A. when sebaceous glands multiply

    B. only when the patient is allergic to the liner used

    C. only when a suspension system is used

    D. when sebaceous glands are plugged

6. Heterotopic ossification

    A. is another name for bone spur.

    B. is when new bone forms at the end of the bone in an amputated limb.

    C. is when bone develops in soft tissue.

    D. describes the situation when an epidermoid cyst forms granulation tissue.

7. A thigh cast with pylon and foot attached is a traditional form of

    A. a definitive prosthesis.

    B. a test socket.

    C. a shrinker sock.

    D. an immediate postoperative prosthesis.

8. A patient who has the ability for more than basic ambulation skills with a prosthesis and who will use the prosthesis with a high energy or stress level is a description for what K level?

   A. K0

   B. K2

   C. K3

   D. K4

9. A patient who doesn't have the potential to safely transfer either with or without assistance and for whom a prosthesis will not improve mobility is at what K level?

   A. K0

   B. K2

   C. K3

   D. K4

10. A patient who will be using the prosthesis for some activities more than simple walking such as activities that require variable cadence is what K level?

   A. K0

   B. K2

   C. K3

   D. K4

11. A patient who can be described as a low-level community ambulatory would fit what K level?

   A. K1

   B. K2

   C. K3

   D. K4

12. A patient who uses his or her prosthesis for household ambulation only is what K level?

A. K1

B. K2

C. K3

D. K4

13. The way in which the prosthesis is held to the residual limb is called the _____ method.

A. suspension

B. propulsion

C. capillary

D. device

14. SACH stands for

A. solid ankle contained heel.

B. solid ankle cushion heel.

C. soft ankle contained heel.

D. soft ankle cushion heel.

15. A Lisfranc amputation is

A. a transmetatarsal amputation.

B. a transtarsal disarticulation.

C. a tarsometatarsal disarticulation.

D. a transtarsal amputation.

16. A Chopart amputation is

   A. a great toe amputation.

   B. a transmetatarsal amputation.

   C. a transtarsal disarticulation.

   D. a transmetatarsal disarticulation.

17. Which of the following is not a partial foot amputation?

   A. Chopart

   B. Lisfranc

   C. Pirogoff

   D. Syme

18. Single-axis, multiaxis, and dynamic response are categories of what?

   A. prosthetic feet

   B. prosthetic sockets

   C. prosthetic knees

   D. prosthetic suspension

19. The two traditional common foot types for Syme amputation are

   A. specially designed solid ankle cushion heel and specially designed dynamic response.

   B. specially designed solid ankle cushion heel and specially designed multiaxis.

   C. standard solid ankle cushion heel and standard dynamic response.

   D. specially designed solid ankle cushion heel and specially designed corset suspension.

20. A Boyd amputation can be considered a variation of a

   A. Lisfranc amputation.

   B. Syme amputation.

   C. Chopart amputation.

   D. transmetatarsal amputation.

21. A transtibial plug fit socket allows

    A. distal contact in all cases.

    B. distal contact most of the time.

    C. no distal contact.

    D. use of distal contact as needed.

22. A standard length for a transtibial amputation would be

    A. 100% of tibial length.

    B. 10% of tibial length.

    C. 50% of tibial length.

    D. 85% of tibial length.

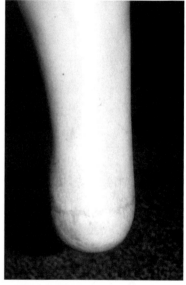

From Bucholz RW, Heckman JD. *Rockwood & Green's Fractures in Adults.* 5th ed. Philadelphia, PA: Lippincott Williams & Wilkins; 2001.

23. Types of transtibial socket designs include

    A. plug fit, patellar tendon bearing, total surface bearing, and hydrostatic.

    B. plug fit, patellar tendon bearing, total surface bearing, and dynamic response.

    C. plug fit, patellar tendon bearing, total surface bearing, and multiaxis.

    D. plug fit, patellar tendon bearing, total surface bearing, and cushion interface.

24. The plug fit design for transtibial prosthesis sockets is

    A. the main socket type used in the United States.

    B. the most technically advanced type of socket.

    C. a socket type that may still be used in some countries.

    D. the ideal socket type.

25. Pressure-tolerant areas of a transtibial residual limb include which of the following?

    A. the patellar tendon, fibular shaft, medial tibial flare, and gastrocnemius

    B. the patellar tendon, patella, and gastrocnemius

    C. the patellar tendon, fibular shaft, fibular head, and gastrocnemius

    D. the patellar tendon, fibular shaft, hamstring tendons, and gastrocnemius

26. Pressure-sensitive areas of a transtibial residual limb include which of the following?

    A. distal fibula, patella, and hamstring tendons

    B. distal fibula, medial tibial flare, and gastrocnemius

    C. distal fibula, fibular head, and fibular shaft

    D. distal fibula, patellar tendon, and gastrocnemius

27. Regarding suspension in transtibial prostheses:

    A. Suspension is not used.

    B. There is only one type of suspension used.

    C. Suction suspension is the best kind.

    D. There are several types of suspension systems, and the best kind depends on the particular patient.

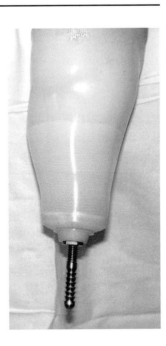

28. One negative feature of the joint and corset suspension system is that it is

A. very light.

B. a system that can only be used in men.

C. heavy.

D. extremely expensive.

29. Persons with transtibial amputations have gait patterns that are

A. uniform.

B. similar within the age groupings of young, middle aged, and older adults.

C. similar within one gender (all males are similar to other males and all females are similar to other females).

D. quite different from person to person depending on a number of factors.

30. Myodesis is

A. the suturing of muscle to bone.

B. the same as myoplasty.

C. the suturing of muscle to muscle.

D. the suturing of either muscle to bone or muscle to muscle.

31. Is use of myoplasty only sufficient with regard to a transfemoral amputation?

A. Yes

B. No

C. It is adequate for women, children, and older adults only.

D. It is adequate for most people older than 65 years.

32. The two traditional designs for transfemoral prosthesis sockets are what?

A. sacral containment and rectangular

B. sacral containment and quadrilateral

C. ischial containment and rectangular

D. ischial containment and quadrilateral

33. Suspension methods for a transfemoral prosthesis include

   A. suction, hoses, and belts.

   B. belts, liners, and suction.

   C. suction and liners only.

   D. belts, liners, and hoses.

34. Do manual locking knees allow normal gait mechanics?

   A. No, patients with this knee type are only able to transfer.

   B. No, patients with this knee type have abnormal gait mechanics.

   C. Yes, all patients walk with normal gait mechanics with this type of knee.

   D. Yes, most patients walk with normal gait mechanics with this type of knee.

35. What is an advantage of a manual locking knee?

   A. Patients don't require any training for proper safe use with these knees.

   B. They allow a normal gait pattern.

   C. They are the most cosmetically appealing knee.

   D. They are very stable.

36. Which of the following environments is a microprocessor knee not well suited for?

   A. office type environment

   B. working as a taxi driver

   C. door-to-door sales

   D. working in a muddy, swamp-like environment

37. Can individuals with translumbar amputation (hemicorporectomy) ambulate with a prosthesis?

    A. No, ambulation is not possible with this level of amputation.

    B. All individuals with translumbar amputation can walk with any prosthesis.

    C. Some individuals with translumbar amputation can be fitted with appropriate components to achieve some ambulation.

    D. No, individuals with translumbar amputation don't desire to ambulate.

38. What are "stubbies"?

    A. Stubbies are a type of training prosthesis for bilateral amputees.

    B. Stubbies are a type of training prosthesis for unilateral amputees.

    C. Stubbies are a type of training prosthesis for either bilateral or unilateral amputees.

    D. There is no such thing as stubbies.

39. Regarding "stubbies," why are feet initially mounted backward?

    A. There is no such thing as stubbies.

    B. to help decrease the risk of falling

    C. The feet on stubbies are never mounted backward.

    D. The main reason is to allow the patient to practice walking backward.

40. Treatment for phantom limb pain is

    A. varied.

    B. not generally needed.

    C. usually worse than the pain itself.

    D. worse in those with congenital limb deficiency.

41. Why use an upper limb orthotic?

    A. to correct structural deformities

    B. to protect part of the body

    C. to improve function

    D. all of the above

42. When walking, persons with unilateral transtibial amputation usually have a _____ rate of oxygen consumption compared to persons without amputation.

    A. lower

    B. higher

    C. variable

    D. similar

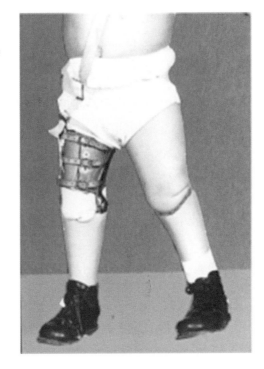

43. Are certain prostheses specific to use in and around the water?

    A. yes

    B. no

    C. Under certain conditions, younger amputees may use prostheses designed for water use.

    D. Prostheses designed for water use are mainly used by competitive swimmers and divers.

44. In transverse limb deficiencies, there is

    A. normal development up to the point of the limb deficiency and then no development after the point of the deficiency.

    B. abnormal development up to the point of the limb deficiency and then no development after the point of the deficiency.

    C. normal development up to the point of the limb deficiency and then abnormal development after the point of the deficiency.

    D. either A or C

45. Longitudinal limb deficiencies can refer to

    A. the absence of pigment in the arms or legs.

    B. poor quality bone matrix resulting in multiple fractures.

    C. when an organ is missing from the body.

    D. when a bone is missing in a limb.

46. Lack of fibula due to a longitudinal limb deficiency is

    A. usually a stand-alone deformity.

    B. usually a condition that exists in association with other deformities.

    C. usually due to a known specific cause.

    D. both B and C

47. Lack of the tibia due to longitudinal limb deficiency is

    A. often caused by exposure to heavy metals during pregnancy.

    B. the most common deficiency of the lower limbs.

    C. one of the most common deficiencies of the lower limbs.

    D. extremely rare.

48. Peripheral vascular disease is the main cause of lower limb amputation.

    A. no, trauma is

    B. no, infection is

    C. yes

    D. both A and B

49. Most upper limb amputations are of

  A. both arms.

  B. one arm.

  C. one forearm.

  D. one or more fingers.

50. The four types of upper limb prostheses are

  A. hybrid system, externally powered system, body-powered system, and passive system.

  B. hybrid system, externally powered system, body-powered system, and hybrid plus system.

  C. internally powered system, externally powered system, body-powered system, and passive system.

  D. hybrid system, externally powered system, body-powered system, and electrically powered system.

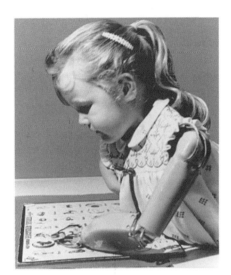

51. What part of a prosthesis could be considered as equivalent to a hand?

  A. the socket

  B. the hook

  C. the terminal device

  D. both B and C

52. What term is often used to describe the remaining part of the body from which part of a limb has been amputated?

  A. the remainder

  B. the residual limb

  C. the sound limb

  D. a below-knee amputation

53. A figure of 8 harness contains which of the following parts?

A. crosspoint and axilla loop

B. axilla loop and crossbow lock

C. crossbow lock, shoulder loop, and shoulder buckle

D. shoulder loop and axilla loop

54. Partial hand prostheses are

A. necessary for use of the limb.

B. commonly used.

C. rarely used.

D. both A and B

55. Phantom limb sensation and pain will likely _____ over time after an amputation.

A. increase

B. remain the same

C. plateau

D. decrease

56. In selecting a level for amputation:

A. Objective criteria such as vascular studies are the main information used.

B. Clinical judgment in association with clinical data is used.

C. The longest limb length possible is the best due to decreased psychological trauma.

D. The patient's wishes should be the primary consideration regardless of other data.

57. Amputations related to diabetes account for _____ amputations than those related to trauma.

    A. about the same number of

    B. fewer

    C. a small amount more

    D. significantly more

58. Problems during the stance phase of walking can be grouped as

    A. hip instability, ankle/foot instability, and knee instability.

    B. hip instability and toe instability.

    C. hip instability and trunk instability.

    D. trunk/pelvis instability, hip instability, and knee instability.

59. Normal walking on a flat surface generally occurs at about

    A. 1 mph.

    B. 1.3 mph.

    C. 1 to 1.5 mph.

    D. 3 mph.

60. A rigid removable dressing helps with

    A. preventing injury to the residual limb.

    B. edema control.

    C. residual limb shaping.

    D. all of the above

61. Desensitization techniques are an _____ part of treatment postamputation.

    A. important

    B. unnecessary

    C. unhelpful

    D. intimidating

62. Patients with amputation can achieve improved emotional support through

A. peer counseling.

B. support groups for those with amputations.

C. psychological counseling as needed.

D. all of the above

63. Orthotics may be used for positioning in the treatment of conditions including

A. nerve injuries, burns, spinal cord injuries, and brain injuries.

B. eczema and psoriasis.

C. dysplastic nevi.

D. lipomas, dermatitis, and scars.

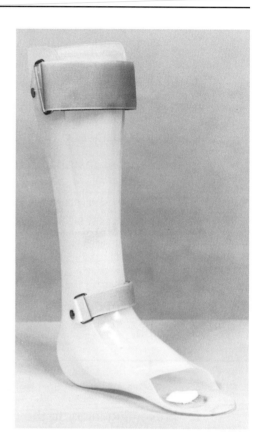

64. Shoe components include

A. upper, sole, heel, trim, and casing.

B. casing, trim, and upper.

C. upper and sole.

D. all of the above

65. Walker types include

    A. hemi-walker, rolling walker, and folding walker.

    B. sliding walker, prong walker, and folding walker.

    C. sliding walker, prong walker, and hemi-walker.

    D. hemi-walker, rolling walker, folding walker, and sliding walker.

66. Cane components include

    A. handle, neck, base, and prongs.

    B. handle, neck, and feet.

    C. head, neck, and feet.

    D. handle, shaft, and rubber tip.

67. Canes may be prescribed for

    A. improved stability and pain reduction.

    B. edema management and pain reduction.

    C. pain reduction and shortness of breath.

    D. all of the above

68. A shoe heel's purpose includes which of the following?

    A. to absorb shock

    B. to decrease shoe wear

    C. none of the above

    D. both A and B

69. Runners are more likely to have which of the following?

    A. pronated foot

    B. supinated foot

    C. pronated and supinated foot

    D. polydactyly

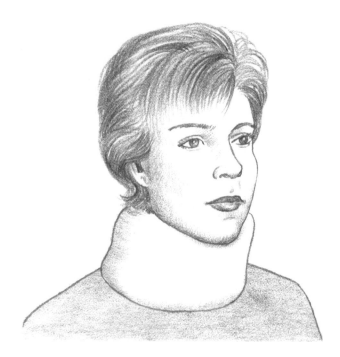

70.   Soft collar braces

    A.   provide significant stabilization from C2 to C7.

    B.   provide significant stabilization from C4 to C7.

    C.   provide significant stabilization from C4 to T2.

    D.   do not provide significant cervical spine motion restriction.

ANSWER KEY WITH EXPLANATIONS

1. The correct answer is A.

Verrucous hyperplasia is a condition in which the distal end of a residual limb appears like a wart. It is thought to be related to a close fit of the prosthesis above the distal end of the residual limb combined with lack of pressure at the actual distal end of the residual limb, with resultant vascular congestion that eventually leads to the condition, although the exact pathophysiology is not well elucidated.

2. The correct answer is A.

Depression and other psychological conditions should be considered in patients with new amputation. Beyond an initial adjustment period related to the limb loss, a significant percentage of patients can continue on to develop chronic depression. The circumstances of traumatic amputation may also lend themselves to the development of posttraumatic stress disorder (PTSD).

3. The correct answer is A.

Hyperhidrosis is a skin condition that often affects patients with amputation who use a prosthesis as the suspension and liner materials covering the residual limb trap heat. Use of antiperspirants and a nylon sheath under the liner may be helpful.

4. The correct answer is B.

Epidermoid cysts are firm, round nodules that may develop in the popliteal fossa area of patients with transtibial amputation who use a prosthesis and at the upper thigh of patients with transfemoral amputation who use a prosthesis. These cysts occur due to plugging of the sebaceous glands. They may be tender and can drain if ruptured. Usual treatment includes decreasing pressure on the area including adjusting prosthesis fit and topical and/or oral antifungal and/or antibacterial medication. Incision and drainage may be used if necessary.

5. The correct answer is D.

Epidermoid cysts are firm, round nodules that occur due to plugging of the sebaceous glands. They are common in patients with amputation due to the pressure of the prosthesis. They may be tender and can drain if ruptured. Usual treatment includes decreasing pressure on the area including adjusting prosthesis fit and topical and/or oral antifungal and/or antibacterial medication. Incision and drainage may be used if necessary.

6. The correct answer is C.

Heterotopic ossification refers to the development of bone spontaneously in soft tissue, commonly after a traumatic amputation. When bone grows at the end of a bone that has been amputated, that would be referred to as a bone spur.

7. The correct answer is D.
IPOP stands for immediate postoperative prosthesis, which may be used in patients with transtibial amputation. A traditional form is a thigh cast with a pylon and foot attached.

8. The correct answer is D.
Functional levels for prosthesis use are K0, K1, K2, K3, and K4. The K levels are based on potential function. K4 refers to activity exceeding basic ambulation, such as that of a child, athlete, or active adult. K4 activity means that the prosthesis may endure high impact or stress levels.

9. The correct answer is A.
Functional levels for prosthesis use are K0, K1, K2, K3, and K4. The K levels are based on potential function. K0 can refer to a patient without the ability/potential to safely use a prosthesis with or without assistance. A patient with severe dementia with amputation may fall into this category.

10. The correct answer is C.
Functional levels for prosthesis use are K0, K1, K2, K3, and K4. The K levels are based on potential function. A patient who will be using the prosthesis for some activities more than simple walking such as activities that require variable cadence is K3.

11. The correct answer is B.
Functional levels for prosthesis use are K0, K1, K2, K3, and K4. The K levels are based on potential function. A patient who can be described as a low-level community ambulatory would fit K level 2.

12. The correct answer is A.
Functional levels for prosthesis use are K0, K1, K2, K3, and K4. The K levels are based on potential function. A patient who uses his or her prosthesis for household ambulation only is K level 1.

13. The correct answer is A.
The way in which the prosthesis is held to the residual limb is called the suspension method. Suction, a sleeve, or a liner may be used. Depending on a patient's anatomy and activity needs, additional suspension methods such as a belt may be used.

14. The correct answer is B.
SACH stands for solid ankle cushion heel, referring to a type of prosthetic foot. This foot type has been available since the 1950s. It is widely used and considered a basic foot type. They are not flexible but are durable and relatively inexpensive.

15. The correct answer is C.
A Lisfranc amputation is a tarsometatarsal disarticulation, a type of partial foot amputation.

16. The correct answer is C.
A Chopart amputation is a transtarsal disarticulation, a type of partial foot amputation.

17. The correct answer is D.
A Syme amputation is an ankle disarticulation, removing the foot; in that sense, it is not a partial foot amputation. A Pirogoff amputation is a variation of the Syme amputation; however, it allows part of the calcaneus to remain. Chopart amputation is a transtarsal disarticulation. Lisfranc amputation is a tarsometatarsal disarticulation.

18. The correct answer is A.
Single-axis, multiaxis, and dynamic response are categories of prosthetic feet. The other major category of prosthetic feet is solid ankle cushion heel (SACH).

19. The correct answer is A.
The two traditional common foot types for Syme amputation are specially designed solid ankle cushion heel and specially designed dynamic response foot.

20. The correct answer is B.
A Syme amputation is an ankle disarticulation, removing the foot. A Boyd amputation can be considered a variation of the Syme amputation; however, it allows part of the calcaneus to remain. Chopart amputation is a transtarsal disarticulation. Lisfranc amputation is a tarsometatarsal disarticulation.

21. The correct answer is C.
A transtibial plug fit socket allows no distal contact. It is basically a hollow cylinder shaped to approximate the shape of the residual limb, and the distal end of the socket is open. This design is no longer used in the United States. It can be considered a less advanced socket type.

22. The correct answer is C.
A standard length for a transtibial amputation is 35% to 50% of the length of the tibia. Longer lengths are not associated with improved function.

23. The correct answer is A.
Types of transtibial socket designs include plug fit, patellar tendon bearing, total surface bearing, and hydrostatic. The plug fit socket allows no distal contact. It is basically a hollow cylinder shaped to approximate the shape of the residual limb, and the distal end of the socket is open. This design is no longer used in the United States.

24. The correct answer is C.
A transtibial plug fit socket allows no distal contact. It is basically a hollow cylinder shaped to approximate the shape of the residual limb, and the distal end of the socket is open. This design is no longer used in the United States. It can be considered a less advanced socket type. It may still be in use in some countries.

25. The correct answer is A.
Pressure-tolerant areas of a transtibial residual limb include the patellar tendon, fibular shaft, medial tibial flare, and gastrocnemius.

26. The correct answer is A.
Pressure-sensitive areas of a transtibial residual limb include the distal fibula, patella, and hamstring tendons.

27. The correct answer is D.
Transtibial prostheses can be suspended in different ways including mechanisms within or external to the socket. The best choice depends on the patient and his or her needs.

28. The correct answer is C.
A joint and corset suspension system may be used in patients with transtibial amputation to provide improved knee stability. One negative feature of this design is that it is heavy.

29. The correct answer is D.
Persons with transtibial amputations have gait patterns that vary significantly depending on the individual and are affected by many issues including residual limb length, strength of lower extremities, range of motion, and prosthesis components.

30. The correct answer is A.
Myodesis is the suturing of muscle to bone. It is different than myoplasty, which is defined as suturing muscle to muscle.

31. The correct answer is B.
Optimal transfemoral amputation involves myodesis, suturing muscle to bone, and myoplasty, suturing muscles together, in order to stabilize the femur to help decrease pain and improve function. Use of myoplasty only is not sufficient.

32. The correct answer is D.
The two traditional designs for transfemoral prosthesis sockets are the ischial containment socket and the quadrilateral socket.

33. The correct answer is B.
Suspension methods for a transfemoral prosthesis include belts, liners, and suction.

34. The correct answer is B.
Patients using a manual locking knee do not have normal gait mechanics. Instead, they have a straight leg gait. The primary positive feature of a manual locking knee is that it is very stable.

35. The correct answer is D.
The main advantage of the manual locking knee is that it provides a great deal of stability.

36. The correct answer is D.
Microprocessor knees are not ideal for conditions such as a muddy, swampy area due to risk of malfunction.

37. The correct answer is C.
Individuals with translumbar amputation (hemicorporectomy) don't normally use ambulation as their main mode of mobility. Some persons with this type of amputation can be fitted with appropriate prostheses in order to ambulate with a swing-to pattern using a walker.

38. The correct answer is A.
"Stubbies" are a type of training prosthesis for bilateral amputees. They are basically a socket attached to a short pylon and then a foot. There is no knee. Feet are first mounted backward to shift the patient's center of mass backward, which helps decrease the risk of falling back. As the patient progresses with use, he or she will have the height increased, feet turned back to the front, and knees added to the prostheses. This is a challenging process that can take some time.

39. The correct answer is B.
"Stubbies" are a type of training prosthesis for bilateral amputees. They are basically a socket attached to a short pylon and then a foot. There is no knee. Feet are first mounted backward to shift the patient's center of mass backward, which helps decrease the risk of falling back. As the patient progresses with use, he or she will have the height increased, feet turned back to the front, and knees added to the prostheses. This is a challenging process that can take some time.

40. The correct answer is A.
Phantom limb pain treatment varies and includes medication use, psychological treatments such as mental visualization, acupuncture, use of physical therapy modalities such as ultrasound, and even procedures such as steroid injection. Most patients with amputation do experience some phantom pain. Phantom pain usually decreases over time and is not known to occur in the limb loss of those individuals born with limb deficiency.

41. The correct answer is D.
Upper limb orthotics are used for various reasons including to correct structural deformities, to protect part of the body, and to improve function.

42. The correct answer is D.
Persons with unilateral transtibial amputation usually have a similar rate of oxygen consumption compared to persons without amputation. They may self-select a slower walking speed that leads to a similar rate of oxygen consumption as a comparable person without amputation.

43. The correct answer is A.
Certain prostheses are specific to use in and around water. They may be worn in the shower, when swimming, or for other activities in and around the water. Persons with amputation who wish to use their prosthesis in the water will need a dedicated device, parts cannot be switched back and forth between land and water use.

44. The correct answer is A.

In transverse limb deficiencies, there is normal development up to the point of the limb deficiency and then no development after the point of the deficiency. This is a type of congenital limb deficiency.

45. The correct answer is D.

Longitudinal limb deficiencies can refer to when a bone is missing in a limb. This is a type of congenital limb deficiency.

46. The correct answer is B.

Lack of fibula due to a longitudinal limb deficiency is usually a condition that exists in association with other deformities, including foot deformity, tibial bowing, and limited hip range of motion. The cause is generally not known.

47. The correct answer is C.

Lack of the tibia due to longitudinal limb deficiency is one of the most common deficiencies of the lower limbs; it's considered to be the third most common congenital lower limb deficiency. The most common congenital lower limb deficiency is fibular longitudinal deficiency. The second most common congenital lower limb deficiency is proximal femoral focal deficiency (PFFD), which can be classified depending on how the acetabulum and femur are involved.

48. The correct answer is C.

Peripheral vascular disease is the main cause of lower limb amputation, being related to more than two-thirds of lower extremity amputation.

49. The correct answer is D.

Most acquired (noncongenital) upper limb amputations are related to trauma. Of acquired upper limb amputations, amputation of one or more fingers is the most common type.

50. The correct answer is A.

The four types of upper limb prostheses are hybrid system, externally powered system, body-powered system, and passive system. A hybrid system uses both external power and the patient's body (joint movement and muscle strength). A passive system tends to be primarily cosmetic but can help provide counterweight for balance/stability.

51. The correct answer is D.

The terminal device in an upper extremity prosthesis can be considered equivalent to a hand. There are different types of terminal devices: passive and active. Passive terminal devices can be cosmetic or functional, with the cosmetic type looking like a hand and the functional type being used to perform a certain function(s). Active terminal devices move in some way. A hook is a terminal device in the active terminal device category.

52. The correct answer is B.

The term *residual limb* is often used to describe the remaining part of the body from which part of a limb has been amputated and can be considered an appropriate term to use in the vast majority of settings.

53. The correct answer is A.
A figure of 8 harness is a suspension method for upper extremity prostheses. It contains parts including the crosspoint, also known as the O ring, the axilla loop, the control attachment strap, and the anterior support strap.

54. The correct answer is C.
Partial hand prostheses are rarely used. Prosthetic devices for partial hand amputation at this point generally don't work well and don't provide significant cosmetic appeal.

55. The correct answer is D.
Phantom limb sensation/pain is common after an amputation and can vary in character. This phenomena will likely decrease over time after a patient's amputation, often within several months.

56. The correct answer is B.
When selecting the optimal amputation level for a patient, many factors are considered. Ultimately, the physician makes a clinical judgment based on the clinical data, which will include patient history including previous functional level and goals, medical issues including cognitive status, vascular health and skin integrity, and appropriate limb length based on many factors. Of course, the patient must consent to the procedure, but the clinical provider must determine whether a certain level of amputation will likely provide a viable and medically appropriate result for the patient and determine the appropriate residual limb length. The clinical provider(s) must appropriately educate the patient to allow the medical team to reach the most appropriate result for that patient, with the patient's consent.

57. The correct answer is D.
Amputations related to diabetes account for significantly more amputations than those related to trauma. Persons with diabetes also often have concomitant medical conditions such as hypertension which can place an individual into the category of amputation related to peripheral vascular disease as well.

58. The correct answer is A.
Problems during the stance phase of walking can be grouped as hip instability, ankle/foot instability, and knee instability.

59. The correct answer is D.
Normal walking on a flat surface generally occurs at about 3 mph, or about 1 to 1.3 m/s. This is the speed at which walking is most efficient on a level surface, and for most people, a comfortable walking rate would be the same as that speed which is most energetically efficient.

60. The correct answer is D.
Use of a rigid removable dressing postamputation helps with preventing injury to the residual limb, edema control, and residual limb shaping. Because this type of dressing can be removed, it allows the surgical wound to be monitored easily and the residual limb manipulated and massaged easily to help reduce edema and decrease uncomfortable sensations.

61. The correct answer is A.

Desensitization techniques are an important part of treatment postamputation. These techniques include tapping and massaging the residual limb, including self-massage.

62. The correct answer is D.

Patients with amputation can achieve improved emotional support through peer counseling, support groups for those with amputations, and psychological counseling as needed. Loss of a limb involves a grieving process, and it should be expected that an adjustment-type period of depression may occur. It is not uncommon for patients to go on to develop persistent depression. If the amputation event involved trauma, other psychological issues such as posttraumatic stress disorder may also occur.

63. The correct answer is A.

Orthotics may be used for positioning in the treatment of conditions including nerve injuries, burns, spinal cord injuries, and brain injuries.

64. The correct answer is C.

The primary components of a shoe are the sole and the upper. Most shoes also have a heel. Shoes may have many internal and external modifications. External modifications can be made to the sole and/or the heel.

65. The correct answer is A.

Generally, the types of walkers include the hemi-walker, rolling walker, folding walker, and forearm walker. Walkers may be modified to meet a patient's specific needs including being made of lightweight materials or being more durable for safe use by heavier patients.

66. The correct answer is D.

In general, cane components include the handle, the shaft, an adjusting mechanism for the handle, a mechanism to adjust the cane height, and a rubber tip at the bottom of the cane. Canes may include additional features to meet a patient's specific needs including prongs for a wider base of support/improved stability or more durable construction for safe use by heavier patients.

67. The correct answer is A.

Canes may be prescribed for various conditions for purposes including improving stability/reducing the likelihood of falls and decreasing pain by reducing the load placed on a painful joint.

68. The correct answer is D.

The purpose of the heel of a shoe is to decrease wear on the shoe and to absorb shock.

69. The correct answer is A.

Issues with pronation are a common problem in runners and can be associated with other problems including plantar fasciitis, Achilles tendonitis, and patellofemoral syndrome.

70. The correct answer is D.

Soft collar braces do not provide significant cervical spine motion restriction. Their primary purpose is to act as a reminder to limit motion. They may be given as a comfort measure for patients. The device may help retain body heat which may help reduce muscle spasm. This action, as well as helping avoid excess movement in the injured area, may help somewhat in decreasing pain and improving healing.

Board Review Points ("Pearls") for Amputee Rehabilitation, Prosthetics, and Orthotics

General Amputation Information

- Depression and other psychological conditions should be considered in patients with new amputation. Beyond an initial adjustment period related to the limb loss, a significant percentage of patients can continue on to develop chronic depression. The circumstances of traumatic amputation may also lend themselves to the development of PTSD.
- Phantom limb pain treatment varies and includes medication use, psychological treatments such as mental visualization, acupuncture, use of physical therapy modalities such as ultrasound, and even procedures such as steroid injection. Most patients with amputation do experience some phantom pain. Phantom pain usually decreases over time and is not known to occur in the limb loss of those individuals born with limb deficiency.
- Functional levels for prosthesis use are K0, K1, K2, K3, and K4. The K levels are based on potential function. K0 can refer to a patient without the ability/potential to safely use a prosthesis with or without assistance. A patient with severe dementia with amputation may fall into this category. A patient who uses his or her prosthesis for household ambulation only is K level 1. A patient who can be described as a low-level community ambulatory would fit K level 2. A patient who will be using the prosthesis for some activities more than simple walking such as activities that require variable cadence is K3. K4 refers to activity exceeding basic ambulation, such as that of a child, athlete, or active adult. K4 activity means that the prosthesis may endure high impact or stress levels.

Lower Extremity Amputation/Prostheses

- IPOP stands for immediate postoperative prosthesis, which may be used in patients with transtibial amputation. A traditional form is a thigh cast with a pylon and foot attached.
- The way in which the prosthesis is held to the residual limb is called the suspension method. Suction, a sleeve, or a liner may be used. Depending on a patient's anatomy and activity needs, additional suspension methods such as a belt may be used.
- The two traditional designs for transfemoral prosthesis sockets are the ischial containment socket and the quadrilateral socket.

- Types of transtibial socket designs include plug fit, patellar tendon bearing, total surface bearing, and hydrostatic. The plug fit socket allows no distal contact. It is basically a hollow cylinder shaped to approximate the shape of the residual limb, and the distal end of the socket is open. This design is no longer used in the United States.
- Single-axis, multiaxis, and dynamic response are categories of prosthetic feet. The other major category of prosthetic feet is SACH.

Upper Extremity Amputation/Prostheses

- The four types of upper limb prostheses are hybrid system, externally powered system, body-powered system, and passive system. A hybrid system uses both external power and the patient's body (joint movement and muscle strength). A passive system tends to be primarily cosmetic but can help provide counterweight for balance/stability.
- A figure of 8 harness is a suspension method for upper extremity prostheses. It contains parts including the crosspoint, also known as the O ring, the axilla loop, the control attachment strap, and the anterior support strap.
- The terminal device in an upper extremity prosthesis can be considered equivalent to a hand. There are different types of terminal devices: passive and active. Passive terminal devices can be cosmetic or functional, with the cosmetic type looking like a hand and the functional type being used to perform a certain function(s). Active terminal devices move in some way. A hook is a terminal device in the active terminal device category.
- Partial hand prostheses are rarely used. Prosthetic devices for partial hand amputation at this point generally don't work well and don't provide significant cosmetic appeal.

Gait Cycle

- Persons with unilateral transtibial amputation usually have a similar rate of oxygen consumption compared to persons without amputation. They may self-select a slower walking speed that leads to a similar rate of oxygen consumption as a comparable person without amputation.
- Normal walking on a flat surface generally occurs at about 3 mph, or about 1 to 1.3 m/s. This is the speed at which walking is most efficient on a level surface, and for most people, a comfortable walking rate would be the same as that speed which is most energetically efficient.
- Problems during the stance phase of walking can be grouped as hip instability, ankle/foot instability, and knee instability.

Orthotics/Assistive Devices

- Orthotics may be used for positioning in the treatment of conditions including nerve injuries, burns, spinal cord injuries, and brain injuries.
- The primary components of a shoe are the sole and the upper. Most shoes also have a heel, whose purpose is to decrease wear on the shoe and to absorb shock. Shoes may have many internal and external modifications. External modifications can be made to the sole and/or the heel.

- Generally, the types of walkers include the hemi-walker, rolling walker, folding walker, and forearm walker. Walkers may be modified to meet a patient's specific needs including being made of lightweight materials or being more durable for safe use by heavier patients.
- In general, cane components include the handle, the shaft, an adjusting mechanism for the handle, a mechanism to adjust the cane height, and a rubber tip at the bottom of the cane. Canes may include additional features to meet a patient's specific needs including prongs for a wider base of support/improved stability or more durable construction for safe use by heavier patients.

REFERENCES & SUGGESTED READINGS

Andrews KL, Nanos KN, Hoskin TL. Determining K-levels following transtibial amputation. *Int J Phys Med Rehabil*. 2017;5:398.

Bosmans JC, Geertzen JH, Post WJ, van der Schans, Dijkstra PU. Factors associated with phantom limb pain: a 3½ year prospective study. *Clin Rehabil*. 2010;24(5):444-453.

Braddom RL, Chan L, Harrast ME, et al, eds. *Physical Medicine and Rehabilitation*. 4th ed. St. Louis, MO: Saunders; 2011.

Cowley E, Marsden J. The effects of prolonged running on foot posture: a repeated measures study of half marathon runners using a foot posture index and navicular height. *J Foot Ankle Res*. 2013;6:20.

Cuccurullo SJ. *Physical Medicine and Rehabilitation Board Review*. 2nd ed. New York, NY: Demos Medical; 2010.

Dehner C, Hartwig E, Strobel P, et al. Comparison of the relative benefits of 2 versus 10 days of soft collar cervical immobilization after acute whiplash injury. *Arch Phys Med Rehabil*. 2006;87(11):1423-1427.

den Bakker FM, Holtslag HR, van den Brand JGH. Pirogoff amputation for foot trauma: an unusual amputation level: a case report. *J Bone Joint Surg Am*. 2010;92(14):2462-2465.

Hanspal RS, Nieveen R. Water activity limbs. *Prosthet Orthot Int*. 2002;26(3):218-225.

Jarvis HL, Bennett AM, Twiste M, Phillip RD, Etherington J, Baker R. Temporal spatial and metabolic measures of walking in highly functional individuals with lower limb amputations. *Arch Phys Med Rehabil*. 2017;98(7):1389-1399.

O'Young BJ, Young M, Stiens SA, eds. *Physical Medicine and Rehabilitation Secrets*. 3rd ed. St. Louis, MO: Mosby; 2007.

Pirouzi G, Abu Osman NA, Eshraghi A, Ali H, Gholizadeh H, Wan Abas WAB. Review of the socket design and interface pressure measurement for transtibial prosthesis. *ScientificWorldJournal*. 2014;2014(2014):849073. doi:10.1155/2014/849073.

Richardson C, Kulkarni J. A review of the management of phantom limb pain: challenges and solutions. *J Pain Res*. 2017;10:1861-1870.

Safari MR, Meier MR. Systematic review of effects of current transtibial prosthetic socket designs—part 1: qualitative outcomes. *J Rehabil Res Dev*. 2015;52(5):491-508.

Shin JY, Roh SG, Lee NH, et al. Influence of epidemiology and patient behavior-related predictors on amputation rates in diabetic patients: systemic review and meta-analysis. *Int J Low Extrem Wounds*. 2017;16(1):14-22.

Tosun B, Buluc L, Gok U, Unal C. Boyd amputation in adults. *Foot Ankle Int*. 2011;32(11):1063-1068.

Wheeless' Textbook of Orthopedics. Foot and ankle amputation. http://www.wheelessonline.com/ortho/foot_and_ankle_amputation. Accessed September 2, 2017.

General Rehabilitation

1. Which of the following is true regarding physical therapy exercise for a 55-year-old male patient with rate-controlled intermittent atrial fibrillation?

   A. He should only participate in weight training.

   B. He should only participate in range-of-motion activities.

   C. He should not exercise.

   D. He should be able to participate in exercise including general aerobic activity.

2. A 68-year-old female on your subacute rehabilitation service is being discharged home. She asks if she can have a deep tissue massage next week. She has a history of deep venous thrombosis (DVT) 1 year ago, but venous Doppler last week was negative. You tell her which of the following?

   A. No, it is contraindicated for the rest of her life.

   B. Yes, if she has no current DVT.

   C. No, she must wait 3 years.

   D. Yes, if the massage therapist does not massage the legs.

3. Contraindications to manual lymph drainage (MLD) include

   A. congestive heart failure.

   B. kidney failure.

   C. organ transplant.

   D. both A and B

4. Your 66-year-old rehabilitation inpatient is offered the pneumococcal vaccine. He's never had it before and he has a mild cold. Can he have the vaccine, and if so, should he wait until he no longer has the cold?

   A. He can have the vaccine, and he can have it now.

   B. He can have the vaccine only after he's over his cold.

   C. He should wait until age 70 years to have the vaccine per Centers for Disease Control and Prevention (CDC) guidelines.

   D. He can have the vaccine after he is discharged from the rehabilitation hospital to prevent hospital acquired infection.

5. Your 50-year-old patient with spinal cord injury (SCI) has an area of redness on his heel. When you press on the skin, the redness remains. He may have

   A. unstageable pressure ulcer.

   B. stage 1 pressure ulcer.

   C. stage 2 pressure ulcer.

   D. stage 3 pressure ulcer.

6. You receive a 50-year-old patient with spinal cord injury (SCI) from another facility. On intake, you notice a dark scabbed area on his heel. He may have

   A. unstageable pressure ulcer.

   B. stage 1 pressure ulcer.

   C. stage 2 pressure ulcer.

   D. stage 3 pressure ulcer.

7. Your 50-year-old patient with spinal cord injury (SCI) has an area of redness on his heel and the top layer of skin is torn off. He has

   A. unstageable pressure ulcer.

   B. stage 1 pressure ulcer.

   C. stage 2 pressure ulcer.

   D. stage 3 pressure ulcer.

8. There are _____ pressure ulcer stages and _____.

    A. four; no other categories

    B. five; two other common designations

    C. five; no other categories

    D. four; two other common designations

9. Your 50-year-old patient with spinal cord injury (SCI) with very dark skin has a darkened area over her ischial area. When you touch it the color does not change. What could this be?

    A. deep tissue injury

    B. stage 1 pressure ulcer

    C. stage 2 pressure ulcer

    D. both A or B

10. Hypercalcemia related to immobilization is _____, affecting perhaps up to _____ of hospitalized patients.

    A. common; 30%

    B. common; 75%

    C. rare; 10%

    D. rare; 2%

11. A 35-year-old female is admitted to general rehabilitation after a serious car accident in which her immediate family was killed. She often asks how her immediate family members are doing. In what stage of grief may she be in?

    A. bargaining

    B. acceptance

    C. denial

    D. anger

12. A 28-year-old female patient on the general rehabilitation ward is pregnant and wants to use nicotine patches. Your best approach might be to

 A. prescribe the nicotine patches as one would for a nonpregnant patient.

 B. advise her that nicotine patches are contraindicated in pregnancy.

 C. consult with OB-GYN regarding the patient's request.

 D. prescribe the nicotine patches at half the dose of a nonpregnant patient.

---

13. A patient's head and neck are burned. What percentage of the total body surface area is this?

 A. 10%

 B. 12%

 C. 9%

 D. 8%

---

14. A patient's head, neck, and right leg are burned. What percentage of the total body surface area is this?

 A. 27%

 B. 20%

 C. 25%

 D. 30%

---

15. A patient's right arm and right leg are burned. What percentage of the total body surface area is this?

 A. 27%

 B. 20%

 C. 25%

 D. 30%

16. In the geriatric inpatient rehabilitation population, delirium that occurs in the setting of preexisting dementia

    A. has no significant effect on functional outcome.

    B. is a weak risk for decline in functional outcome.

    C. is a moderate risk for decline in functional outcome.

    D. is a strong risk for decline in functional outcome.

17. Ms. S., a 70-year-old female, was admitted to inpatient rehabilitation for a short stay posthip replacement. She was previously fully independent in activities of daily living and was working as a certified public accountant (CPA). When you come in to assess her on Monday morning, she is distracted by the elves behind you and when asked states she is in Rome. What's going on?

    A. delirium caused by lack of sleep and pain

    B. delirium caused by urinary tract infection

    C. acute psychotic break

    D. both A and B

18. Ms. J., a 78-year-old inpatient rehabilitation patient admitted postmyocardial infarction, notices some knee pain after physical therapy. What would be a good treatment for her?

    A. acetaminophen

    B. ice/heat, massage, knee sleeve (compression brace)

    C. oxycodone

    D. both A and B

19. Which of the following is true regarding the use of timed voiding in the inpatient rehabilitation setting for managing urinary incontinence in adults?

   A. Timed voiding has strong scientific evidence for its efficacy and is considered the treatment of choice.

   B. Timed voiding has been shown to decrease the length of the rehabilitation stay and decrease costs.

   C. Research does not provide strong evidence as to the effectiveness of this intervention, but it is widely practiced in the rehabilitation setting.

   D. Timed voiding is no longer considered an appropriate intervention due to increased risk of urinary tract infection.

20. Ms. T. is an 80-year-old patient on the inpatient rehabilitation ward post-stroke. Can she drive when she leaves the rehabilitation hospital?

   A. no, not for 6 months poststroke

   B. yes

   C. no, not without further evaluation

   D. no, not for 2 months poststroke

ANSWER KEY WITH EXPLANATIONS

1. The correct answer is D.

In general, exercise including aerobic exercise, is considered safe in persons with rate-controlled intermittent atrial fibrillation and can help decrease risk associated with common comorbid conditions such as obesity and hypertension. Of course, he should be evaluated if he starts to experience concerning symptoms such as chest pain or shortness of breath.

2. The correct answer is B.

In a patient with previous history of DVTs with no current DVT, deep tissue massage by a professional is generally considered safe. As per routine, the patient should share her relevant medical history and any concerns with her massage therapist.

3. The correct answer is D.

MLD is used in lymphedema management and is contraindicated in conditions including congestive heart failure and renal failure.

4. The correct answer is A.

The CDC recommends pneumococcal vaccination to all individuals 65 years or older, with the only contraindications being allergy to the vaccine or any component of the vaccine, or also, in the case of the PCV13 vaccine, if the individual had a severe allergic reaction to any vaccine containing diphtheria toxoid after having been vaccinated with either PCV13 or PCV7. Mild cold symptoms are not actually a contraindication to receiving the vaccine. (Reference: Centers for Disease Control and Prevention. Vaccines and preventable diseases. https://www.cdc.gov/vaccines/vpd/pneumo/hcp/recommendations.html. Accessed September 9, 2017.)

5. The correct answer is B.

The hallmark of stage 1 pressure ulcer is redness that does not turn white when pressure is applied.

6. The correct answer is A.

An unstageable pressure ulcer is one in which the extent of the ulcer is unknown due to it being covered by scab/dead tissue.

7. The correct answer is C.

When the skin barrier is broken but not through the whole thickness of the skin into deeper structures, that is a stage 2 pressure ulcer.

8. The correct answer is D.

Pressure ulcer categories are stage 1, stage 2, stage 3, and stage 4. There are two other common designations: unstageable and deep tissue injury.

9. The correct answer is D.

Deep tissue injury can occur in either skin that is intact or not intact. Discoloration in the area can appear differently depending on the skin color of the patient. Based on the information given, it is not entirely clear if the patient has a stage 1 pressure ulcer or a deep tissue injury.

10. The correct answer is D.

Hypercalcemia related to immobilization is rare. A 2012 study by Malberti noted the all-cause prevalence of hypercalcemia in adult inpatients has been reported as up to 3%. (Reference: Malberti F. Treatment of immobilization-related hypercalcaemia with denosumab. *Clin Kidney J*. 2012;5[6]:491-495.)

11. The correct answer is C.

In light of a recent tragedy, your patient does not seem to be acknowledging what occurred. Although there may be other issues you should investigate, she may be in the stage of grief called "denial."

12. The correct answer is C.

Despite some non-US research finding that nicotine patches are okay for use during pregnancy (Reference: Berlin I, Grange G, Jacob N, et al. Nicotine patches in pregnant smokers: randomised, placebo controlled, multicentre trial of efficacy. *BMJ*. 2014;348:g1622.), the American Congress of Obstetricians and Gynecologists recommends caution when determining whether use of these products are appropriate. It would probably be best to request OB-GYN consult to provide their input in this situation. (Reference: American Congress of Obstetricians and Gynecologists. Tobacco, alcohol and drugs and pregnancy. https://www.acog.org/Patients/FAQs/Tobacco-Alcohol-Drugs-and-Pregnancy#help. Accessed September 1, 2017.)

13. The correct answer is C.

Wallace's 1951 study (Reference: Wallace AB. The exposure treatment of burns. *Lancet*. 1951;1[6653]:501-504.) discusses burn percents based on body areas. The head and neck is considered 9%. (References: Chemical Hazards Emergency Medical Management. Burn triage and treatment—thermal injuries. https://chemm.nlm.nih.gov/burns.htm. Accessed September 1, 2017; and Hettiaratchy S, Papini R. Initial management of a major burn: II—assessment and resuscitation. *BMJ*. 2004;329[7457]:101-103.)

14. The correct answer is A.

Wallace's 1951 study (Reference: Wallace AB. The exposure treatment of burns. *Lancet*. 1951;1[6653]:501-504.) discusses burn percents based on body areas. The head and neck is considered 9%. Each leg is considered 18%. Therefore, 9 + 18 is 27%. (References: Chemical Hazards Emergency Medical Management. Burn triage and treatment—thermal injuries. https://chemm.nlm.nih.gov/burns.htm. Accessed September 1, 2017; and Hettiaratchy S, Papini R. Initial management of a major burn: II—assessment and resuscitation. *BMJ*. 2004;329[7457]:101-103.)

15. The correct answer is A.

Wallace's 1951 study (Reference: Wallace AB. The exposure treatment of burns. *Lancet*. 1951;1[6653]:501-504.) discusses burn percents based on body areas. Each arm is 9%. Each leg is 18%. Therefore, 9 + 18 is 27%. (References: Chemical Hazards Emergency Medical Management. Burn triage and treatment—thermal injuries. https://chemm.nlm.nih.gov/burns.htm. Accessed September 1, 2017; and Hettiaratchy S, Papini R. Initial management of a major burn: II—assessment and resuscitation. *BMJ*. 2004;329[7457]:101-103.)

16. The correct answer is D.

A 2014 prospective cohort study by Morandi et al. that evaluated 2,642 elderly patients being treated in inpatient rehabilitation found that the presence of delirium on admission occurring in patients with preexisting dementia was associated with an odds ratio of 15.5 for dependence in walking (with the confidence interval 5.6 to 42.7). (Reference: Morandi A, Davis D, Fick DM, et al. Delirium superimposed on dementia strongly predicts worse outcomes in rehabilitation inpatients. *J Am Med Dir Assoc*. 2014;15[5]:349-354.) An odds ratio that big, whose confidence interval does not cross 1, is a strong or even very strong risk factor for the outcome. (Reference: Rosenthal JA. Qualitative descriptors of strength of association and effect size. *J Soc Serv Res*. 1996;21[4]:37-59.) (The number 1 is important because it is the "null value" for the odds ratio, at which the risk for the outcome is the same for the exposed and the nonexposed groups.) The confidence interval would likely be smaller (more precise) if the study included more patients.

17. The correct answer is D.

Given the patient was independent in activities and continued to work as a CPA prior to admission, this scenario would represent an acute change in mental status. Delirium with a possible single or multifactorial underlying cause would be most likely. An infection workup; review and adjustment of pain medications and other medications; regular reorientation to place, time, and event; adequate hydration; and sleep hygiene measures are in order.

18. The correct answer is B.

Not knowing the rest of your patient's medical history, ice/heat, massage, and a knee sleeve would be ideal, to avoid the use of medications. Acetaminophen is often considered a first-line medication for treatment of pain in geriatric patients, so D could be considered an acceptable answer, assuming no contraindications to the use of acetaminophen. A multidisciplinary approach to pain management in the older adults can help decrease complications.

19. The correct answer is C.

Timed voiding is often done in inpatient rehabilitation wards. Unfortunately, we do not currently have good evidence to support its use. A 2004 Cochrane Database Systematic Review did find a lower percent incontinent of those in the group receiving daily checks using timed voiding versus control but still concluded that the data was not of high enough quality and there was not enough data to provide support in favor or against the use of timed voiding. (Reference: Ostaszkiewicz J, Johnston L, Roe B. Timed voiding for the management of urinary incontinence in adults. *Cochrane Database Syst Rev*. 2004;[1]:CD002802.)

20. The correct answer is C.

Depending on the nature and severity of the stroke, patients likely should have speech therapy evaluation to provide information on cognitive deficits and then proceed to driver's rehabilitation to provide a more in depth assessment of the appropriateness of driving and what modifications may be needed to drive safely. There is no particular set time line in the United States as to when a particular patient can start driving again poststroke.

Board Review Points ("Pearls") for General Rehabilitation

- Pressure ulcer categories are stage 1, stage 2, stage 3, and stage 4. There are two other common designations: unstageable and deep tissue injury.
- Wallace's 1951 study (Reference: Wallace AB. The exposure treatment of burns. *Lancet*. 1951;1[6653]:501-504.) discusses burn percents based on body areas. The head and neck is considered 9%. Each arm is 9%. Each leg is 18%. (References: Chemical Hazards Emergency Medical Management. Burn triage and treatment—thermal injuries. https://chemm.nlm.nih.gov/burns.htm. Accessed September 1, 2017; and Hettiaratchy S, Papini R. Initial management of a major burn: II—assessment and resuscitation. *BMJ*. 2004;329[7457]:101-103.)
- In general, exercise including aerobic exercise is considered safe in persons with rate-controlled intermittent atrial fibrillation and can help decrease risk associated with common comorbid conditions such as obesity and hypertension.
- The CDC recommends pneumococcal vaccination to all individuals 65 years or older, with the only contraindications being allergy to the vaccine or any component of the vaccine, or also, in the case of the PCV13 vaccine, if the individual had a severe allergic reaction to any vaccine containing diphtheria toxoid after having been vaccinated with either PCV13 or PCV7. (Reference: Centers for Disease Control and Prevention. Vaccines and preventable diseases. https://www.cdc.gov/vaccines/vpd/pneumo/hcp/recommendations.html. Accessed September 9, 2017.)

REFERENCES & SUGGESTED READINGS

American Congress of Obstetricians and Gynecologists. Tobacco, alcohol and drugs and pregnancy. https://www.acog.org/Patients/FAQs/Tobacco-Alcohol-Drugs-and -Pregnancy#help. Accessed September 1, 2017.

Berlin I, Grange G, Jacob N, et al. Nicotine patches in pregnant smokers: randomised, placebo controlled, multicentre trial of efficacy. *BMJ*. 2014;348:g1622.

Braddom RL, Chan L, Harrast ME, et al, eds. *Physical Medicine and Rehabilitation*. 4th ed. St. Louis, MO: Saunders; 2011.

Cano-Torres E, González-Cantú A, Hinojosa-Garza G, Castilleja-Leal F. Immobilization induced hypercalcemia. *Clin Cases Miner Bone Metab*. 2016;13(1):46-47.

Centers for Disease Control and Prevention. Vaccines and preventable diseases. https://www .cdc.gov/vaccines/vpd/pneumo/hcp/recommendations.html. Accessed September 9, 2017.

Chemical Hazards Emergency Medical Management. Burn triage and treatment—thermal injuries. https://chemm.nlm.nih.gov/burns.htm. Accessed September 1, 2017.

Hettiaratchy S, Papini R. Initial management of a major burn: II—assessment and resuscitation. *BMJ*. 2004;329(7457):101-103.

Jabr FI. Massive pulmonary emboli after legs massage. *Am J Phys Med Rehabil*. 2007;86(8):691.

Kaye AD, Baluch A, Scott JT. Pain management in the elderly population: a review. *Ochsner J*. 2010;10(3):179-187.

Malberti F. Treatment of immobilization-related hypercalcaemia with denosumab. *Clin Kidney J*. 2012;5(6):491-495.

Malmo V, Nes BM, Amundsen BH, et al. Aerobic interval training reduces the burden of atrial fibrillations in the short term—a randomized trial. *Circulation*. 2016;133:466-473.

Morandi A, Davis D, Fick DM, et al. Delirium superimposed on dementia strongly predicts worse outcomes in older rehabilitation inpatients. *J Am Med Dir Assoc*. 2014;15(5):349-354.

National Pressure Ulcer Advisory Panel. NPUAP pressure injury stages. http://www.npuap .org/resources/educational-and-clinical-resources/npuap-pressure-injury-stages/. Accessed September 1, 2017.

Newman L. Elisabeth Kübler-Ross. *BMJ*. 2004;329(7466):627.

Ostaszkiewicz J, Johnston L, Roe B. Timed voiding for the management of urinary incontinence in adults. *Cochrane Database Syst Rev*. 2004;(1):CD002802.

Physiopedia. Manual lymph drainage. https://www.physio-pedia.com/Manual_lymph_drainage. Accessed September 1, 2017.

Rosenthal JA. Qualitative descriptors of strength of association and effect size. *J Soc Serv Res*. 1996;21(4):37-59.

Wallace AB. The exposure treatment of burns. *Lancet*. 1951;1(6653):501-504.

Pediatric Rehabilitation

1. Corrective bracing in adolescent idiopathic scoliosis is generally recommended for those

   A. with back pain.

   B. skeletally mature with frontal spine curvature of at least 20 degrees.

   C. skeletally immature with progression of the curve deformity.

   D. planning on participating in sports-related activities.

2. Which spine disorder is best characterized by curve deformity, irregular vertebral endplates, three or more wedged vertebral bodies, and Schmorl nodes in skeletally immature individuals?

   A. juvenile ankylosing spondylitis

   B. diffuse idiopathic skeletal hyperostosis (DISH)

   C. Scheuermann disease

   D. congenital scoliosis

3. A 6-year-old male with no prior medical history is brought by his parents to your office with low back pain and refusal to walk for 1 week. He has no known history of trauma or recent illness and reached developmental milestones appropriate for his age. Review of systems is otherwise negative. Physical examination reveals loss of lumbar lordosis, paravertebral muscle spasm, and restricted lumbar forward flexion with pain. Muscle tone, sensation, motor strength, and deep tendon reflexes are all normal. Lumbar spine radiographs are unremarkable. Blood cultures and purified protein derivative (PPD) of tuberculin are negative. White blood count (WBC) and erythrocyte sedimentation rate (ESR) are elevated. The most likely etiology is

   A. infectious.

   B. autoimmune.

   C. sprain/strain.

   D. malignancy.

4. A consulting physiatrist examining a newborn female with a suspected unilateral hip dislocation grasps the affected limb with thumb at the lesser trochanter and fingers at the greater trochanter. The examiner flexes the affected limb at the knee and abducts the hip while the finger over the greater trochanter gently pushes the femur anteriorly and feels a "clunk" as the hip reduces back into the acetabulum. Which physical examination maneuver does this best describe?

   A. passive hip abduction

   B. Galeazzi test

   C. Ortolani test

   D. Barlow test

5. A 3-month-old female with suspected developmental dysplasia of the hip (DDH) is referred to your office. Your physical and ultrasound examinations confirm a left hip dislocation that is easily reducible but remains unstable. What is the best initial recommendation for this patient?

   A. dynamic flexion-abduction orthosis (Pavlik harness)

   B. static abduction splint or spica cast

   C. orthopedic surgery referral for open reduction

   D. observation

6. A 10-year-old female accompanied by her parents presents to your office complaining of episodic muscle cramps in her thighs and behind her knees that only occur in the evening and at night, resolve spontaneously, and are relieved by massaging the affected areas. There is no significant past medical history. Family history is negative for limb movement disorders. Review of systems is otherwise negative. Physical examination is unremarkable. Plain radiographs and laboratory blood tests are normal. The most likely diagnosis is

A. restless legs syndrome (RLS).

B. akathisia.

C. patellofemoral pain syndrome.

D. growing pains.

7. Legg-Calvé-Perthes disease is

A. displacement of the proximal femoral epiphysis off of the femoral neck.

B. chronic stress reaction in the femoral neck.

C. transient synovitis of the hip joint.

D. avascular necrosis of the femoral epiphysis.

8. The best initial treatment for stable nonacute slipped capital femoral epiphysis (SCFE) is

A. conservative, consisting of physical therapy.

B. conservative, consisting of observation and serial radiographs until resolution.

C. surgical, consisting of fixation by a single pin.

D. surgical, consisting of total joint arthroplasty.

9. Which of the following is NOT a factor contributing to poor prognosis in a pediatric patient with Legg-Calvé-Perthes disease?

A. loss of height in the lateral one-third of the femoral epiphysis

B. delayed skeletal maturation

C. older age at onset with involvement of more than 50% of the femoral head

D. abduction contracture

10. The minimum radiographic curve angle measurement diagnostic of idiopathic scoliosis in adolescents and children is

A. 10 degrees.

B. 20 degrees.

C. 30 degrees.

D. 45 degrees.

11. Which ossification center is the first to appear in the pediatric elbow?

A. olecranon

B. capitellum

C. radius

D. trochlea

12. What is the proposed mechanism of injury in "Little League elbow" in skeletally immature throwers?

A. repetitive overuse

B. medial (valgus) tension and lateral (varus) compression at the elbow

C. traction forces on the medial apophysis

D. all of the above

13. In the skeletally immature pediatric population, which structure is most vulnerable to repetitive stress injury primarily due to tensile forces?

A. apophysis

B. epiphyseal (growth) plate

C. diaphysis

D. metaphysis

14. A 12-year-old male soccer player with no significant past medical history presents to your office with a 4-week history of right inferior knee pain. He denies any history of direct injury. Physical examination reveals point tenderness over the tibial tubercle. The lateral radiograph of the right knee demonstrates fragmentation of the tibial tubercle. Typical management of this condition consists of

    A. immobilization in a long leg cylinder cast for 6 weeks.

    B. arthroscopic debridement of loose bone fragments.

    C. brief rest, ice, analgesics, knee strap, and stretching exercises.

    D. corticosteroid injection.

15. A 14-year-old female sprinter presents with acute onset of left hip pain during a race. There is focal tenderness to palpation over the left anterior inferior iliac spine (AIIS). Anteroposterior (AP) radiograph of the pelvis confirms an avulsion fracture at the AIIS. This injury involves which muscle attachment?

    A. rectus femoris

    B. sartorius

    C. iliopsoas

    D. tensor fasciae latae

16. Right-sided congenital muscular torticollis is suspected in a 2-month-old infant presenting to your office. The typical head/neck posture in this condition is best described as

    A. head/neck fully extended and chin rotated toward the left.

    B. head/neck tilted to the right and chin rotated toward the left.

    C. head/neck tilted to the left and chin rotated toward the right.

    D. head/neck tilted to the right and chin rotated toward the right.

17.   You are consulted to evaluate a left foot deformity in a newborn male. On physical examination, you observe that the left ankle is plantarflexed, the hindfoot is inverted and internally rotated, the forefoot is adducted and supinated, and there is a medial skin crease on the plantar aspect of the midfoot. The deformity is rigid on passive range of motion testing. What is your diagnosis?

A. talipes calcaneovalgus

B. congenital vertical talus

C. metatarsus adductus

D. talipes equinovarus

18.   Which type of lumbar spondylolisthesis is associated with a higher risk of progression and neurologic involvement in children and adolescents?

A. degenerative

B. isthmic

C. dysplastic

D. pathologic

19.   A 15-year-old female gymnast presents with a 1-week history of severe axial right-sided low back pain, exacerbated by performing backbends and walkovers. She recently increased her number of training hours in preparation for a competition. On examination, there is tenderness over the right lower lumbar posterior elements and pain with lumbar extension. Anteroposterior (AP), lateral, and oblique lumbar radiographs are negative. Single-photon emission computed tomography (SPECT) imaging shows increased uptake at the right L5 pars interarticularis. Computed tomography (CT) shows intact marrow and bone cortex in the right L5 pars interarticularis. Which of the following best describes the pathology?

A. spondylolysis

B. spondylolisthesis

C. spondylosis

D. stress reaction

20. Which of the following spine structures is derived from the embryonic notochord in humans?

A. vertebral body

B. spinal cord

C. nucleus pulposus

D. annulus fibrosis

21. Iridocyclitis ("anterior uveitis") most commonly is associated with which clinical subtype of juvenile idiopathic arthritis (JIA) (juvenile rheumatoid arthritis)?

A. pauciarticular (oligoarticular)

B. enthesitis-related

C. systemic

D. psoriatic

22. Which clinical subtype of juvenile idiopathic arthritis (JIA) (juvenile rheumatoid arthritis) is most likely to involve the hip joint?

A. pauciarticular (oligoarticular)

B. polyarticular

C. systemic

D. psoriatic

23. Which of the following is a similarity between juvenile idiopathic arthritis (JIA) (juvenile rheumatoid arthritis) and adult forms of rheumatoid arthritis (RA)?

A. Both commonly involve large joints.

B. Both diseases have a female predominance.

C. Rheumatoid nodules are common in both.

D. Both diseases commonly involve the cervical spine.

24. Macrophage activation syndrome (MAS) is a complication most commonly associated with which clinical subtype of juvenile idiopathic arthritis (JIA) (juvenile rheumatoid arthritis)?

   A. pauciarticular (oligoarticular)

   B. enthesitis-related

   C. systemic

   D. psoriatic

25. Which of the following is NOT a poor prognostic factor in juvenile idiopathic arthritis (JIA) (juvenile rheumatoid arthritis)?

   A. rheumatoid factor (RF)-negative status

   B. unremitting (prolonged active) course

   C. hip involvement

   D. polyarticular joint involvement

26. Cerebral palsy occurs due to a brain injury that happens

   A. before birth.

   B. around the time of birth.

   C. both A and B

   D. any time in life.

27. Issues that commonly occur in individuals with cerebral palsy include

   A. abnormal gait.

   B. seizures.

   C. mental retardation.

   D. all of the above

28. Spina bifida occulta is

A. a neural tube defect resulting in extrusion of matter through the skin.

B. not a neural tube defect.

C. a neural tube defect resulting in lack of development of the rib cage.

D. a neural tube defect resulting in abnormal spine formation.

29. Spinal muscular atrophy involves pathology of the

A. motor neurons of the anterior horn cells.

B. motor neurons of the posterior horn cells.

C. sensory neurons of the anterior horn cells.

D. sensory neurons of the posterior horn cells.

30. At 3 months old, a startled infant spreads its arms out and then brings them back in, crying. What reflex is this, and is it normal?

A. tonic neck and it's abnormal

B. tonic neck and it's normal

C. Moro and it's normal

D. Moro and it's abnormal

31. An individualized education plan (IEP) is designed for students who

A. meet criteria for special education services.

B. don't speak English as a first language.

C. use crutches due to a tibial fracture.

D. meet criteria for an academic scholarship.

32. A thin teenage pediatric patient with normal facies presents by himself with height of 6 ft 5 in and scoliosis. What condition may he have?

A. Angelman syndrome

B. Marfan syndrome

C. Hunter syndrome

D. Klinefelter syndrome

33. Your tall teenage pediatric patient presents distraught. His girlfriend is pregnant, and he says he knows she must have been cheating. What condition may be in his medical history?

A. Angelman syndrome

B. Marfan syndrome

C. Hunter syndrome

D. Klinefelter syndrome

34. All the following are lysosomal storage diseases, EXCEPT

A. Tay-Sachs disease.

B. phenylketonuria.

C. Hurler syndrome.

D. Gaucher disease.

35. Risk factors for development of autism spectrum disorders include

A. older parents.

B. siblings with autism spectrum disorder.

C. particular medications taken during pregnancy.

D. all of the above

36. _____ is the most common type of muscular dystrophy in children.

A. Myotonic muscular dystrophy

B. Becker muscular dystrophy

C. Duchenne muscular dystrophy

D. Limb-girdle muscular dystrophy

37. Common causes of traumatic brain injury (TBI) in infants and children include

A. motor vehicle accidents.

B. child abuse.

C. falls.

D. all of the above

38. Of the following pediatric brain and spinal cord tumors, which is the most common malignant condition?

    A. glioma

    B. medulloblastoma

    C. astrocytoma

    D. ependymoma

39. You are seeing an otherwise healthy child with normal examination and no concerning family history, as follow-up for a mild concussion in your pediatric musculoskeletal/general rehabilitation clinic, and note a functional heart murmur. Should your patient's caregivers be worried?

    A. No, this can be a normal finding.

    B. Yes, this patient needs immediate referral for an echocardiogram.

    C. Yes, this patient requires immediate inpatient admission.

    D. Yes, this patient requires immediate referral to a pediatric cardiologist.

40. You are the team physician for your daughter's high school basketball team. It's time for presports participation physicals, and your daughter is worried her best friend with a small persistent atrial septal defect (ASD) and no pulmonary hypertension won't be able to play with her. You say which of the following?

    A. Yes, your friend can't participate at all. It's for her own safety.

    B. Yes, your friend can't play team sports. She can practice shooting hoops with you though.

    C. She should be able to play.

    D. Your friend wouldn't be able to keep up. She probably shouldn't even come to games in case it's too much excitement.

41. Cystic fibrosis is an _____ condition.

    A. autosomal recessive

    B. X-linked recessive

    C. autosomal dominant

    D. X-linked dominant

42. Compared to adults, pediatric patients generally experience

    A. equivalent pain management.

    B. better pain management.

    C. worse pain management.

    D. no pain at all.

43. A generally healthy, normal-appearing, 12-year-old female patient on the pediatric rehabilitation floor is wheelchair-reliant without clear etiology. Sufficient workup at the acute medical hospital prior to coming to inpatient rehabilitation found no medical cause. Of note, the patient's parents have recently divorced. There is no indication that the patient's apparent motor deficit is intentional. What condition might this patient have?

    A. malingering

    B. Angelman syndrome

    C. Duchenne muscular dystrophy

    D. conversion disorder

44. At your academic inpatient rehabilitation hospital, you are conducting a study as a physician researcher. You want to include a 9-year-old male patient on the pediatrics floor. Can this patient give informed consent to participate in the study?

    A. no, he cannot without the permission of his guardians

    B. yes, he can in all cases

    C. no, but he can be forced to participate

    D. yes, but only if you, the physician researcher, explain the study in detail

45. Is a wheelchair-reliant 9-year-old child disabled because he or she cannot work?

    A. No, 9-year-old children aren't expected to work, so work participation is not a criteria of disability.

    B. Yes, he or she should be able to work.

    C. Yes, if reasonable accommodation cannot be provided.

    D. No, employers must provide reasonable accommodations.

ANSWER KEY WITH EXPLANATIONS

1. The correct answer is C.

According to the 2011 International Scientific Society on Scoliosis Orthopaedic and Rehabilitation Treatment (SOSORT) guidelines, corrective bracing is recommended for skeletally immature individuals with a frontal plane curve above 20 degrees and/or curve progression of 5 degrees or greater between examinations. The brace is typically worn until the individual reaches skeletal maturity and then is gradually weaned off. The greatest risk of scoliosis progression occurs during the adolescent growth spurt and decreases once skeletal maturity is reached. It is not common for adolescents with idiopathic scoliosis to have associated back pain; those with back pain should be evaluated for other etiologies and treated accordingly. An individual with idiopathic scoliosis can participate in sports activities most of the time; participation in sports activity alone does not constitute a requirement for corrective bracing.

2. The correct answer is C.

Scheuermann disease/kyphosis most commonly involves the thoracic spine and predominantly affects adolescent males with characteristic vertebral body wedging and endplate abnormalities creating a progressive rigid kyphotic deformity. Ankylosing spondylitis is a seronegative spondyloarthropathy in juveniles and younger adults characterized by chronic inflammation in the axial skeleton leading to pathologic spine immobility (ankylosis) with changes including vertebral body squaring and marginal syndesmophyte formation creating the appearance of a "bamboo" spine. DISH is a noninflammatory disorder in adults with characteristic spinal ligament ossification and bridging osteophytes at multiple vertebral levels causing pathologic spine immobility. Congenital scoliosis refers to a structural spinal curve deformity resulting from embryonic developmental anomalies in vertebral body segmentation or formation (the most common being a hemivertebrae) and can coexist with other genetic disorders.

3. The correct answer is A.

The clinical presentation for this pediatric patient is most suggestive of lumbar discitis; however, osteomyelitis is also in the differential diagnosis. The etiology of discitis is most likely infectious with a hematogenous source due to the rich vascular supply of the vertebral endplates in children that decreases with age. Radiographs are usually negative in the first 3 weeks but can later show disc space narrowing and endplate sclerosis. Blood cultures are usually negative. ESR is usually elevated. A common causative organism is *Staphylococcus aureus*. Discitis usually responds well to antibiotics and rest. Imaging via magnetic resonance imaging (MRI) is appropriate to support the diagnosis and rule out other causes. Bone scan can also confirm the diagnosis. Guillain-Barré syndrome (autoimmune) or a spinal tumor (malignancy) can present similarly but are less likely in the absence of weakness and other neurologic or systemic symptoms. Sprain/strain injury is less likely given no clear history of trauma and usually does not involve elevation in WBC or ESR.

4. The correct answer is C.

Ortolani test is used to determine if a dislocated hip in a newborn or infant can be reduced. Passive hip abduction can be used to evaluate for a hip dislocation if restriction is noted on one or both sides with maximal abduction of each hip, but it does not involve attempting to relocate the hip. Galeazzi test evaluates for a unilateral hip dislocation by flexing the bilateral hips and comparing each side for a relative shortening of the affected limb as evidenced by lower knee height level. Barlow test evaluates for hip instability by applying lateral or posterior pressure over the lesser trochanters while the hips are held in a flexed and adducted position; a positive test is indicated by the hip dislocating or subluxing over the posterior acetabular rim.

5. The correct answer is A.

The Pavlik harness is used in neonates and infants with early DDH to encourage gradual spontaneous reduction and stabilization of the hip by maintaining hip flexion and preventing adduction while allowing joint movement with a failure rate of 10% or less in this age group if initiated promptly. There is a risk of avascular necrosis with hip bracing, and the Pavlik harness is usually not prescribed in children older than 6 months and in those whose hips are irreducible. The condition is more difficult to treat beyond age 6 months and would next entail a trial of splinting or a spica cast, followed by eventual surgical intervention for those who failed a trial of closed reduction. Early detection and treatment of DDH is essential to prevent the need for extensive corrective surgery; thus, early treatment (not observation) is recommended in most cases.

6. The correct answer is D.

Growing pains are a benign, self-limiting condition of uncertain etiology that affect the pediatric population and are most commonly in the thighs, calves, or behind the knees. The cramping or throbbing pain typically occurs at the end of the day or night and can wake the child up from sleep. RLS can often be misdiagnosed as growing pains, but the difference between the conditions is that the unpleasant leg sensations in RLS are accompanied by an urge to move the legs and are relieved by movement. RLS is also a persistent condition and can continue to affect a person into adulthood. RLS has a primary genetic link and, secondarily, can be caused by iron deficiency. Akathisia is a side effect of antipsychotic drugs manifested by restlessness and an urge to move the body. Patellofemoral pain syndrome presents as anterior knee pain that typically worsens with physical activity and prolonged bent-knee positioning.

7. The correct answer is D.

Legg-Calvé-Perthes disease predominantly affects male children between the ages of 4 and 10 years and is characterized by avascular necrosis of the femoral epiphysis with variable radiographic findings depending on the disease stage; femoral head sclerosis, fragmentation, reossification, or remodeling can be seen. Slipped capital femoral epiphysis is characterized by displacement of the femoral head on the femoral neck to varying degrees in preadolescent to adolescent. A chronic stress reaction is a precursor to a stress fracture of the hip. Transient synovitis of the hip is a benign and self-limited disorder that must be distinguished from a septic hip.

8. The correct answer is C.

SCFE is displacement of the proximal femoral epiphysis off of the femoral neck, occurring predominantly in preadolescent-adolescent males with obesity as a risk factor. The treatment is almost always surgical as SCFE will continue to be painful and progress further if left untreated and increase the chances of developing avascular necrosis, premature osteoarthritis, and functional abnormalities. Thus, observation is not advised, and physical therapy will not correct the slip. The consensus of orthopedic surgeons still favors single pin fixation in situ for stable nonacute SCFE although alternative surgical techniques have been developed. For unstable SCFE, urgent gentle reduction, decompression, and internal fixation are favored. Some surgically treated patients with SCFE will eventually require future hip arthroplasty.

9. The correct answer is B.

Delayed skeletal maturation has been found in children with Legg-Calvé-Perthes disease and might have etiologic significance; however, it does not indicate a poor prognosis. Disease onset in children with younger bone age actually allows more time for femoral epiphysis reossification and remodeling, and often, the femoral head retains its spherical shape by the time the individual reaches skeletal maturity. The prognosis is generally good in children who present with the disease at an earlier age (younger than 6 years) with less than 50% of femoral head involvement. Some factors for poor prognosis include loss of height in the lateral one-third of the femoral epiphysis ("lateral pillar collapse"), hip abduction contracture ("stiff hip"), and older age at diagnosis with >50% involvement of the femoral head.

10. The correct answer is A.

The Scoliosis Research Society (SRS) criteria for radiographic idiopathic scoliosis is a spine curve of minimum 10 degrees in the frontal/coronal plane measured typically on standing spine radiographs using the Cobb angle measurement technique. Of note, there can be a margin of error of ±5 degrees in the measurement. Axial rotation is measured at the apical vertebrae. Additional clinical assessment to rule out congenital or acquired disease and functional causes is important. Observation and interval follow-up radiographs monitor if there is progression of the curve with more frequent follow-up during the pubertal growth spurt. The risk of further progression in adulthood for idiopathic scoliosis increases in curves greater than 30 degrees. Curves greater than 40 to 45 degrees generally require surgical management as these will likely continue to progress in adulthood with serious secondary health complications.

11. The correct answer is B.

The widely used mnemonic CRITOE can be used to describe the order of appearance of the secondary ossification centers in the pediatric elbow: capitellum, radius, internal (medial) epicondyle, trochlea, olecranon, external (lateral) epicondyle. The capitellum develops as a single smooth ossification center at an age range of typically 3 months to 2 years. It is important to be able to identify the typical chronology and appearance of elbow ossification centers as they can be confused with fractures. Contralateral radiographs are recommended for comparison when unilateral injury is suspected.

12. The correct answer is D.

"Little League elbow" describes a spectrum of elbow repetitive overuse injuries in skeletally immature individuals who participate in throwing sports. The mechanism of injury involves valgus stress on the medial structures and compression of the lateral structures of the elbow during the throwing. The repetitive contraction of the flexor-pronator muscle mass produces traction forces on the apophysis of the medial humeral epicondyle which can lead to microtrauma and inflammation. Thus, the common manifestation of "Little League elbow" is medial epicondylitis/apophysitis. This can progress to fragmentation or avulsion at the medial epicondyle. The secondary compression of the lateral structures from valgus stress can lead to osteochondritis dissecans of the capitellum, posterior impingement, and radiocapitellar compression.

13. The correct answer is A.

The apophysis is a cartilaginous secondary ossification center in skeletally immature individuals, where muscle origins and tendon insertions occur. The apophysis cartilage is most vulnerable to overuse injury from repetitive tensile forces, causing microfractures and inflammation (i.e., apophysitis). This is further exacerbated during periods of rapid growth when muscle and tendon inflexibility occur. Examples of these apophyseal injuries include Sever disease (posterior calcaneus), Osgood-Schlatter disease (tibial tuberosity), Sinding-Larsen-Johansson syndrome (inferior patella), and Little League elbow (medial humeral epicondyle). Stress injury to the epiphyseal plates can occur due to compression, tension, or shear depending on the mechanical forces on the long bone from the repetitive activity. Diaphyseal and metaphyseal stress injuries are not common in skeletally immature individuals; injuries to these regions usually represent fractures due to acute trauma.

14. The correct answer is C.

The clinical presentation is most consistent with Osgood-Schlatter disease, a generally self-limited disease characterized by traction apophysitis of the tibial tubercle at the patellar tendon insertion site. This condition usually resolves by the time the individual reaches skeletal maturity and responds to conservative symptomatic management. Immobilization is rarely required for Osgood-Schlatter disease. Osteochondritis dissecans of the femoral condyle is a separate, unrelated condition that does require immobilization in symptomatic individuals. Surgical management is rarely required for Osgood-Schlatter disease. Corticosteroid injections generally are not recommended as there is a risk of subcutaneous atrophy.

15. The correct answer is A.

The rectus femoris muscle originates at the AIIS. The sartorius and tensor fasciae latae muscles originate at the anterior superior iliac spine (ASIS). The iliopsoas inserts on the lesser trochanter. Apophyseal avulsion fractures at the AIIS typically occur in adolescent athletes (mostly in running and kicking sports) due to sudden, forceful eccentric contraction of the rectus femoris muscle while the hip is hyperextended and the knee flexed. Management is conservative in cases of nondisplaced or minimally displaced fractures.

16. The correct answer is B.
Unilateral fibrosis and shortening of the sternocleidomastoid (SCM) muscle occur in congenital muscular torticollis, causing an abnormal head/neck posture in the direction of the typical muscle contraction. When contracting alone, the SCM normally flexes the head/neck to the ipsilateral side and simultaneously rotates it to the contralateral side. Thus, right-sided torticollis would appear as the head/neck tilted to the right and the chin rotated toward the left side. The opposite is true for left-sided torticollis, where the head would appear tilted toward the left and the chin rotated toward the right side. Thorough evaluation should be undertaken to rule out other causes of torticollis, and the bilateral hips should be examined as developmental hip dysplasia can coexist in some children with congenital muscular torticollis.

17. The correct answer is D.
Talipes equinovarus (also known as congenital clubfoot) occurs in 1 out of 1,000 births with a male predominance and is characterized by fixed ankle plantarflexion (equinus), hindfoot inversion (varus), and forefoot adduction (metatarsus adductus). It requires prompt orthopedic treatment, consisting of a trial of serial casting followed by surgery for any residual deformity. Talipes calcaneovalgus (calcaneovalgus foot) is a self-limited, semiflexible deformity where there the ankle is dorsiflexed and the hindfoot is everted. Congenital vertical talus (rocker bottom foot) is a rigid deformity where the ankle/hindfoot is plantarflexed and the midfoot joints are dislocated dorsally. Metatarsus adductus is a common, self-limited, and flexible deformity where the forefoot metatarsals are medially deviated (adducted) with a normal hindfoot and ankle; the rigid variant of the condition (metatarsus varus) requires more aggressive treatment.

18. The correct answer is C.
Dysplastic spondylolisthesis occurs when there is congenital malformation of the L5-S1 posterior elements and sacrum, allowing anterior slippage of the L5 vertebral body over the sacrum without a pars interarticularis defect. Although dysplastic spondylolisthesis is not as common as isthmic spondylolisthesis in children and adolescents, the dysplastic form has a higher risk of progression and more frequent associated neurologic symptoms. The degenerative and pathologic types of spondylolisthesis generally are not found in children and adolescents.

19. The correct answer is D.
The clinical presentation and imaging studies support a diagnosis of an active stress reaction or "prelysis" involving the right L5 pars interarticularis. Repetitive stress leads to local bone remodeling and increased uptake of radioactive tracer on SPECT, indicating a metabolically active lesion. The accompanying CT scan is negative for overt pars interarticularis fracture or defect (i.e., spondylolysis); hence, a stress reaction is the most appropriate description. A true spondylolysis would describe a scenario where the CT scan would show a fracture of the pars interarticularis, whether incomplete or complete. Spondylolisthesis refers to a forward slip of one vertebral body on the one below it; the imaging was negative for this finding. Spondylosis refers to degenerative changes in the lumbar spine that typically occur in adults.

20. The correct answer is C.

The nucleus pulposus of the intervertebral disc is derived from the notochord. The annulus fibrosis of the intervertebral disc is derived from mesenchyme. The vertebral body develops from sclerotomes. The neural tube develops into the spinal cord.

21. The correct answer is A.

The pauciarticular (oligoarticular) form of JIA involves one to four joints during the first 6 months of the disease and comprises the largest JIA clinical subtype. Pauciarticular JIA carries the risk of asymptomatic iridocyclitis and, if untreated, can lead to chronic ocular disease and vision loss. Iridocyclitis has been associated with positive serum antinuclear antibodies (ANA). Acute symptomatic iridocyclitis can be found in enthesitis-related arthritis.

22. The correct answer is B.

The polyarticular form of JIA involves five or more joints during the first 6 months of the disease and consists of rheumatoid factor–positive and rheumatoid factor–negative subgroups. Polyarticular JIA is known for more frequent hip joint involvement than other types, which sometimes can present as stiffness, rather than pain. Hip joint involvement is also commonly seen in enthesitis-related arthritis.

23. The correct answer is B.

The majority of patients with JIA are female. Most subtypes of JIA have sex ratios showing females more affected than males; the exceptions are systemic JIA (1:1 F:M ratio), enthesitis-related arthritis (1:7 F:M ratio), and undifferentiated arthritis (1:1 F:M ratio). Adult forms of RA also have a female predominance (2:1 F:M ratio). JIA more frequently involves large joints and the cervical spine than adult RA. Rheumatoid nodules are more common in adult RA than JIA.

24. The correct answer is C.

The systemic form of JIA, also known as Still disease, presents with arthritis in one or more joints accompanied or preceded by a fever of at least 2 weeks duration, documented to be daily for at least 3 days with one or more of the following: evanescent rash, lymphadenopathy, hepatosplenomegaly, and/or serositis. MAS is an uncommon but life-threatening complication of systemic JIA characterized by abnormal macrophage and T-cell proliferation with phagocytosis of mature and immature blood cells (hemophagocytosis), creating pancytopenia and coagulopathy. Clinical manifestations can include neurologic symptoms, hemorrhage, and hepatomegaly. Laboratory test can show pancytopenia, elevated liver enzymes, hypofibrinogenemia, and bone marrow aspirate showing hemophagocytosis.

25. The correct answer is A.

JIA occurs before age 16 years with arthritis lasting more than 6 weeks in one or more joints. Early identification, treatment, and rehabilitation can improve functional outcomes. Remission is possible for all disease subtypes, but those with polyarticular (five or more joints affected during the first 6 months) rheumatoid-positive disease tend to have a lower chance of remission when the course is unremitting. Hip joint arthritis can lead to significant disability in patients with JIA and poor functional outcomes.

26. The correct answer is C.
Cerebral palsy is a condition that occurs due to a brain injury that may happen at any time before, at the time of, or shortly after birth.

27. The correct answer is D.
Individuals with cerebral palsy often have additional issues related to their condition including difficulty with ambulation, seizures/epilepsy, mental retardation, as well as other problems.

28. The correct answer is D.
Spina bifida occulta is a type of neural tube defect in which the formation of the spine is abnormal, but the deficit is hidden by skin, hence the term *occulta*, meaning "hidden" in Latin.

29. The correct answer is A.
There are various forms of the condition spinal muscular atrophy. The motor neurons of the anterior horn cells are affected in all forms. Presentation and prognosis varies depending on the form.

30. The correct answer is C.
The Moro, or startle, reflex is a primitive reflex that normally disappears by about 6 months of age. It involves the baby spreading its arms out and then bringing them back in, usually crying.

31. The correct answer is A.
An IEP is designed for students who meet criteria for special education services. Although being on crutches due to chronic gait abnormalities may contribute to a child qualifying for special education services, an otherwise healthy child with a tibial fracture using crutches, who is expected to heal without long-term disability, is unlikely to be assessed for need for an IEP.

32. The correct answer is B.
Although patients with Klinefelter syndrome may be tall, the further information including the presence of scoliosis makes Marfan syndrome more likely in this patient. Over 50% of patients with Marfan syndrome may have scoliosis. Angelman syndrome is associated with significant mental retardation and other features making it unlikely a teenager with that syndrome would present by himself. Hunter syndrome is associated with typical facial characteristics which this patient is lacking.

33. The correct answer is D.
Although patients with Marfan syndrome tend to be tall, that syndrome is not significantly associated with infertility. Patients with Klinefelter syndrome are generally infertile without special assistance. The presentation of this patient is inconsistent with history of Angelman syndrome or of Hunter syndrome.

34. The correct answer is B.

Of the conditions listed, phenylketonuria is not classified as a lysosomal storage disease. Phenylketonuria results from a deficiency of the enzyme that breaks down the amino acid phenylalanine, resulting in increased levels which can lead to issues such as mental retardation.

35. The correct answer is D.

Risk factors for development of autism spectrum disorders include being born to older parents, having siblings with autism spectrum disorder, and particular medications taken during pregnancy, such as valproic acid. (Reference: Christensen J, Grønborg TK, Sørensen MJ, et al. Prenatal valproate exposure and risk of autism spectrum disorders and childhood autism. *JAMA.* 2013;309[16]:1696-1703.)

36. The correct answer is C.

Duchenne muscular dystrophy is the most common type of muscular dystrophy in children. Myotonic muscular dystrophy is the most common adult muscular dystrophy. Duchenne muscular dystrophy is an X-linked recessive disorder. Females generally do not exhibit signs/symptoms of the condition.

37. The correct answer is D.

TBI can be a significant cause of disability and even death. Common causes of TBI in infants and children include intentional injury (child abuse) and unintentional injuries such as falls and motor vehicle accidents.

38. The correct answer is B.

Of pediatric brain tumors, medulloblastoma is the most common malignancy. This condition is thought to comprise about 15% to 20% of pediatric brain tumors.

39. The correct answer is A.

Another name for a "functional murmur" is an "innocent murmur." They are relatively common in children and may disappear over time. This finding is not a cause for concern and would not in itself necessitate referral for further evaluation or inpatient admission.

40. The correct answer is C.

The 2015 guidelines from the American Heart Association and the American College of Cardiology state that "[i]t is recommended that athletes with small defects (<6 mm), normal right-sided heart volume, and no pulmonary hypertension should be allowed to participate in all sports *(Class I; Level of Evidence C)* . . . It is recommended that athletes with a large ASD and no pulmonary hypertension should be allowed to participate in all sports *(Class I; Level of Evidence C).*" Therefore, barring other issues, your daughter's best friend should be able to play on the high school basketball team. (Reference: Van Hare GF, Ackerman MJ, Evangelista JA, et al; for the American Heart Association Electrocardiography and Arrhythmias Committee of the Council on Clinical Cardiology, Council on Cardiovascular Disease in the Young, Council on Cardiovascular and Stroke Nursing, Council on Functional Genomics and Translational Biology, and the American College of Cardiology. Eligibility and disqualification recommendations for competitive athletes with cardiovascular abnormalities: task force 4: congenital heart disease: a scientific statement from the American Heart Association and American College of Cardiology. *Circulation.* 2015;132[22]:e281-e291.)

41. The correct answer is A.

Cystic fibrosis is an autosomal recessive condition. Carriers, individuals with one identified copy of the gene, are unlikely to exhibit symptoms.

42. The correct answer is C.

Compared to adults, pediatric patients generally experience worse pain management. Barriers include difficulties in medical providers assessing pediatric patients' pain levels due to lack of understanding of pain presentation in this population. (Reference: Ramira ML, Instone S, Clark MJ. Pediatric pain management: an evidence-based approach. *Pediatr Nurs.* 2016;42[1]:39-46, 49.)

43. The correct answer is D.

This patient may have conversion disorder. The diagnosis of malingering generally includes the criteria that the patient is consciously aware of "faking" their deficits, which it does not appear this patient is doing. Angelman syndrome would present with characteristic appearance and mannerisms which this patient does not have. Duchenne muscular dystrophy would be expected to present with recognizable symptoms earlier in development. The patient's age, gender, and the presence of a precipitating life stressor are also in line with common presentation of this condition.

44. The correct answer is A.

In general, law states that minors (usually defined as those younger than 18 years) cannot give informed consent to participate in research. Therefore, this 9-year-old patient is unable to give informed consent. In general, if both parents agree, and the patient gives his approval, called "assent," then the patient may participate. However, the patient may also dissent, and in that case, his dissent should also be respected.

45. The correct answer is A.

Definitions of disability vary, but in general, a common way to think about whether an individual is "disabled" is whether they are able to meet their expected role(s) in society given their age and other considerations. So when we ask if a child can be considered "disabled" due to not being able to work, an appropriate answer would be no because working is not a usual societal role for a child.

Board Review Points ("Pearls") for Pediatric Rehabilitation

Pediatric Musculoskeletal Medicine

- Growing pains are a benign, self-limiting condition of uncertain etiology that affect the pediatric population and are most commonly in the thighs, calves, or behind the knees. The cramping or throbbing pain typically occurs at the end of the day or night and can wake the child up from sleep. RLS can often be misdiagnosed as growing pains, but the difference between the conditions is that the unpleasant leg sensations in RLS are accompanied by an urge to move the legs and are relieved by movement. RLS is also a persistent condition and can continue to affect a person into adulthood. RLS has a primary genetic link and, secondarily, can be caused by iron deficiency. Akathisia is a side effect of antipsychotic drugs manifested by restlessness and an urge to move the body. Patellofemoral pain syndrome presents as anterior knee pain that typically worsens with physical activity and prolonged bent-knee positioning.

- The SRS criteria for radiographic idiopathic scoliosis is a spine curve of minimum 10 degrees in the frontal/coronal plane measured typically on standing spine radiographs using the Cobb angle measurement technique. Of note, there can be a margin of error of ±5 degrees in the measurement. Axial rotation is measured at the apical vertebrae. Additional clinical assessment to rule out congenital or acquired disease and functional causes is important. Observation and interval follow-up radiographs monitor if there is progression of the curve with more frequent follow-up during the pubertal growth spurt. The risk of further progression in adulthood for idiopathic scoliosis increases in curves greater than 30 degrees. Curves greater than 40 to 45 degrees generally require surgical management as these will likely continue to progress in adulthood with serious secondary health complications.

- The nucleus pulposus of the intervertebral disc is derived from the notochord. The annulus fibrosis of the intervertebral disc is derived from mesenchyme. The vertebral body develops from sclerotomes. The neural tube develops into the spinal cord.

- JIA occurs before age 16 years with arthritis lasting more than 6 weeks in one or more joints. Early identification, treatment, and rehabilitation can improve functional outcomes. Remission is possible for all disease subtypes, but those with polyarticular (five or more joints affected during the first 6 months) rheumatoid-positive disease tend to have a lower chance of remission when the course is unremitting. Hip joint arthritis can lead to significant disability in patients with JIA and poor functional outcomes.

Pediatric Neurologic Disorders

- Cerebral palsy is a condition that occurs due to a brain injury that may happen at any time before, at the time of, or shortly after birth. Individuals with cerebral palsy often have additional issues related to their condition including difficulty with ambulation, seizures/epilepsy, and mental retardation as well as other problems.

- Risk factors for development of autism spectrum disorders include being born to older parents, having siblings with autism spectrum disorder, and particular medications taken during pregnancy, such as valproic acid. (Reference: Christensen J, Grønborg TK, Sørensen MJ, et al. Prenatal valproate exposure and risk of autism spectrum disorders and childhood autism. *JAMA.* 2013;309[16]:1696-1703.)

General Pediatric Rehabilitation

- In general, law states that minors (usually defined as those younger than 18 years) cannot give informed consent to participate in research/procedures. In general, if both parents agree, and the patient gives his or her approval, called "assent," then the patient may participate. However, the patient may also dissent, and in that case, the child's dissent should also be respected.

■ Definitions of disability vary, but in general, a common way to think about whether an individual is "disabled" is whether they are able to meet their expected role(s) in society given their age and other considerations. So when we ask if a child can be considered "disabled" due to not being able to work, an appropriate answer would be no because working is not a usual societal role for a child.

REFERENCES & SUGGESTED READINGS

American Cancer Society. Types of brain and spinal cord tumors in children. http://www.cancer .org/cancer/braincnstumorsinchildren/detailedguide/brain-and-spinal-cord-tumors-in -children-typesof-brainand-spinal-tumors. Accessed December 26, 2016.

Atteritano M, David A, Bagnato G, et al. Haemophagocytic syndrome in rheumatic patients: a systematic review. *Eur Rev Med Pharmacol Sci*. 2012;16(10):1414-1424.

Bernhardt DT. Knee and leg injuries. In: Birrer RB, Griesemer BA, Cataletto M, eds. *Pediatric Sports Medicine for Primary Care*. Philadelphia, PA: Lippincott Williams & Wilkins; 2002:411-414.

Braddom RL, Chan L, Harrast ME, et al, eds. *Physical Medicine and Rehabilitation*. 4th ed. St. Louis, MO: Saunders; 2011.

Brown R, Husain M, McHugh K, Novelli V, Jones D. Discitis in young children. *J Bone Joint Surg Br*. 2001;83(1):106-111.

Campbell RS, Grainger AJ, Hide IG, Papastefanou S, Greenough CG. Juvenile spondylolysis: a comparative analysis of CT, SPECT, and MR. *Skeletal Radiol*. 2005;34:63-73.

Centers for Disease Control and Prevention. Facts about ASD. https://www.cdc.gov/ncbddd /autism/facts.html. Accessed December 26, 2016.

Christensen J, Grønborg TK, Sørensen MJ, et al. Prenatal valproate exposure and risk of autism spectrum disorders and childhood autism. *JAMA*. 2013;309(16):1696-1703.

Frontera WR, DeLisa JA, Gans B, et al, eds. *DeLisa's Physical Medicine & Rehabilitation: Principles and Practice*. 5th ed. Philadelphia, PA: Lippincott Williams & Wilkins; 2010.

Galen JO, Hicks JE, Gerber LH. Rehabilitation of the patient with rheumatic fiseases. In: Frontera WR, DeLisa JA, Gans B, et al, eds. *DeLisa's Physical Medicine & Rehabilitation: Principles and Practice*. 5th ed. Philadelphia, PA: Lippincott Williams & Wilkins; 2010:1061-1065.

Ganley TJ, Spiegel DA, Gregg JR, et al. Overuse injuries to the physes in young athletes: a clinical and basic science review. *Univ Penn Orthop J*. 1998;11:27-35.

Houghton KM. Review for the generalist: evaluation of pediatric hip pain. *Pediatr Rheumatol Online J*. 2009;7:10. http://www.ped-rheum.com/content/7/1/10.

Isdale IC. Hip disease in juvenile rheumatoid arthritis. *Ann Rheum Dis*. 1970;29:603-608.

Negrini S, Aulisa AG, Aulisa L, et al. 2011 SOSORT guidelines: orthopaedic and rehabilitation treatment of idiopathic scoliosis during growth. *Scoliosis*. 2012;7:3. http://scoliosisjournal .com/content/7/1/3.

Larson AN, McIntosh AL, Trousdale RT, Lewallen DG. Avascular necrosis most common indication for hip arthroplasty in patients with slipped capital femoral epiphysis. *J Pediatr Orthop*. 2010;30(8):767-773.

LeBlanc KE. Scoliosis. In: Birrer RB, Griesemer BA, Cataletto M, eds. *Pediatric Sports Medicine for Primary Care*. Philadelphia, PA: Lippincott Williams & Wilkins; 2002:222-225.

Loder RT, Dietz FR. What is the best evidence for the treatment of slipped capital femoral epiphysis. *J Pediatr Orthop*. 2012;32(suppl 2):S158-S165.

Lonstein JE. Spondylolisthesis in children: cause, natural history, and management. *Spine*. 1999;24(24):2640-2648.

Maheswaran M, Kushida CA. Restless legs syndrome in children. *MedGenMed*. 2006;8(2):79. http://www.ncbi.nlm.nih.gov/pmc/articles/PMC1785221/.

Malina RM. Growth and maturation applications to children and adolescents in sports. In: Birrer RB, Griesemer BA, Cataletto M, eds. *Pediatric Sports Medicine for Primary Care*. Philadelphia, PA: Lippincott Williams & Wilkins; 2002:39-58.

National Institute of Child Health and Human Development. Klinefelter syndrome (KS): other facts. https://www.nichd.nih.gov/health/topics/klinefelter/conditioninfo/pages/faqs.aspx. Accessed December 26, 2016.

Paul SM. Scoliosis and other spinal deformities. In: Frontera WR, DeLisa JA, Gans B, et al, eds. *DeLisa's Physical Medicine & Rehabilitation: Principles and Practice*. 5th ed. Philadelphia, PA: Lippincott Williams & Wilkins; 2010:883-906.

Prieur AM, Chèdeville G. Prognostic factors in juvenile idiopathic arthritis. *Curr Rheumatol Rep*. 2001;3(5):371-378.

Rab GT. Pediatric orthopedic surgery. In: Skinner HB, ed. *Current Diagnosis & Treatment in Orthopedics*. 4th ed. New York, NY: Lange Medical; 2006:589-637.

Ramira ML, Instone S, Clark MJ. Pediatric pain management: an evidence-based approach. *Pediatr Nurs*. 2016;42(1):39-46, 49.

Rossi R, Alexander M, Cuccurullo S. Pediatric rehabilitation. In: Cuccurullo SJ, ed. *Physical Medicine & Rehabilitation Board Review*. 2nd ed. New York, NY: Demos Medical; 2010:645-803.

Rostom S, Amine B, Bensabbah R, Abouga R, Hajjaj-Hassouni N. Hip involvement in juvenile idiopathic arthritis. *Clin Rheumatol*. 2008;27(6):791-794.

Shaw JL, O'Connor FG. Elbow injuries. In: Birrer RB, Griesemer BA, Cataletto M, eds. *Pediatric Sports Medicine for Primary Care*. Philadelphia, PA: Lippincott Williams & Wilkins; 2002:350-366.

Simon LM. Thigh, hip, and pelvis injuries. In: Birrer RB, Griesemer BA, Cataletto M, eds. *Pediatric Sports Medicine for Primary Care*. Philadelphia, PA: Lippincott Williams & Wilkins; 2002:385-396.

Simon LM, Jih W, Buller JC. Back pain and injuries. In: Birrer RB, Griesemer BA, Cataletto M, eds. *Pediatric Sports Medicine for Primary Care*. Philadelphia, PA: Lippincott Williams & Wilkins; 2002:222-225.

Tripathy S, Sen R, Dhatt S, Goyal T. Legg-Calve-Perthes disease current concepts. *WebmedCentral Orthop*. 2010;1(11):WMC001173.

Van Hare GF, Ackerman MJ, Evangelista JA, et al; for the American Heart Association Electrocardiography and Arrhythmias Committee of the Council on Clinical Cardiology, Council on Cardiovascular Disease in the Young, Council on Cardiovascular and Stroke Nursing, Council on Functional Genomics and Translational Biology, and the American College of Cardiology. Eligibility and disqualification recommendations for competitive athletes with cardiovascular abnormalities: task force 4: congenital heart disease: a scientific statement from the American Heart Association and American College of Cardiology. *Circulation*. 2015;132(22):e281-e291.

Zukotynski K, Curtis C, Grant F, Micheli L, Treves T. The value of SPECT in the detection of stress injury to the pars interarticularis in patients with low back pain. *J Orthop Surg Res*. 2010;5:13. http://www.josr-online.com/content/5/1/13.

Traumatic Brain Injury

1. A major cause of traumatic brain injury in those 65 years or older is

   A. falling.

   B. gunshot wound.

   C. abuse/violence.

   D. unknown cause.

2. Which of the following is not a common traumatic brain injury (TBI) severity measure?

   A. length of loss of consciousness

   B. the Glasgow Coma Scale

   C. presence of limb paresthesia

   D. length of posttraumatic amnesia

3. Who is not normally considered a part of the traumatic brain injury (TBI) interdisciplinary care team for a patient with severe brain injury?

   A. the spouse

   B. the rehabilitation physician

   C. the rehabilitation nurse

   D. the psychologist

4. After a severe traumatic brain injury (TBI), increase in sympathetic activation can result in

A. decreased sweating.

B. hypotension.

C. bradycardia.

D. tachycardia.

5. When should a swallowing evaluation be performed in a patient with traumatic brain injury (TBI)?

A. 5 days after the injury

B. upon triage at the emergency department

C. upon admission to the acute care hospital

D. when the patient is medically stable and alert

6. Pituitary dysfunction can occur in

A. mild traumatic brain injury (TBI).

B. moderate TBI.

C. severe TBI.

D. all of the above

7. After traumatic brain injury (TBI), _____ may occur as an adverse effect of the injury.

A. improved cognition

B. stable mood

C. delayed gastric emptying

D. both A and B

8. _____ may occur after traumatic brain injury (TBI).

A. Abnormal tone

B. Heterotopic ossification

C. Seizures

D. all of the above

9. Heterotopic ossification involves the formation of bone in

   A. an abnormal location.

   B. soft tissue.

   C. both A and B

   D. the skeletal system during fetal development.

10. It is _____ that muscle contracture refers to, in part, shortening of the muscle. This condition _____ treated with stretching, bracing, medications, or even surgery.

   A. true; should be

   B. true; should not be

   C. not true; should be

   D. not true; should not be

11. Injury related to direct blow to the head would best be classified as

   A. secondary traumatic brain injury (TBI).

   B. primary TBI.

   C. initial TBI.

   D. acute TBI.

12. In the context of traumatic brain injury (TBI), DAI refers to

   A. primary focal brain injury.

   B. primary brain injury.

   C. primary diffuse brain injury.

   D. secondary brain injury.

13. Focal brain injuries include all of the following, EXCEPT

   A. DAI.

   B. epidural hematoma.

   C. subdural hematoma.

   D. penetrating trauma.

14. For evaluation of new closed head mild traumatic brain injuries, _____ would not normally be used.

A. skull x-ray

B. brain magnetic resonance imaging (MRI)

C. both A and B

D. head computed tomography (CT)

15. Electroencephalography (EEG) is very useful in evaluation of mild traumatic brain injury (TBI) in _____ patients.

A. 50% of

B. few if any

C. 30% to 50% of

D. the majority of

16. In severe traumatic brain injury (TBI), studies have found that both longer duration of loss of consciousness and posttraumatic amnesia are associated with worse functional recovery.

A. no

B. This is true for loss of consciousness but not posttraumatic amnesia.

C. yes

D. This is true for posttraumatic amnesia but not loss of consciousness.

17. Which of the following functional measures is specific to those with brain injury?

A. Mayo-Portland Adaptability Inventory

B. Community Integration Questionnaire

C. A, B, and D

D. Craig Handicap Assessment and Reporting Technique

18. _____ is a warning sign that mild traumatic brain injury (TBI) requires further evaluation.

   A. Headache

   B. Nausea

   C. A and B

   D. Seizure

19. Do patients with traumatic brain injury (TBI) have a high metabolic demand and require appropriate nutrition for improved outcomes?

   A. No, patients with TBI have a lower metabolic demand than those without TBI.

   B. No, patients with TBI have the same metabolic demand as those without TBI.

   C. No, patients with TBI don't require special attention to nutrition.

   D. yes

20. A negative aspect of the use of an indwelling Foley catheter in a patient with traumatic brain injury (TBI) is that

   A. it increases the risk of falls.

   B. a confused patient may pull out the catheter.

   C. the presence of an indwelling catheter means that bladder training cannot be performed.

   D. both B and C

21. The association between traumatic brain injury (TBI) and subsequent development of Alzheimer-type dementia is

   A. significant only for moderate and severe TBI.

   B. significant for mild, moderate, and severe TBI.

   C. nonexistent.

   D. described by an odds ratio of 15 to 20.

22. Do posttraumatic stress disorder (PTSD) and traumatic brain injury (TBI) have similar symptoms?

A. yes

B. no

C. only in 25% of cases

D. in about 75% of cases

23. A diagnosis of postconcussion syndrome must include history of head injury

A. in all cases.

B. if a patient can remember it.

C. with seizures.

D. unless the injury was due to blast exposure.

24. A patient with a history of traumatic brain injury (TBI) experiences involuntary stiffening of his arm but can still talk and respond appropriately during the event. This is most likely

A. an absence seizure.

B. a simple partial seizure.

C. a generalized tonic clonic seizure.

D. an absence or generalized tonic clonic seizure.

25. Fatigue is a _____ symptom after traumatic brain injury (TBI) and _____ related to the TBI.

A. rare; is usually

B. rare; may be

C. common; may be

D. common; is always

ANSWER KEY WITH EXPLANATIONS

1. The correct answer is A.

The major causes of traumatic brain injury differ in the different age groups. Among those individuals aged 65 years and older, falls are a primary etiology. Information from National Vital Statistics System Mortality Data found that falls were not as significant a causal factor in younger age groups as compared to those 65 years and older. (Reference: Centers for Disease Control and Prevention. Percent distributions of TBI-related deaths by age group and injury mechanism—United States, 2006–2010. https://www.cdc.gov /traumaticbraininjury/data/dist_death.html. Accessed June 20, 2017.)

2. The correct answer is C.

Common measures to assess the severity of TBI include the Glasgow Coma Scale and presence and duration of posttraumatic amnesia and loss of consciousness. The Glasgow Coma Scale measures motor, verbal, and eye response to create a score corresponding to severity of brain injury. The presence of paresthesia in the limbs is not commonly used to grade the severity of a brain injury.

3. The correct answer is A.

Although the patient's spouse plays an important role in providing support postinjury, he or she is not usually considered a part of the interdisciplinary care team for the patient in the sense that the spouse's primary role is not to provide specific medical evaluation and treatment. Rehabilitation physicians; nurses; therapists including physical, occupational, and speech therapists; and psychologists are all integral parts of the care team for patients with severe brain injuries. Other providers may also provide care for the patient including recreational and vocational therapists, neurosurgeons, neurologists, and others, depending on the patient's needs.

4. The correct answer is D.

After severe TBI, activation of the sympathetic nervous system can result in tachycardia, increased diaphoresis, hypertension, and other symptoms. These are signs of autonomic dysregulation postinjury.

5. The correct answer is D.

Issues with swallowing are common after a TBI, especially with increased severity of injury. In general, a complete swallowing evaluation should be performed when the patient is medically stable and generally alert, although initial evaluations may be performed earlier. As swallowing status changes, further assessments may be needed by speech therapy.

6. The correct answer is D.

Pituitary dysfunction, specifically hypopituitarism, can occur in mild, moderate, or severe TBI.

7. **The correct answer is C.**
Although depending on the severity of the TBI, certainly a patient may experience stable mood and improved cognition as part of the natural recovery from the injury, the only answer choice that indicates a possible adverse effect of TBI is C, delayed gastric emptying.

8. **The correct answer is D.**
A myriad of additional issues may arise after TBI including abnormal tone, seizures, and heterotopic ossification.

9. **The correct answer is C.**
Heterotopic ossification refers to the development of bone in an abnormal body site, usually in the soft tissue. It may occur after traumatic brain injury (TBI).

10. **The correct answer is A.**
Muscle contracture describes a deficit in normal range of motion due in part to muscle shortening. Muscle contracture and associated spasticity is treated with passive and active stretching, bracing, medications, and possibly even surgery. This condition can affect maintenance of adequate hygiene and can contribute to pain and functional impairment, so it should be treated if possible.

11. **The correct answer is B.**
TBI is often categorized as primary injury versus secondary injury, with primary injury referring to brain injury that occurs at the time of the injury event, and secondary injury referring to injury that occurs as subsequent processes unfold. Of course, descriptive terms such as initial or acute injury may be used but are not the correct answer in this case as the question did not discuss timeline/history.

12. **The correct answer is C.**
In the context of TBI, DAI stands for diffuse axonal injury, referring to injury not limited to focal areas of the brain. DAI is a descriptor for a type of primary brain injury; therefore, it would be appropriate to call it a primary diffuse brain injury.

13. **The correct answer is A.**
DAI refers to diffuse axonal injury, by definition a diffuse brain injury. Epidural and subdural hematomas and trauma related to penetration of the skull by an object would be more focal processes.

14. **The correct answer is C.**
Current guidelines for evaluation of new closed head mild traumatic brain injuries indicate that skull x-ray and brain MRI would not normally be used. Noncontrast head CT would be appropriate for patients with Glasgow Coma Scale scores of 14 or 15 under certain conditions such as severe headache. (Reference: Jagoda AS, Bazarian JJ, Brunes JJ Jr, et al. Clinical policy: neuroimaging and decision making in adult mild traumatic brain injury in the acute setting. *Ann Emerg Med*. 2008;52[6]:714-718.)

15. The correct answer is B.

Because there are no particularly clear EEG findings commonly associated specifically with mild TBI either acutely or over time, EEG is not generally considered very useful in the evaluation of mild TBI.

16. The correct answer is C.

In severe TBI, studies have found that both longer duration of loss of consciousness and posttraumatic amnesia are associated with worse functional recovery.

17. The correct answer is C.

There are many functional measures that can be used to assess those with traumatic brain injury (TBI). The Mayo-Portland Adaptability Inventory, Community Integration Questionnaire, and Craig Handicap Assessment and Reporting Technique all target assessment of those with brain injury.

18. The correct answer is D.

Seizure is a warning sign that mild TBI requires further evaluation. Headache and nausea are common usual features of mild TBI.

19. The correct answer is D.

Patients with TBI have a higher metabolic demand and require appropriate nutrition for improved outcomes.

20. The correct answer is D.

If possible, it is good to remove an indwelling Foley catheter to reduce the risk of urinary tract infection as well as the risk of injury if a confused patient accidently pulls out the catheter. Removal of a urinary catheter allows for bladder training. Although it is possible that the catheter tubing may predispose to falls in an ambulatory patient, on the other hand, the presence of a urinary catheter means the patient is not getting up from bed specifically for urination, and in that sense, decreases the risk of falls.

21. The correct answer is A.

Current literature finds a significant association for moderate to severe TBI and subsequent development of Alzheimer-type dementia years later. The association between mild TBI and future Alzheimer dementia is not clear. An odds ratio of 15 to 20 would indicate a very strong association between moderate to severe TBI and Alzheimer dementia, and current literature does not indicate an association this strong.

22. The correct answer is A.

PTSD and TBI have similar symptoms including sleep and memory impairment and irritability.

23. The correct answer is A.

In general, the diagnosis of postconcussion syndrome must include history of head injury in all cases. Specific features of the head injury, and associated symptoms, vary depending on the criteria used.

24. The correct answer is B.

The best answer regarding the patient's seizure type is simple partial seizure because he or she does not lose consciousness and is able to respond appropriately. Generally, absence and generalized tonic clonic seizures would include an alteration in consciousness.

25. The correct answer is C.

Fatigue is a common symptom after TBI and may be related to the TBI; however, as fatigue is a common nonspecific symptom overall, other possible causes must be evaluated.

Board Review Points ("Pearls") for Traumatic Brain Injury

- The major causes of traumatic brain injury differ in the different age groups. Among those individuals aged 65 years and older, falls are a primary etiology. Information from National Vital Statistics System Mortality Data found that falls were not as significant a causal factor in younger age groups as compared to those 65 years and older. (Reference: Centers for Disease Control and Prevention. Percent distributions of TBI-related deaths by age group and injury mechanism—United States, 2006–2010. https://www.cdc.gov/traumaticbraininjury/data/dist_death.html. Accessed June 20, 2017.)

- Common measures to assess the severity of traumatic brain injury include the Glasgow Coma Scale and presence and duration of posttraumatic amnesia and loss of consciousness. The Glasgow Coma Scale measures motor, verbal, and eye response to create a score corresponding to severity of brain injury. The presence of paresthesia in the limbs is not commonly used to grade the severity of a brain injury.

- Traumatic brain injury is often categorized as primary injury versus secondary injury, with primary injury referring to brain injury that occurs at the time of the injury event, and secondary injury referring to injury that occurs as subsequent processes unfold.

- After severe TBI, activation of the sympathetic nervous system can result in tachycardia, increased diaphoresis, hypertension, and other symptoms. These are signs of autonomic dysregulation postinjury.

- Issues with swallowing are common after a TBI, especially with increased severity of injury. In general, a complete swallowing evaluation should be performed when the patient is medically stable and generally alert, although initial evaluations may be performed earlier. As swallowing status changes, further assessments may be needed by speech therapy.

- Pituitary dysfunction, specifically hypopituitarism, can occur in mild, moderate, or severe TBI.

- A myriad of additional issues may arise post-TBI including abnormal tone, seizures, and heterotopic ossification.

REFERENCES & SUGGESTED READINGS

Braddom RL, Chan L, Harrast ME, et al, eds. *Physical Medicine and Rehabilitation*. 4th ed. St. Louis, MO: Saunders; 2011.

Centers for Disease Control and Prevention. Percent distributions of TBI-related deaths by age group and injury mechanism—United States, 2006–2010. https://www.cdc.gov /traumaticbraininjury/data/dist_death.html. Accessed June 20, 2017.

Comprehensive Epilepsy Center. Seizure types. http://epilepsy.yale.edu/care/information/types.aspx. Accessed July 9, 2017.

Jagoda AS, Bazarian JJ, Brunes JJ Jr, et al. Clinical policy: neuroimaging and decision making in adult mild traumatic brain injury in the acute setting. *Ann Emerg Med*. 2008;52(6):714-718.

Kung WM, Tsai SH, Chiue WT, et al. Correlation between Glasgow Coma score components and survival in patients with traumatic brain injury. *Injury*. 2011;42(9):940-944.

Olsen AB, Hetz RA, Xue H, et al. Effects of traumatic brain injury on intestinal contractility. *Neurogastroenterol Motil*. 2013;25(7):593-e463.

Zasler ND, Katz DI, Zafonte RD, Arciniegas DB, Bullock MR, Kreutzer JS. *Brain Injury Medicine: Principles and Practice*. 2nd ed. New York, NY: Demos Medical; 2013.

Neuromuscular Disorders and Other Neurologic Conditions

Types of Multiple Sclerosis

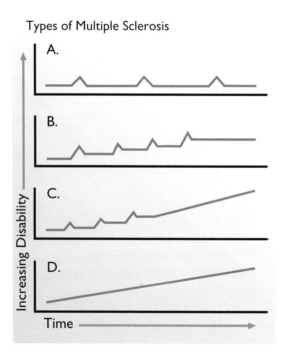

Adapted with permission from the Anatomical Chart Company. *Understanding Multiple Sclerosis Anatomical Chart*. Philadelphia, PA: Lippincott Williams & Wilkins; 2006.

1. Which of the given graphs best depicts the secondary progressive form of multiple sclerosis (MS)?

   A. A

   B. B

   C. C

   D. D

2. Which type of multiple sclerosis (MS) typically develops much later in life than the other forms, equally affects males and females, and often starts with motor weakness?

   A. relapsing-remitting

   B. secondary progressive

   C. primary progressive

   D. progressive-relapsing

3. Regarding magnetic resonance imaging (MRI) findings in multiple sclerosis (MS):

   A. Clinical symptoms and physical examination findings are better indicators of disease activity than abnormal MRI findings.

   B. The classic MRI findings are T2 hypointense cortical lesions.

   C. Enhancing lesions seen on T1 weighted images after gadolinium represent active blood–brain barrier breakdown.

   D. The presence of MRI lesions in isolated cases of optic neuritis does not increase the future risk of developing MS.

4. Which diagnostic test is LEAST helpful in establishing a diagnosis of multiple sclerosis (MS)?

   A. magnetic resonance imaging (MRI)

   B. electromyography

   C. evoked potentials

   D. cerebrospinal fluid (CSF) studies

5. Regarding prognostic factors for multiple sclerosis (MS):

   A. There is a better prognosis for those with complete recovery from first attack.

   B. There is a better prognosis for men and those at older age at diagnosis.

   C. There is a worse prognosis in women who become pregnant while having MS.

   D. There is a worse prognosis for those with MS who carry the human leukocyte antigen (HLA) DR2 allele.

6. The use of intravenous (IV) methylprednisolone in multiple sclerosis (MS) is best for

   A. treating acute exacerbations.

   B. immunomodulation to prevent disease progression and relapse.

   C. managing secondary complications.

   D. none of the above

7. Which multiple sclerosis drug was associated with cases of progressive multifocal leukoencephalopathy (PML)?

   A. interferon beta

   B. glatiramer acetate

   C. mitoxantrone

   D. natalizumab

8. A 28-year-old female presents with newly diagnosed relapsing-remitting multiple sclerosis (MS) with no current residual functional disability. Which of the following statements is true?

   A. A first-line drug to recommend starting would be ACTH.

   B. A first-line drug to recommend starting would be in the interferon beta class.

   C. A first-line drug to recommend starting would be mitoxantrone.

   D. No drug therapy is recommended until she develops first signs of disability.

9. A reason for decreased efficacy with long-term use of the interferon drug class for relapsing form of multiple sclerosis (MS) is

   A. antidrug neutralizing antibodies.

   B. disease mutation into a medication resistant form of MS.

   C. conversion to Devic disease.

   D. immunosuppression.

10. All of the following are oral treatments for multiple sclerosis (MS), EXCEPT

   A. fingolimod.

   B. dimethyl fumarate.

   C. teriflunomide.

   D. alemtuzumab.

11. Those with multiple sclerosis (MS) commonly experience

   A. depression.

   B. fatigue.

   C. cognitive impairment.

   D. all of the above

12. Your patient with multiple sclerosis reports symptoms of frequent, unexplained, and uncontrollable bouts of crying and laughing. These symptoms most likely are consistent with

   A. a medication side effect.

   B. pseudobulbar affect.

   C. adjustment disorder.

   D. early signs of dementia.

13. Starting drug therapy with dalfampridine 10 mg twice daily in your patient with multiple sclerosis would best aid in

   A. decreasing symptoms of nocturia.

   B. reducing tremor.

   C. improving walking.

   D. mitigating fatigue.

14. Which of the following options is the best outpatient rehabilitation option for a patient with multiple sclerosis (MS) with mild to moderate disability?

   A. energy conservation techniques to manage fatigue

   B. steam room sessions to reduce muscle pain and spasms

   C. anaerobic interval training to improve endurance

   D. high-intensity, high-repetition weight lifting to improve muscle strength

15. What percentage of amyotrophic lateral sclerosis (ALS) is familial in origin?

   A. 5%

   B. 10%

   C. 15%

   D. 20%

16. Which lifestyle factor increases risk of developing amyotrophic lateral sclerosis (ALS)?

   A. alcohol use

   B. cigarette smoking

   C. crash dieting

   D. sedentary lifestyle

17. Which neurotransmitter has been implicated directly in the pathogenesis of amyotrophic lateral sclerosis (ALS)?

   A. dopamine

   B. serotonin

   C. norepinephrine

   D. glutamate

18. Which of the following is a poor prognostic factor for amyotrophic lateral sclerosis (ALS)?

   A. male sex

   B. younger age at diagnosis

   C. early bulbar dysfunction

   D. muscle atrophy and distal limb weakness at onset

19. A patient with the diagnosis of amyotrophic lateral sclerosis would be LEAST likely to have which finding on physical examination?

   A. brisk reflexes

   B. muscle atrophy

   C. fasciculations

   D. sensory loss

20. Which feature represents a variant phenotype of amyotrophic lateral sclerosis (ALS)?

    A. frontotemporal dementia

    B. limb-girdle spasticity

    C. facioscapulohumeral atrophy

    D. vertebrobasilar insufficiency

21. Your 60-year-old male patient with amyotrophic lateral sclerosis (ALS) diagnosed 1 year ago presents with frequent nighttime awakenings, vivid dreams, morning headache, and daytime somnolence. Your best clinical recommendation is

    A. to practice good sleep hygiene by avoiding distractions before bedtime and going to sleep at the same time every night.

    B. to refer him to behavioral health because poor sleep is a sign he is having trouble coming to terms with his diagnosis.

    C. to refer him immediately for pulmonary testing as this could be an early sign of respiratory failure.

    D. to prescribe zolpidem to aid in establishing a more regular sleep–wake cycle.

22. Your 58-year-old male patient who was newly diagnosed with amyotrophic lateral sclerosis (ALS) is asking whether he should take riluzole. Which of the following is true?

    A. Riluzole has shown modest effects in slowing disease progression in ALS.

    B. Riluzole is inexpensive and coverage is universal among prescription plans.

    C. Riluzole has been shown in a systematic review to prolong ALS median survival by 3 years.

    D. Lithium carbonate is a better option; it has level A recommendations based on studies showing significant increase in survivorship compared to riluzole.

23. Regarding rehabilitation therapy for patients with amyotrophic lateral sclerosis (ALS):

    A. Aerobic exercise is contraindicated.

    B. Muscle strengthening exercises show no benefit.

    C. Multidisciplinary approach is necessary.

    D. Dysarthria improves with orofacial and articulation exercises.

24. Which type of spinal muscular (SMA) or spinobulbar muscular atrophy (SBMA) is an X-linked recessive disorder affecting the androgen receptor gene with notable complications of testicular atrophy, decreased fertility, and gynecomastia?

    A. SMA type 1

    B. SMA type 2

    C. SMA type 3

    D. SBMA

25. Which rapidly progressive hereditary lower motor neuron disorder occurs in infancy and leads to death by age 2 years?

    A. Werdnig-Hoffmann disease

    B. Kugelberg-Welander disease

    C. progressive muscular atrophy

    D. primary lateral sclerosis

26. Paralytic poliomyelitis primarily affects which spine nervous system structure?

    A. dorsal root ganglions

    B. anterior horn cells

    C. nerve roots

    D. corticospinal tracts

27. Which is a common risk factor for cerebral palsy (CP)?

A. male sex

B. advanced maternal age

C. low birth weight

D. folate deficiency

28. A child with a level 3 mobility on the Gross Motor Functional Classification System (GMFCS) demonstrates

A. use of power wheelchair indoors and outdoors.

B. walking using assistive device indoors.

C. total dependence in wheelchair mobility.

D. walking without an assistive device.

29. A young child with cerebral palsy (CP) has the best prognosis of walking if he or she

A. does not have ataxia.

B. has conductive education.

C. retains three or more primitive reflexes at 18 to 24 months.

D. is able to sit independently by age 2 years.

30. Which rehabilitation therapeutic approach to treating cerebral palsy (CP) aims to normalize tone and reduce primitive reflexes by hands-on positioning and movement facilitation?

A. reflex locomotion (Vojta)

B. patterning (Doman-Delacato)

C. sensorimotor (Rood)

D. neurodevelopmental (Bobath)

31. Which type of cerebral palsy is associated with neonatal hyperbilirubinemia?

A. dyskinetic

B. spastic

C. hypotonic

D. all of the above

32. The parents of a 7-year-old male have brought him into your office for a second opinion. The child was diagnosed with cerebral palsy at age 5 years after he started having difficulty walking. Before that time, the child had reached his developmental milestones without delay. The parents have noticed his walking has been progressively worsening since his diagnosis, and he is also dropping objects. Physical examination reveals areflexia in the lower limbs, upper and lower limb ataxia, speech dysarthria, thoracic scoliosis, and lower extremity muscle weakness. You tell the parents this child's symptom constellation is

  A. consistent with cerebral palsy and deficits should stabilize over the next 2 years with no further progression.

  B. consistent with cerebral palsy and further functional decline is expected.

  C. inconsistent with cerebral palsy and requires further work up, including genetic testing.

  D. consistent with a traumatic brain injury and requires neuroimaging.

33. A distinguishing difference between Duchenne muscular dystrophy (DMD) and Becker muscular dystrophy (BMD) is

  A. DMD is due to mutation in the dystrophin gene.

  B. DMD is associated with cardiac complications.

  C. BMD shows elevation in creatine kinase (CK) levels.

  D. BMD shows ability to ambulate into adolescence.

34. Which muscle group shows the earliest signs of weakness in Duchenne muscular dystrophy (DMD)?

  A. finger flexors

  B. neck flexors

  C. knee flexors

  D. hip girdle

35. An example of a classic compensation a child with Duchenne muscular dystrophy (DMD) will develop in response to pelvic girdle muscle weakness is

  A. flatback.

  B. Gower sign.

  C. heel walking.

  D. scissor gait.

36. Special consideration in the rehabilitation and management of Duchenne muscular dystrophy (DMD) should include all of the following, EXCEPT

   A. effective airway clearance for pulmonary insufficiency.

   B. nutrition assessment.

   C. bracing to prevent progression of scoliosis.

   D. contracture prevention and management.

37. Which type of strengthening exercise has been shown in studies to have potential for muscle damage in patients with myopathy?

   A. eccentric

   B. isokinetic

   C. isometric

   D. isotonic

38. Which inflammatory myopathy has the highest rate of associated malignancy?

   A. dermatomyositis

   B. polymyositis

   C. inclusion body myositis

   D. drug-induced

39. Which inflammatory myopathy is more common in those older than age 50 years with a characteristic pattern of proximal and distal muscle weakness?

   A. dermatomyositis

   B. polymyositis

   C. inclusion body myositis

   D. all of the above

40. Which are involuntary, slow, writhing, snakelike movements?

   A. tremor

   B. ballismus

   C. chorea

   D. athetosis

41. All of the following prescription drugs can cause dyskinesia, EXCEPT

    A. haloperidol.

    B. valbenazine.

    C. levodopa.

    D. metoclopramide.

42. Of the tremor descriptions listed, which is most likely to be benign in etiology (i.e., not associated with a significant neurologic disorder)?

    A. tremor present at rest

    B. tremor present with movement

    C. tremor present with sustained posture

    D. both A and B

43. Tobacco smoking and coffee drinking are protective for which neurologic disorder?

    A. multiple sclerosis

    B. amyotrophic lateral sclerosis

    C. Alzheimer disease

    D. Parkinson disease

44. The primary cellular lesion in Parkinson disease involves which basal ganglia brain structure?

    A. caudate

    B. pars compacta

    C. subthalamic nucleus

    D. globus pallidus

45. Where is the substantia nigra located?

    A. midbrain

    B. cerebellum

    C. cerebrum

    D. spinal cord

46. Regarding symptomatology or clinical findings in Parkinson disease (PD):

A. The symptoms at onset are typically bilateral and symmetrical.

B. The presence of muscle weakness is a diagnostic criterion.

C. The postural reflexes are increased and cause hyperkinesia.

D. The tremor is increased by fatigue and inhibited by sleep.

47. Which of the following is true regarding treatment in Parkinson disease (PD)?

A. Carbidopa is added to levodopa to enhance neural reuptake of dopamine.

B. Amantadine is the most effective drug in the treatment of PD.

C. Deep brain stimulation (DBS) is the surgical treatment of choice for advanced PD.

D. Antihypertensive medication is useful in treating autonomic symptoms.

48. A helpful strategy in the gait training of a patient with Parkinson disease would be teaching how to

A. step to the rhythm of music.

B. keep feet close to the ground.

C. take short quick steps.

D. pivot when turning.

49. Which is an example of an "on phase," "peak dose" finding with levodopa medication treatment for Parkinson disease?

A. chorea

B. akinesia

C. depression

D. rigidity

50. The Parkinson disease drug, bromocriptine, mechanism of action is

A. dopamine precursor.

B. dopamine agonist.

C. anticholinergic.

D. catechol O-methyltransferase (COMT) inhibitor.

ANSWER KEY WITH EXPLANATIONS

1. The correct answer is C.
Graph C depicts secondary progressive MS. Graphs A and B depict "benign" and relapsing-remitting forms of multiple sclerosis. Graph D depicts primary progressive MS.

2. The correct answer is C.
The primary progressive form of MS (10% cases) typically develops much later in life than the other forms, equally affects males and females, and often starts with motor weakness. Those with the more common forms of MS are 2 times more likely to be female than male. The relapsing-remitting type of MS is the most common initial presentation and often starts with optic neuritis or sensory paresthesias. Those with MS who have the secondary progressive form may initially have had the relapsing-remitting form but have gone on to develop a more continuously progressive course over time. The progressive-relapsing form of MS (less than 5% cases) starts off with progressive worsening and later in its course manifests as episodic relapses.

3. The correct answer is C.
The enhancing lesions on T1 weighted images after gadolinium represent active disease and breakdown of the blood–brain barrier. Lesions seen via MRIs better track disease activity than presence of clinical symptoms and physical examination findings (active lesions often seen in absence of clinical relapse symptoms). The classic MRI finding is T2 hyperintense periventricular white matter lesions. T1 hypointense "black hole" lesions represent areas of brain atrophy where there has been considerable axon loss. In cases of isolated optic neuritis, the finding of lesion(s) on MRI increases the chance of developing MS.

4. The correct answer is B.
Electromyography and standard limb nerve conduction studies in many cases are normal as the disease primarily affects the central nervous system. MRI findings are part of the diagnostic criteria for MS. Evoked potentials (visual, brainstem, or sensory) can measure central nervous system activity and show slowing of central conduction. Lumbar puncture with CSF testing can reveal nonspecific findings of immune system activity, namely the presence of oligoclonal bands and/or immunoglobulin G (IgG).

5. The correct answer is A.
There is a better prognosis for females, younger age at diagnosis, complete recovery from first attack, and normal magnetic resonance imaging (MRI) at presentation. There is a worse prognosis for males, older age at diagnosis, and lesions on MRI at presentation. In addition, those with more frequent relapses and worse disability in general tend to have a worse prognosis. The time during pregnancy has a reduced rate of relapse but does not affect prognosis. Those with HLA DR2 allele have been suggested to be more susceptible to developing MS but not related to prognosis.

6. The correct answer is A.
Short-term therapy with IV methylprednisolone has scientific evidence for efficacy over placebo in treating acute exacerbations of MS. It does not affect disease progression or relapse rate. It is not used to manage MS complications as long-term steroid use actually can cause its own set of complications.

7. The correct answer is D.
Natalizumab was voluntarily withdrawn by its manufacturer in 2004 after reported PML. The medication was later reinstated in 2006 under a strict monitoring protocol. There is potential liver toxicity from using interferon beta; thus, liver enzymes should be monitored. Glatiramer acetate has been associated with transient postinjection reaction that can include symptoms of chest pain. Mitoxantrone has been associated with dose-dependent cardiotoxicity and leukemia.

8. The correct answer is B.
The updated July 2016 National Multiple Sclerosis Society publication on the current recommendations for disease-modifying therapy (DMT) states that timely initiation of DMT is recommended after diagnosis of relapsing MS in any age group. Recommendations indicate controlling the disease early in its course can lessen disability and reduce relapses. An example of first-line drugs for relapsing MS would be the interferon beta class (1a, 1b). ACTH has been used in the past for acute exacerbations. Mitoxantrone is the only agent approved for secondary progressive MS.

9. The correct answer is A.
Neurologists treating MS monitor for antidrug neutralizing antibodies to interferons which can decrease treatment efficacy. Devic disease (neuromyelitis optica) is a necrotizing myelitis that involves spinal cord (lesions that span more than three spinal levels) and the optic nerve.

10. The correct answer is D.
Oral U.S. Food and Drug Administration (FDA)-approved medications recently have emerged on the drug market for treatment of MS. Fingolimod was the first oral MS medication approved. Alemtuzumab is an infusion.

11. The correct answer is D.
All answer choices are common MS-related symptoms.

12. The correct answer is B.
Pseudobulbar affect (sometimes referred to as *emotional incontinence*) is recognized to be secondary to brain injury or neurologic disorder. It can be seen in patients with multiple sclerosis. Pharmacologic options for this condition include dextromethorphan-quinidine and amitriptyline.

13. The correct answer is C.
Dalfampridine is a potassium channel blocker shown to improve walking speed in phase 3 clinical trials. It is contraindicated in those with seizures and renal impairment.

14. The correct answer is A.

Energy conservation strategies are important in the rehabilitation plan for a patient with MS as fatigue is a major symptom that greatly impacts daily activities. It is known that people with MS can experience worsening of their neurologic symptoms in hot environments and with elevated core body temperatures as would occur in the setting of excessive heat or excessively strenuous exercise. Considering the mentioned factors, steam room sessions, anaerobic exercise, and high-intensity/repetition weight lifting are not the best ideas. Aerobic exercise in general is indicated for ambulatory patients with MS with proper precautions and avoiding exercising muscles to the point of fatigue. Rehabilitation evaluation for balance, coordination, and need for assistive devices are also important, as falls are common in the population with MS.

15. The correct answer is B.

10% of ALS cases are familial, commonly with autosomal dominant inheritance. Mutations in SOD1 are the most common. Familial ALS has been known to have earlier onset than sporadic ALS (about 10 years earlier).

16. The correct answer is B.

Cigarette smoking has been found to increase the risk of developing sporadic ALS.

17. The correct answer is D.

Elevated glutamate levels have been found in brains with ALS as well as reduced γ-aminobutyric acid (GABA) activity, implying a possible imbalance between excitatory and inhibitory neurotransmitters.

18. The correct answer is C.

Poor prognostic factor for ALS include female sex, older age at diagnosis, early bulbar dysfunction, and early pulmonary dysfunction (forced vital capacity [FVC] less than 90% predicted at diagnosis and decline within 6 months of diagnosis). Muscle atrophy and distal limb weakness in general are common symptoms of ALS.

19. The correct answer is D.

Amyotrophic lateral sclerosis is a motor neuron disease characterized by presence of both upper and lower motor neuron abnormal physical examination findings with preservation of sensory function.

20. The correct answer is A.

A small portion of patients with ALS also have concomitant frontotemporal dementia (more likely to be found in those with bulbar symptoms at onset). A population in the Western pacific islands also has an ALS variant with concomitant parkinsonism and dementia. Although there is controversy, some experts have called progressive muscular atrophy (lower motor neuron [LMN] disorder), primary lateral sclerosis (upper motor neuron [UMN] disorder), progressive bulbar palsy, and brachial amyotrophic diplegia (LMN affecting upper limbs) "variants" of ALS as well. Of note, there is also an inherited juvenile form of ALS as well with a slower progression and more favorable prognosis than adult ALS.

21. The correct answer is C.

Most of the patient population with ALS will develop pulmonary dysfunction at some point in the disease course. These symptoms are early indicators of respiratory failure and should be evaluated and addressed to mitigate further pulmonary complications. It is also important to initiate an honest discussion about present and future options for respiratory failure. Nighttime noninvasive ventilation might be an option to relieve symptoms in this particular case and has shown benefit in studies to slow rate of forced vital capacity (FVC) decline and lengthen survival.

22. The correct answer is A.

Riluzole is the U.S. Food and Drug Association (FDA)-approved medication for ALS. It has shown modest increase in median survival of 2 to 3 months and/or time to tracheostomy. The American Academy of Neurology recommends offering option of riluzole to patients with ALS (level A recommendations). Although the medication is covered by some Medicare prescription plans, the coverage varies depending on geographic area and type of plan. Out of pocket, the medication can be expensive. Lithium carbonate has insufficient evidence to support its use in ALS.

23. The correct answer is C.

ALS is a progressive and fatal disease in the majority of cases. The multifaceted complications that arise during each stage of the disease require a multidisciplinary approach by a team of physicians, rehabilitation therapists (physical, occupational, respiratory, and speech), palliative care specialists, spiritual support personnel, and behavioral health providers. In the earlier stages of the disease, there are studies showing the benefits of moderate aerobic exercise and strengthening exercises for patients with ALS. Dysarthria in ALS often does not respond well to traditional orofacial and articulation exercises. Instead, adaptive strategies are taught and augmented communication aids and devices are provided.

24. The correct answer is D.

SBMA is also known as Kennedy disease. It is an X-linked recessive (i.e., phenotype expressed in males) disorder that manifests with progressive spinal and bulbar muscle atrophy as well as characteristics of androgen insensitivity.

25. The correct answer is A.

Infants with spinal muscular atrophy (SMA) type 1 (Werdnig-Hoffmann disease) will present with severe weakness and hypotonia; they will have poor feeding and respiratory deterioration leading to death by age 2 years. SMA type 3 (Kugelberg-Welander disease) has proximal greater than distal muscle weakness; the typical onset is between 5 and 15 years with a slower progression in its course and less complications than seen in SMA type 2. Progressive muscular atrophy is a sporadic lower motor neuron disease with onset later in adulthood. Primary lateral sclerosis is a sporadic upper motor neuron disease of adulthood.

26. The correct answer is B.
Paralytic poliomyelitis damages and destroys anterior horn cells of the spinal cord, causing weakness and other characteristic lower motor neuron signs. Sensation is spared.

27. The correct answer is C.
Prematurity and low birth weight are risk factors for CP. There is no known risk from being either male or female. Well-known maternal risk factors for CP include mental retardation, seizure disorder, and hyperthyroidism. Advanced maternal age is a risk factor for Down syndrome, and not CP. Maternal iodine deficiency can lead to development of endemic cretinism with CP. Folate deficiency is associated with neural tube defects, and not CP.

28. The correct answer is B.
At level 3 on the GMFCS, the child walks with assistive mobility devices with limitations walking outdoors (e.g., outdoors, child might use manual wheelchair). At level 2, the child walks without assistive devices in most settings with limitations outdoors. At level 4, the child has limited self-mobility using assistive device at home and relies on powered mobility or is transported by wheelchair in the community or outdoors. At level 5, there is very limited self-mobility and dependent on being transported by push wheelchair.

29. The correct answer is D.
Molnar's classic 1976 study of children with CP found that independent sitting by the age of 2 years was predictive of ambulation. Badell-Ribera (1985) found crawling by 1.5 to 2 years to be a good prognostic indicator of ambulation. Poor prognostic indicator is retaining three or more primitive reflexes at 18 to 24 months. Seventy-five percent of children with spastic CP will ambulate. Those with hemiplegia have best chance of independent ambulation, followed by those with diplegia, and then quadriplegia. Those with isolated ataxia usually are ambulatory. Conductive education is an integrated physical movement and education program performed in a classroom setting and does not have sufficient evidence to support or refute its efficacy.

30. The correct answer is D.
The question stem describes the Bobath system of neurodevelopmental therapeutic management for CP, which is the most widely used approach. Vojta stimulates points to induce reflexive posture and movement patterns (such as reflex creeping) with the goal of early intervention to prevent and treat motor impairments. Doman-Delacato is a controversial treatment protocol using repeated passive movement patterns to improve mobility, communication, intelligence, and motor coordination. Rood uses sensory stimulation to activate motor response with philosophy that postural stability comes before movement.

31. The correct answer is A.
The dyskinetic (specifically athetoid) type of cerebral palsy can occur as a result of neonatal hyperbilirubinemia progressing to kernicterus. This is also associated with sensorineural hearing loss.

32. The correct answer is C.
The child's clinical constellation of symptoms is consistent with a neurodegenerative condition. Specifically, these symptoms are suggestive of Friedreich ataxia, an autosomal recessive disorder characterized by progressive ataxia. Cerebral palsy and traumatic brain injury are not neurodegenerative conditions; the neurologic deficits associated with these conditions remain stable and do not progress.

33. The correct answer is D.
The distinguishing difference between DMD and BMD is that those with BMD are able to ambulate well into their adolescent years because BMD has a slower progression. Both DMD and BMD involve mutation in the gene for the muscle cytoskeletal protein, dystrophin. In DMD, there is absence of dystrophin. Whereas in BMD, there is either a reduction in amount of dystrophin of (20% to 80%) or an abnormal protein molecular weight. Thus, BMD typically has milder manifestations than DMD. Unlike DMD, BMD does not have serious cognitive or pulmonary manifestations. Both DMD and BMD have significant cardiac complications (cardiomyopathy with electrophysiologic abnormalities). Both DMD and BMD show elevated CK levels.

34. The correct answer is B.
The neck flexors show the earliest sign of weakness in DMD followed by shoulder and hip girdle muscles.

35. The correct answer is B.
Gower sign is a classic compensation for pelvic girdle muscle weakness whereby a child rises from seated position on the floor to standing—starting with both hands and feet on the ground, leaning toward upper body to push up with knees extended, and walking hands up the legs to the thighs until upright. This can be seen in other neuromuscular disorders where there is pelvic girdle muscle weakness. In addition, the child will develop increased lumbar lordosis in response to the hip extensor weakness. Myopathic gait involves toe walking to compensate for hip and knee extensor weakness. Scissor gait is characteristic of cerebral palsy as a result of muscle spasticity and is not found in myopathies like DMD.

36. The correct answer is C.
Pulmonary complications, malnutrition, scoliosis, and contractures are rehabilitation considerations for patients with DMD. Of note, the updated rehabilitation and orthopedic literature shows that the scoliosis progression in DMD is NOT prevented with bracing. Surgery is the definitive management for progressive scoliosis.

37. The correct answer is A.
Research has shown eccentric exercise has potential to cause muscle damage in those with myopathy; caution is advised.

38. The correct answer is A.
Dermatomyositis is an inflammatory myopathy associated with characteristic dermatologic manifestations. It is the most rapidly progressive myositis. It is associated with up to 6 times increase in rate of associated malignancy (usually occult). Screening for malignancy is especially important in this population.

39. The correct answer C.
Inclusion body myositis (IBM) is an inflammatory myopathy most common older than age 50 years. Unlike dermatomyositis and polymyositis, IBM involves both distal and proximal muscles in a characteristic progressive pattern: quadriceps femoris, forearm flexors, flexor digitorum profundus, and the finger extensors.

40. The correct answer is D.
All answer choices describe types of involuntary movements. Athetosis is distinguished from the other answer choices as slow, nonrhythmic "writhing," "snakelike" movements. Tremor is (typically rapid of varying frequency oscillations) rhythmic muscle contraction, often described as "shaking." Chorea is rapid, nonrhythmic, "jerking," "dance-like" movement of the distal limb (greater than proximal) musculature. Ballismus is rapid, "flinging," "thrashing," "violent" movement of the proximal limb (greater than distal) musculature.

41. The correct answer is B.
Valbenazine is the first U.S. Drug and Food Administration (FDA)-approved drug to treat tardive dyskinesia (TD); thus, it does not cause it. Haloperidol, a neuroleptic dopamine antagonist, is known for complication of developing TD. Metoclopramide, an antiemetic dopamine antagonist, is also known for causing acute dystonia or TD. Levodopa treatment itself is widely known to cause dyskinesia in those receiving long-term treatment for Parkinson disease (commonly chorea and dystonia) via proposed complex interactions involving the indirect pathway to the subthalamic nucleus.

42. The correct answer is C.
Essential tremor and physiologic tremor are postural tremors; they are most often benign. Tremor at rest is associated with Parkinson disease. Tremor with movement can occur in the setting of cerebellar disease.

43. The correct answer is D.
Yes, smoking and coffee drinking can reduce the risk of Parkinson disease. (*authors do not endorse starting smoking because of this.*)

44. The correct answer is B.
Almost every medical student and medical resident knows the substantia nigra is the basal ganglia brain structure involved in the pathology of Parkinson disease. This question was meant to take it one step further in case the pesky examiners want more detail: The pars compacta is the structure within the substantia nigra that contains the dopaminergic neurons. Damage to these dopamine-producing neurons is thought to lead to the primary signs and symptoms of Parkinson disease.

45. The correct answer is A.
The substantia nigra is located in the midbrain. Other structures of the basal ganglia reside in the cerebrum.

46. The correct answer is D.

The resting tremor is characteristic of PD that is inhibited by activity and sleep and increased by fatigue and stress. PD symptoms at onset commonly involve only one side of the body (called *asymmetric onset*). PD is thought to negatively impact motor control and coordination causing slowing of movement. Thus, muscle weakness is not a diagnostic criterion because the pathophysiology of PD does not directly damage the upper or lower motor neuron pathways. Postural reflexes are decreased or lost in PD, leading to falls. Bradykinesia, hypokinesia, and akinesia all represent movement slowing to varying degrees seen in PD.

47. The correct answer is C.

The subthalamic nucleus is a commonly targeted brain region for DBS which is reserved for advanced PD, refractory to pharmacologic treatment. Carbidopa inhibits the conversion of levodopa to dopamine peripherally (i.e., in the body), so there is more levodopa available to cross the blood–brain barrier and be converted to dopamine. Despite its side effects and dosing issues, levodopa still remains the most effective PD pharmacologic treatment. Amantadine is most often used to treat symptoms of dyskinesias. Orthostatic hypotension is common in PD; thus, antihypertensive medication will not help.

48. The correct answer is A.

Verbal/auditory cueing, visual cueing, counting, and stepping to the rhythm of music are helpful strategies in gait training to prevent the "freezing" phenomenon. Taking longer steps and lifting the legs is helpful to combat the "festination" phenomenon. Impairment of postural reflexes make falls likely when making sudden turns. Therefore, turning using a wide arc of multiple steps is advised to enhance safety and reduce falls.

49. The correct answer is A.

During the peak effects of a levodopa medication dose, patients may experience drug-induced dyskinesias, such as chorea. When the drug effects wear off, the typical Parkinson disease symptoms predominate. With long-term use of levodopa, these motor fluctuations can become more unpredictable and distressing to the patients and their caregivers.

50. The correct answer is B.

Bromocriptine is considered a dopamine agonist. Levodopa is considered a dopamine precursor. Benztropine is considered an anticholinergic. Entacapone is considered a COMT inhibitor.

Board Review Points ("Pearls") for Neuromuscular Disorders and Other Neurologic Conditions

Multiple Sclerosis

- The relapsing-remitting type of MS is the most common initial presentation and often starts with optic neuritis or sensory paresthesias. Those with the more common forms of MS are 2 times more likely to be female than male. Those with MS who have the secondary progressive form may initially have had the relapsing-remitting form but have gone on to develop a more continuously progressive course over time. The primary progressive form of MS (10% cases) typically develops much later in life than the other forms, equally affects males and females, and often starts with motor weakness.

- There is a better prognosis for females, younger age at diagnosis, complete recovery from first attack, and normal MRI at presentation. There is a worse prognosis for males, older age at diagnosis, and lesions on MRI at presentation. The time during pregnancy has a reduced rate of relapse but does not affect prognosis.

- The classic MRI finding is T2 hyperintense periventricular white matter lesions. T1 hypointense "black hole" lesions represent areas of brain atrophy where there has been considerable axon loss.

- Energy conservation strategies are important in the rehabilitation plan for a patient with MS as fatigue is a major symptom that greatly impacts daily activities. It is known that people with MS can experience worsening of their neurologic symptoms in hot environments and with elevated core body temperatures as would occur in the setting of excessive heat or excessively strenuous exercise.

Amyotrophic Lateral Sclerosis

- ALS is a motor neuron disease characterized by presence of both UMN and LMN abnormal physical examination findings with preservation of sensory function.

- Cigarette smoking has been found to increase the risk of developing sporadic ALS.

- Poor prognostic factor for ALS include female sex, older age at diagnosis, early bulbar dysfunction, and early pulmonary dysfunction (FVC less than 90% predicted at diagnosis and decline within 6 months of diagnosis).

- Most of the patient population with ALS will develop pulmonary dysfunction at some point in the disease course. Frequent nighttime awakenings, vivid dreams, morning headache, and daytime somnolence are early indicators of respiratory failure.

- Riluzole is the FDA-approved medication for ALS. It has shown modest increase in median survival of 2 to 3 months and/or time to tracheostomy.

Other Motor Neuron Disease

- SBMA is also known as Kennedy disease. It is an X-linked recessive (i.e., phenotype expressed in males) disorder that manifests with progressive spinal and bulbar muscle atrophy as well as characteristics of androgen insensitivity—testicular atrophy, decreased fertility, and gynecomastia.

- Infants with SMA type 1 (Werdnig-Hoffmann disease) will present with severe weakness and hypotonia; they will have poor feeding and respiratory deterioration leading to death by age 2 years. SMA type 3 (Kugelberg-Welander disease) has proximal greater than distal muscle weakness; the typical onset is between 5 and 15 years with a slower progression in its course and less complications than seen in SMA type 2.

- Progressive muscular atrophy is a sporadic LMN disease with onset later in adulthood. Primary lateral sclerosis is a sporadic UMN disease of adulthood.

Cerebral Palsy

- Prematurity and low birth weight are risk factors for CP. Well known maternal risk factors for CP include mental retardation, seizure disorder, and hyperthyroidism.
- At level 2 GMFCS, the child walks without assistive devices in most settings with limitations outdoors. At level 3, the child walks with assistive mobility devices with limitations walking outdoors (e.g., outdoors, child might use manual wheelchair). At level 4, the child has limited self-mobility using assistive device at home and relies on powered mobility or is transported by wheelchair in the community or outdoors. At level 5, there is very limited self-mobility and dependent on being transported by push wheelchair.
- 75% children with spastic CP will ambulate. Those with hemiplegia have the best chance of independent ambulation, followed by those with diplegia, and then quadriplegia. Those with isolated ataxia usually are ambulatory.
- Good prognosis for ambulation: Independent sitting by the age of 2 years was predictive of ambulation; crawling by 1.5 to 2 years
- Poor prognosis for ambulation: retaining three or more primitive reflexes at 18 to 24 months
- The dyskinetic (specifically athetoid) type of cerebral palsy can occur as a result of neonatal hyperbilirubinemia progressing to kernicterus. This is also associated with sensorineural hearing loss.
- The neurologic deficits associated with CP remain stable and do not progress.

Myopathy

- DMD is the most common congenital myopathy with pathophysiology involving absence of dystrophin gene. DMD is progressive with loss of ambulation typically occurring during childhood years. There are associated cardiac, pulmonary, spine deformity, and cognitive manifestations.
- BMD has a slower progression and milder manifestations than DMD in that those with BMD are able to ambulate well into their adolescent years. In BMD, there is either a reduction in amount of dystrophin (20% to 80%) or an abnormal protein molecular weight. Both DMD and BMD have significant cardiac complications (cardiomyopathy with electrophysiologic abnormalities). Both DMD and BMD show elevated CK levels.
- The neck flexors show the earliest sign of weakness in DMD followed by shoulder and hip girdle muscles.
- Myopathic gait involves toe walking to compensate for hip and knee extensor weakness.
- In myopathies, there is some evidence eccentric exercise could damage muscles. In addition, high-resistance exercise programs may lead to overwork weakness. Submaximal resistance training is advised. Do not exercise to exhaustion.
- Dermatomyositis is an inflammatory myopathy associated with characteristic dermatologic manifestations (e.g., heliotrope rash). It is the most rapidly progressive myositis. It is associated with up to 6 times increase in rate of associated malignancy (usually occult). The classic diagnostic pathology found on muscle biopsy is "tubuloreticular endothelial cell inclusions."

- IBM is an inflammatory myopathy most common older than age 50 years. Unlike dermatomyositis and polymyositis, IBM involves both distal and proximal muscles in a characteristic progressive pattern: quadriceps femoris, forearm flexors, flexor digitorum profundus, and the finger extensors. The classic diagnostic pathology found on muscle biopsy are "rimmed vacuoles, intranuclear and cytoplasmic tubulofilamentous inclusions."

Movement Disorders and Parkinson Disease

- Athetosis is slow, nonrhythmic "writhing," and "snakelike."
- Chorea is rapid, nonrhythmic, "jerking," "dance-like" distal limb (greater than proximal).
- Ballismus is rapid, "flinging," "thrashing," "violent" proximal limb (greater than distal). Unilateral ballismus (hemiballismus) from stroke can occur if there is an infarct in the subthalamic nucleus (hemiballismus in right arm caused by lesion left subthalamic nucleus).
- Drug-induced dyskinesias: Haloperidol, metoclopramide, and levodopa are common culprits.
- Essential tremor and physiologic tremor are postural tremors; they are most often benign. Tremor at rest is associated with PD. Tremor with movement can occur in the setting of cerebellar disease.
- Smoking and coffee drinking can reduce the risk of PD.
- Damage to the dopamine-producing cells in the pars compacta of the substantia nigra (in the midbrain) is involved in the pathology of PD.
- PD symptoms: resting tremor, rigidity, bradykinesias, and impaired postural reflexes. Asymmetric onset is common.
- Levodopa is most effective treatment but trouble with long-term use complications ("on-off" phenomenon, dyskinesias, decreased response over time).
- Levodopa is combined with carbidopa. Carbidopa inhibits the peripheral conversion of levodopa to dopamine peripherally (i.e., in the body), so there is more levodopa available to cross the blood–brain barrier and be centrally converted to dopamine.

REFERENCES & SUGGESTED READINGS

American Academy of Neurology. AAN summary of evidence-based guidelines for clinicians. The care of the patient with amyotrophic lateral sclerosis: drug, nutritional, and respiratory therapies. https://www.aan.com/Guidelines/Home/GetGuidelineContent/373. Accessed April 10, 2017.

Archer JE, Gardner AC, Roper HP, Chikermane AA, Tatman AJ. Duchenne muscular dystrophy: the management of scoliosis. *J Spine Surg.* 2016;2(3):185-194. doi:10.21037/jss.2016.08.05.

Badell-Ribera A. Cerebral palsy: postural-locomotor prognosis in spastic diplegia. *Arch Phys Med Rehabil.* 1985;66:614-619.

Bethoux F, Rae-Grant A. Multiple sclerosis. In: Frontera WR, DeLisa JA, Gans B, et al, eds. *DeLisa's Physical Medicine & Rehabilitation: Principles and Practice.* 5th ed. Philadelphia, PA: Lippincott Williams & Wilkins; 2010:625-644.

Campagnolo DI, Vollmer TL. Multiple sclerosis. In: Kirshblum S, Campagnolo DI. *Spinal Cord Medicine.* 2nd ed. Philadelphia, PA: Lippincott Williams & Wilkins Health; 2011:617-631.

Cuccurullo S. *Physical Medicine and Rehabilitation Board Review.* 3rd ed. New York, NY: Demos Medical; 2014.

Darrah J, Watkins B, Chen L, Bonin C. Conductive education intervention for children with cerebral palsy: an AACPDM evidence report. *Dev Med Child Neurol.* 2004;46:187-203. doi:10.1111/j.1469-8749.2004.tb00471.x.

Diamond M, Armento M. Children with disabilities. In: Frontera WR, DeLisa JA, Gans B, et al, eds. *DeLisa's Physical Medicine & Rehabilitation: Principles and Practice.* 5th ed. Philadelphia, PA: Lippincott Williams & Wilkins; 2010:1475-1502.

Foerster BR, Pomper MG, Callaghan BC, et al. 3T MR spectroscopy reveals an imbalance between excitatory and inhibitory neurotransmitters in amyotrophic lateral sclerosis. *JAMA Neurol.* 2013;70(8):1009-1016. doi:10.1001/jamaneurol.2013.234.

Han JJ, Kilmer DD. Myopathy. In: Frontera WR, DeLisa JA, Gans B, et al, eds. *DeLisa's Physical Medicine & Rehabilitation: Principles and Practice.* 5th ed. Philadelphia, PA: Lippincott Williams & Wilkins; 2010:757-780.

Hirschberg R, Sharma N, Scarborough DM. Rehabilitation of persons with Parkinson's disease and other movement disorders. In: Frontera WR, DeLisa JA, Gans B, et al, eds. *DeLisa's Physical Medicine & Rehabilitation: Principles and Practice.* 5th ed. Philadelphia, PA: Lippincott Williams & Wilkins; 2010:645-664.

Hong T, Paneth N. Maternal and infant thyroid disorders and cerebral palsy. *Semin Perinatol.* 2008;32(6):438-445. doi:10.1053/j.semperi.2008.09.011.

Joyce NC, Carter GT, Krivickas LS. Adult motor neuron disease. In: Kirshblum S, Campagnolo DI. *Spinal Cord Medicine.* 2nd ed. Philadelphia, PA: Lippincott Williams & Wilkins Health; 2011:632-650.

Krivickas LS, Carter GT. Adult motor neuron disease. In: Frontera WR, DeLisa JA, Gans B, et al, eds. *DeLisa's Physical Medicine & Rehabilitation: Principles and Practice.* 5th ed. Philadelphia, PA: Lippincott Williams & Wilkins; 2010:717-740.

Lim H, Kim T. Effects of Vojta therapy on gait of children with spastic diplegia. *J Phys Ther Sci.* 2013;25(12):1605-1608. doi:10.1589/jpts.25.1605.

Mastaglia FL, Garlepp MJ, Phillips BA, Zilko PJ. Inflammatory myopathies: clinical, diagnostic and therapeutic aspects. *Muscle Nerve.* 2003;27:407-425. doi:10.1002/mus.10313.

Mazzoni P, Shabbott B, Cortés JC. Motor control abnormalities in Parkinson's disease. *Cold Spring Harb Perspect Med.* 2012;2(6):a009282. doi:10.1101/cshperspect.a009282.

Molnar GE, Gordon SU. Cerebral palsy: predictive value of selected clinical signs of early prognostication of motor function. *Arch Phys Med Rehabil.* 1976;57:153-158.

Multiple Sclerosis Coalition. The use of disease-modifying therapies in multiple sclerosis: principles and current evidence. A consensus paper by the Multiple Sclerosis Coalition. http://www.nationalmssociety.org/getmedia/5ca284d3-fc7c-4ba5-b005-ab537d495c3c/DMT_Consensus_MS_Coalition_color. Accessed April 10, 2017.

Phillips BA, Mastaglia FL. Exercise therapy in patients with myopathy. *Curr Opin Neurol.* 2000;13(5):547-552.

Singer BA. Initiating oral fingolimod treatment in patients with multiple sclerosis. *Ther Adv Neurol Disord.* 2013;6(4):269-275. doi:10.1177/1756285613491520.

U.S. Food and Drug Administration. FDA approves first drug to treat tardive dyskinesia. https://www.fda.gov/NewsEvents/Newsroom/PressAnnouncements/ucm552418.htm. Published April 11, 2017. Accessed April 10, 2017.

Wilkinson I, Lennox G. Multiple sclerosis. In: Wilkinson I, Lennox G. *Essential Neurology.* 4th ed. Malden, MA: Blackwell; 2005:99-110.

Wilkinson I, Lennox G. Parkinsonism, involuntary movements and ataxia. In: Wilkinson I, Lennox G. *Essential Neurology.* 4th ed. Malden, MA: Blackwell; 2005:67-82.

Wood NW. Diagnosing Friedreich's ataxia. *Arch Dis Child.* 1998;78:204-207.

Fundamentals of Rehabilitation Therapy

1. According to the International Classification of Functioning Disability and Health (ICF), *disability*

    A. is entirely created by society and the environment.

    B. is solely a problem limited to the individual person having the disability.

    C. refers to problems in body function or structure such as significant deviation or loss.

    D. includes impairments, activity limitations, and participation restrictions.

2. Which of the following generally is considered an instrumental activity of daily living (IADL)?

    A. meal preparation

    B. bathing

    C. dressing

    D. mobility

3. Which of the following is NOT a Functional Independence Measure (FIM™) category?

    A. Community Integration

    B. Self-Care

    C. Transfers

    D. Sphincter Control

4. The physical therapist on your interdisciplinary team reports your patient upon discharge can ascend and descend stairs safely on his or her own if given verbal cues. The discharge Functional Independence Measure (FIM™) score for this locomotion item would be

A. 4.

B. 5.

C. 6.

D. 7.

5. Regarding sternotomy precautions after coronary artery bypass grafting (CABG):

A. Protocols commonly advise patients to perform exercises lifting their arms above their heads.

B. Most patients are allowed weight lifting up to 20 lb after surgery.

C. They have been researched extensively with high-quality evidence of preventing sternotomy complications.

D. Protocols vary by institution, and there are no universally accepted restrictions.

6. Which of the following would be a reasonable restriction after posterolateral total hip arthroplasty to prevent early dislocation?

A. no weight bearing for 6 weeks

B. immobilization for 3 weeks

C. limiting flexion of the hip to less than 90 degrees

D. keeping legs together at night

7. All the following are Medicare Part A medical necessity documentation requirements for a patient to be admitted to an acute inpatient rehabilitation facility (IRF), EXCEPT

A. admission orders.

B. individualized overall plan of care.

C. preadmission financial disclosure form.

D. postadmission physician examination.

8. Which is an example of a potential intervention to address the participation restriction of unemployment faced by a person with paraplegia caused by spinal cord injury?

A. work space accommodation

B. use of adaptive van

C. antispasticity medication

D. stretching to prevent contractures

9. You are consulted to determine the discharge disposition and rehabilitation needs for a 70-year-old male with chronic obstructive pulmonary disease (COPD) who presents with symptoms of generalized weakness and shortness of breath with minimal exertion. He is on acute care hospital day 40 for admitting diagnosis of sepsis with associated respiratory failure. He is currently on the medical floor, vitals stable, and the hospitalist has determined him to be medically stable for discharge on 2 L continuous oxygen. Prior to hospitalization, he required minimal to moderate assistance from his wife for basic activities of daily living (ADLs). He is currently at total assist level in all assessment areas after 2 weeks of hospital physical therapy (PT)/occupational therapy (OT) with complaints of extreme fatigue and decreased activity tolerance during the 30-minute treatment sessions. There are no wounds, intravenous lines, or infusions needed. Based on the available information, what is the most appropriate recommendation for discharge disposition?

A. long-term acute care facility (LTAC)

B. skilled nursing facility

C. acute inpatient rehabilitation facility

D. home with outpatient therapy

10. Which of these scenarios would meet the medical necessity standards for skilled rehabilitation therapy services under the Centers for Medicare & Medicaid Services (CMS)?

   A. A patient's medical and functional status have been steadily declining after 30 days of inpatient rehabilitation receiving 3 to 4 hours of physical and occupational therapy daily.

   B. A patient received a pictorial pamphlet of daily exercises from a physical therapist that she currently performs under the supervision of a physical therapy assistant.

   C. A patient is participating in a restorative therapy program at the nursing home.

   D. A patient is receiving instruction by a physical therapist on how to perform a maintenance program.

11. Phase 2 of cardiac rehabilitation after myocardial infarction

   A. requires exercise treadmill test prior to initiation.

   B. occurs during acute care hospitalization.

   C. does not include telemetry monitoring.

   D. goals include self-care, ADLs, and household ambulation.

12. Which type of stretching technique includes in sequence (1) passive stretching of a muscle, (2) contraction of the muscle, (3) relaxation of the muscle, and (4) further passive stretching to increase range of motion?

   A. ballistic stretching

   B. static stretching

   C. dynamic stretching

   D. proprioceptive neuromuscular facilitation

13. Vestibular rehabilitation therapy (VRT) is best indicated for

   A. treatment of a progressively worsening vestibular deficit.

   B. Ménière disease.

   C. benign paroxysmal positional vertigo.

   D. migraine headaches.

14. Aquatic therapy would be expected to cause which effect due to external pressure from immersion in water?

   A. increased work of breathing

   B. increased compressive forces on body joints

   C. decreased central blood volume

   D. decreased chest wall pressure

15. An example of heat energy transfer via convection is

   A. whirlpool.

   B. hydrocollator pack.

   C. heating lamp.

   D. ultrasound.

16. Which extremity therapy treatment transfers energy via convection by blowing heat through cellulose beads or pulverized corncobs in a closed machine.

   A. paraffin bath

   B. fluidotherapy

   C. contrast bath

   D. balneotherapy

17. Which gliding massage technique induces muscle relaxation?

   A. friction

   B. pétrissage

   C. effleurage

   D. tapotement

18. Which type of transcutaneous electrical nerve stimulation (TENS) is considered to be "conventional"?

   A. high-frequency, high-intensity

   B. high-frequency, low-intensity

   C. low-frequency, high-intensity

   D. low-frequency, low-intensity

19. Ultrasound

   A. has deeper tissue penetration at high frequencies.

   B. uses radio waves converted to heat.

   C. is a useful treatment for joint pain postarthroplasty.

   D. is a type of diathermy.

20. Which of the following conditions has the best quality scientific evidence for the use of acupuncture?

   A. myofascial trigger points

   B. lumbar radiculopathy

   C. lower limb spasticity in stroke

   D. postoperative nausea and vomiting

21. Which type of paraffin bath technique provides the most intense heat penetration into tissues?

   A. dipping

   B. immersion

   C. brushing

   D. layering

22. All of the following are contraindications for cervical manipulation, EXCEPT

   A. myelopathy.

   B. joint instability.

   C. degenerative joint disease.

   D. vertebrobasilar insufficiency.

23. Which technique places a body part in a passive position of maximal comfort for duration of approximately 90 seconds, shortening the restricted muscle, resetting muscle spindle fiber activity, and reducing pain over tender points?

    A. counterstrain

    B. muscle energy

    C. thrust

    D. myofascial release

24. Cryotherapy can be indicated for which condition?

    A. Raynaud's disease

    B. ischemia

    C. superficial thrombophlebitis

    D. spasticity

25. Regarding thermotherapy:

    A. It is indicated to treat scar tissue adhesions.

    B. Hubbard tank temperature at 46° C is ideal for wounds and burns.

    C. It increases collagen extensibility.

    D. It is contraindicated for collagen vascular disease.

ANSWER KEY WITH EXPLANATIONS

1. The correct answer is D.

The ICF was the result of 10 years of revisions by the World Health Organization to an original classification published in 1980 called the *International Classification of Impairments, Disabilities, and Handicaps*. The ICF was approved in 2001 and provides common framework describing human functioning and disability. The ICF views *disability* as "an umbrella term for impairments, activity limitations, and participations restrictions." These factors are influenced by health conditions and contextual factors (personal and environmental). The medical model (disability is personal, caused by disease) or social model (disability is caused by society) alone are both too limiting. ICF defines *impairments* as problems in body functions or structure, such as significant deviation or loss.

2. The correct answer is A.

All the alternate answer choices—bathing, dressing, and mobility—represent basic activities of daily living (BADLs), which are basic self-care and personal care tasks. The category of IADLs goes beyond basic self-care tasks and describes tasks that allow the individual to live independently by maintaining the home environment or in the community.

3. The correct answer is A.

The six FIM™ categories are Self-Care, Sphincter Control, Transfers, Locomotion, Communication, and Social Cognition.

4. The correct answer is B.

Your patient is at supervision level for locomotion using stairs with corresponding FIM™ of 5; he or she can perform without physical assistance but requires a person to be present for safety and cueing. A score of 4 is minimal assistance (patient performs 75% or more of task). A score of 6 is modified independence (takes extra time or uses assistive device). A score of 7 is complete independence where a person completes the task in a timely and safe manner.

5. The correct answer is D.

At the date of publication, there are no universal consensus regarding sternotomy precautions after CABG and protocols vary by surgeon and institution. The most common sternotomy precautions (restrictions) are no lifting greater than 10 lb of weight after surgery. Many protocols advise against lifting arms over the head or past 90 degrees of shoulder flexion. A literature search could not locate any meta-analyses, systemic reviews, or any high-level scientific evidence of sternotomy precautions preventing complications (*please contact us authors if you find any*). Perhaps, this would be a future research project for you to undertake at your institution.

6. The correct answer is C.

Traditional hip precautions have included limiting flexion of the operative hip to less than 90 degrees, sleeping with abduction pillow (avoiding adduction past midline), and no car transfers. Scientific evidence is conflicting as to whether precautions/restrictions prevent hip dislocation, and recent studies suggest they may not. Most patients are able to bear weight after hip arthroplasty and are encouraged to avoid prolonged bed rest and joint immobilization.

7. The correct answer is C.

At date of publication, Medicare Part A IRF documentation requirements: preadmission screening, post admission physician evaluation, individualized overall plan of care, admission orders, and Inpatient Rehabilitation Facility Patient Assessment Instrument.

8. The correct answer is A.

The International Classification of Functioning Disability and Health describes the interaction among body function and structure, a person's health condition, activity limitations, participation restrictions, and contextual factors (diagram is available online and in *DeLisa's Physical Medicine & Rehabilitation: Principles and Practice*, Chapter 11). Work space accommodation is the most direct intervention for this participation restriction. Use of adaptive van would be intervention to address activity limitation of not being able to drive (to work). Medication would address body function impairment of increased lower extremity tone causing pain. Stretching is a preventative intervention designed to prevent further range of motion impairment.

9. The correct answer is B.

This patient (who has baseline mild to moderate functional impairment) has not progressed from total assist after 2 weeks of hospital-based PT. While he does require ongoing therapy with more than one skilled therapy discipline, he will not be able to tolerate intensive rehabilitation of at least 3 hours daily or 15 hours weekly if he is currently not able to tolerate 30-minute sessions. He is not suitable for LTAC as he is medically stable and does not require daily acute care services for medically complex needs. He has significant functional decline from baseline, and a home discharge would not be safe or logistically feasible. A skilled nursing facility would provide skilled nursing therapy (PT and OT) at a less intensive pace.

10. The correct answer is D.

CMS considers skilled therapists' knowledge medically necessary to design maintenance programs for chronic diagnoses and to properly train the patient and/or caregivers. The patient performing a maintenance program independently or with assistance of non-skilled personnel is not considered medically necessary. Therefore, the scenario with a physical therapy assistant supervising a patient performing exercises and the scenario with the restorative nursing therapy program both cannot be billed as skilled therapy services. The scenario with medical/functional decline despite intensive therapy does not meet "reasonable and necessary" standards as there must be expectation that the patient's condition would improve in a measurable amount of time with continued therapy.

11. The correct answer is A.

Phase 2 of cardiac rehabilitation typically begins 3 weeks after hospital discharge and requires an exercise treadmill test prior to initiation to determine the initial exercise intensity level. Phase 2 includes telemetry monitoring. Goals include progressive cardiac conditioning and usually performed 1 hour 3 times per week.

12. The correct answer is D.

The description is of the proprioceptive neuromuscular facilitation (PNF) contract–relax technique. Ballistic stretching consists of repetitive bouncing movements at a rapid rate. Static stretching requires gradual application of stretch while holding the stretch in end position. Dynamic stretching is moving the muscle through to its maximum range of motion in a series of repetitions.

13. The correct answer is C.

VRT is most often indicated for stable vestibular lesions, vestibular symptoms in traumatic brain injury, benign paroxysmal positional vertigo (BPPV), disequilibrium in older people, and vertigo of unclear etiology. It is not indicated for those with an unstable, progressively worsening deficit. Those with spontaneous, fluctuating episodes like in the case of Ménière disease would benefit less from the therapy. Those with nonvestibular causes of dizziness are less likely to benefit.

14. The correct answer is A.

There is 60% increase in work of breathing during water immersion to neck. The immersion increases chest and abdominal wall pressures due to compression; this leads to decreased lung volumes and increased airway resistance. Venous compression leads to increased central blood volume. During water immersion, water is dispersed which offloads the joints and reduces effects of gravity.

15. The correct answer is A.

Convection refers to the flow of large amounts of molecules over large distances to transfer heat; convection best occurs with liquids or gases. The whirlpool uses fluid flow to transfer heat. Conduction describes direct transfer of heat energy over a small distance between two surfaces in direct contact with different temperature gradients, the hydrocollator pack being a good example. Radiation (conversion) refers to electromagnetic energy being converted to heat as in the example of a heating lamp or ultrasound.

16. The correct answer is B.

The question stem describes fluidotherapy. Paraffin bath transfers heat energy via conduction in a 1:7 ratio of mineral oil to paraffin. Contrast baths use two containers and alternate exposure to cold and heat to produce vasodilation-vasoconstriction, desensitization, and reflex hyperemia. Balneotherapy is a mineral water bath therapy popular in European countries often delivered in spa or retreat settings.

17. The correct answer is C.

Effleurage involves the practitioner's hands gliding over the client's skin and is a type of stroking massage technique. Friction involves pressure applied by the "ball" of the fingers in varying degrees to prevent or break up adhesions. Pétrissage involves the practitioner compressing the client's skin and muscle between his or her fingers, often in kneading motion, to increase circulation and mobilize fluid. Tapotement is percussion massage and is stimulatory.

18. The correct answer is B.

Conventional TENS uses high-frequency, low-intensity stimulation. Electroacupuncture uses low-frequency, high-intensity stimulation. Low-frequency, low-intensity stimulation has been used in wound healing and bone stimulation applications. High-intensity electrostimulation is not well-tolerated by patients.

19. The correct answer is D.

Ultrasound is a type of diathermy (heating therapy) using sound waves to produce heat energy through conversion. The other types of diathermy are shortwave diathermy (uses radio waves) and microwave diathermy (uses microwaves). Ultrasound has deeper tissue penetration at low frequencies and is generally not advised to be used near arthroplasty joints due to concern over potential heat damage to prosthesis. It is contraindicated in those with pacemakers.

20. The correct answer is D.

Numerous high-quality randomized controlled trials, systematic reviews, and meta-analyses suggest effectiveness for acupuncture or acupressure for treatment of nausea and vomiting in postoperative settings as well as for chemotherapy-induced and pregnancy-related nausea and vomiting. The acupuncture point most tested is pericardium 6 (volar wrist 3 finger breaths proximal to the wrist crease). Studies in the other areas have conflicting evidence.

21. The correct answer is B.

Immersion technique is to dip the extremity in the paraffin bath 6 to 10 times and then immerse it in the bath continuously for 20 to 30 minutes. Dipping technique is more common and involves consecutive dipping of the extremity for 7 to 12 times and allowing the paraffin layer to cool between submersions; the extremity is then wrapped and placed in an insulated cover for 20 minutes. Skin temperatures fall more rapidly with the dipping technique as opposed to the immersion technique. The brushing technique brushes the paraffin on larger areas that are difficult to submerge and has less increase in temperature than the other techniques. There is no such thing as the layering technique.

22. The correct answer is C.

Degenerative joint disease is not a contraindication to receiving cervical manipulation. The other choices are either absolute or relative contraindications.

23. The correct answer is A.

The description of the manual therapy technique of counterstrain, used by osteopathic and chiropractic practitioners. Muscle energy involves patient performing active voluntary isometric muscle contractions with practitioner applying a counterforce to relax a muscle. Thrust refers to spinal manipulative therapy. Myofascial release most commonly involves practitioner applying sustained pressure to the muscle and allowing it to release/relax.

24. The correct answer is D.

Cryotherapy can be used to treat spasticity as it reduces muscle tone with prolonged application. Heat therapy can be indicated to treat superficial thrombophlebitis. Cryotherapy is contraindicated in Raynaud's disease and ischemia.

25. The correct answer is C.

Heat (thermotherapy) increases collagen extensibility. It is indicated to treat soft tissue complications of collagen vascular disease and contraindicated for use over scar tissue. Neutral temperatures between 33° and 36° C are well-tolerated for wounds and burns.

Board Review Points ("Pearls") for Fundamentals of Rehabilitation Therapy

- The ICF describes the interaction among body function and structure, a person's health condition, activity limitations, participation restrictions, and contextual factors (diagram is available online and in *DeLisa's Physical Medicine & Rehabilitation: Principles and Practice*, Chapter 11). The ICF views *disability* as "an umbrella term for impairments, activity limitations, and participations restrictions." These factors are influenced by health conditions and contextual factors (personal and environmental). ICF defines *impairments* as problems in body functions or structure such as significant deviation or loss.

- Bathing, dressing, and mobility represent BADLs, which are basic self-care and personal care tasks. The category of IADLs goes beyond basic self-care tasks and describes tasks that allow the individual to live independently by maintaining the home environment or in the community.

- The six FIM™ categories are Self-Care, Sphincter Control, Transfers, Locomotion, Communication, and Social Cognition. The levels are 1 to 7. Level 1 is total assistance, and level 7 is complete independence. A score of 6 is modified independence (takes extra time or uses assistive device). Supervision level has corresponding FIM™ of 5. A score of 4 is minimal assistance (patient performs 75% or more of task). A score of 3 is moderate assistance (patient performs 50% or more of task). A score of 2 is maximal assistance (patient performs 25% or more of task).

- At date of publication, Medicare Part A IRF documentation requirements: preadmission screening, postadmission physician evaluation, individualized overall plan of care, admission orders, and Inpatient Rehabilitation Facility Patient Assessment Instrument.

- Admission to inpatient rehabilitation facility requires ongoing therapy with more than one skilled therapy discipline and intensive rehabilitation of at least 3 hours daily or 15 hours weekly.

- Proprioceptive neuromuscular facilitation contract–relax technique involves passive stretching of a muscle, contraction of the muscle, and relaxation followed by further passive stretching to increase range of motion. Ballistic stretching consists of repetitive bouncing movements at a rapid rate. Static stretching requires gradual application of stretch while holding the stretch in end position. Dynamic stretching is moving the muscle through to its maximum range of motion in a series of repetitions.

- Convection (whirlpool, fluidotherapy) refers to the flow of large amounts of molecules over large distances to transfer heat; convection best occurs with liquids or gases.

- Conduction (paraffin, hydrocollator) describes direct transfer of heat energy over a small distance between two surfaces in direct contact with different temperature gradients.

- Conversion (diathermy therapies, heat lamp) refers to electromagnetic energy being converted to heat as in the example of a heating lamp or ultrasound.

- Massage: Effleurage involves the practitioner's hands gliding over the client's skin and is a type of stroking massage technique. Friction involves pressure applied by the "ball" of the fingers in varying degrees to prevent or break up adhesions.

Pétrissage involves the practitioner compressing the client's skin and muscle between his or her fingers, often in kneading motion, to increase circulation and mobilize fluid. Tapotement is percussion massage and is stimulatory.

- Conventional TENS uses high-frequency, low-intensity stimulation. Electro-acupuncture uses low-frequency, high-intensity stimulation. Low-frequency, low-intensity stimulation has been used in wound healing and bone stimulation applications.

- The three types of diathermy are ultrasound, shortwave diathermy, and micro-wave diathermy. Ultrasound has deeper tissue penetration at low frequencies. It is generally not advised to be used near arthroplasty joints and is contraindicated in those with pacemakers.

- Manual therapy: Counterstrain technique places a body part in a passive position of maximal comfort, resetting muscle spindle fiber activity. Muscle energy involves patient performing active voluntary isometric muscle contractions with practitioner applying a counterforce to relax a muscle. Thrust refers to spinal manipulative therapy. Myofascial release most commonly involves practitioner applying sustained pressure to the muscle and allowing it to release/relax.

REFERENCES & SUGGESTED READINGS

Basford J, Baxter D. Therapeutic physical agents. In: Frontera WR, DeLisa JA, Gans B, et al, eds. *DeLisa's Physical Medicine & Rehabilitation: Principles and Practice*. 5th ed. Philadelphia, PA: Lippincott Williams & Wilkins; 2010:1691-1712.

Bloodworth DM. Cardiovascular conditioning exercise and cardiac rehabilitation. In: Garrison SJ, ed. *Handbook of Physical Medicine and Rehabilitation: The Basics*. 2nd ed. Philadelphia, PA: Lippincott Williams & Wilkins; 2003:96-104.

Cahalin LP, LaPier TK, Shaw DK. Sternal precautions: is it time for change? Precautions versus restrictions—a review of literature and recommendations for revision. *Cardiopulm Phys Ther J*. 2011;22(1):5-15.

Christiansen CH, Rogers SL, Haertl KL. Functional evaluation and management of self-care and other activities of daily living. In: Frontera WR, DeLisa JA, Gans B, et al, eds. *DeLisa's Physical Medicine & Rehabilitation: Principles and Practice*. 5th ed. Philadelphia, PA: Lippincott Williams & Wilkins; 2010:243-288.

Cotter AC, Bartoli L, Rosenfeld J, Schulman R, Seto DJ. Complementary and alternative medicine. In: Frontera WR, DeLisa JA, Gans B, et al, eds. *DeLisa's Physical Medicine & Rehabilitation: Principles and Practice*. 5th ed. Philadelphia, PA: Lippincott Williams & Wilkins; 2010:2119-2134.

Cuccurullo S. *Physical Medicine and Rehabilitation Board Review*. 3rd ed. New York, NY: Demos Publishing; 2014.

Ernst E. Acupuncture—a critical analysis. *J Intern Med*. 2006;259:125–137. doi:10.1111/j.1365-2796.2005.01584.x

Gnatz SM. Acute pain. In: Garrison SJ, ed. *Handbook of Physical Medicine and Rehabilitation: The Basics*. 2nd ed. Philadelphia, PA: Lippincott Williams & Wilkins; 2003:10-23.

Han BI, Song HS, Kim JS. Vestibular rehabilitation therapy: review of indications, mechanisms, and key exercises. *J Clin Neurol*. 2011;7(4):184-196.

King JC, Blankenship KJ, Schalla W, Mehta A. Rehabilitation team function and prescriptions, referrals, and order writing. In: Frontera WR, DeLisa JA, Gans B, et al, eds. *DeLisa's Physical Medicine & Rehabilitation: Principles and Practice*. 5th ed. Philadelphia, PA: Lippincott Williams & Wilkins; 2010:359-386.

Lee A, Chan SK, Fan LT. Stimulation of the wrist acupuncture point PC6 for preventing postoperative nausea and vomiting. *Cochrane Database Sys Rev*. 2015;(11):CD003281. doi:10.1002/14651858.CD003281.pub4.

Solomon B, Brewer C, Brodsky M, Palmer J, Ryder J. Speech, language, swallowing, and auditory rehabilitation. In: Frontera WR, DeLisa JA, Gans B, et al, eds. *DeLisa's Physical Medicine & Rehabilitation: Principles and Practice*. 5th ed. Philadelphia, PA: Lippincott Williams & Wilkins; 2010:413-444.

Stucki G, Kostanjsek N, Üstun B, Ewett T, Ciera A. Applying the ICF in rehabilitation medicine. In: Frontera WR, DeLisa JA, Gans B, et al, eds. *DeLisa's Physical Medicine & Rehabilitation: Principles and Practice*. 5th ed. Philadelphia, PA: Lippincott Williams & Wilkins; 2010:301-324.

Stucki G, Melvin J. The International Classification of Functioning, Disability and Health: a unifying model for the conceptual description of physical and rehabilitation medicine. *J Rehabil Med*. 2007;39(4):286-292.

Ververeli P, Lebby E, Tyler C, Fouad C. Evaluation of reducing postoperative hip precautions in total hip replacement: a randomized prospective study. *Orthopedics*. 2009;32(12):889. doi:10.3928/01477447-20091020-09.

Wieting JM, Andary MT, Holmes TG, Cugalj A, Cross N, Thompson G. Manipulation, massage, and traction. In: Frontera WR, DeLisa JA, Gans B, et al, eds. *DeLisa's Physical Medicine & Rehabilitation: Principles and Practice*. 5th ed. Philadelphia, PA: Lippincott Williams & Wilkins; 2010:1713-1742.

Web Sites

https://www.cdc.gov/nchs/icd/icf.htm
https://oig.hhs.gov/oei/reports/oei-09-97-00121.pdf
https://www.cms.gov/Regulations-and-Guidance/Guidance/Manuals/downloads/bp102c01.pdf
https://www.cms.gov/Outreach-and-Education/Medicare-Learning-Network-MLN /MLNProducts/downloads/Inpatient_Rehab_Fact_Sheet_ICN905643.pdf

Health Policy, Research, and Biostatistics

1. A physician-scientist wants to study the effects of an antidepressant on cognitive function in patients with stroke. He or she plans to use previously collected data from hospital records. What type of study is this?

   A. randomized controlled trial

   B. case-control study

   C. ecologic study

   D. retrospective cohort study

2. A physician-scientist wants to study the effects of an antidepressant on cognitive function in patients with stroke. He or she plans to look at population-level data. What type of study is this?

   A. randomized controlled trial

   B. case-control study

   C. ecologic study

   D. retrospective cohort study

3. A physician-scientist wants to study the effects of an antidepressant on cognitive function in patients with stroke. He or she plans to enroll patients using randomization into one of two groups. One group will receive a placebo, and the other will receive an active antidepressant treatment. Cognitive function will be measured in both groups and then compared. What type of study is this?

   A. randomized controlled trial

   B. case-control study

   C. ecologic study

   D. retrospective cohort study

4. A physician-scientist wants to study the effects of an antidepressant on cognitive function in patients with stroke. He or she will identify patients with stroke with poor cognitive function and then find patients with stroke who are age- and gender-matched controls. He or she will then ascertain which patients used the antidepressant. What type of study is this?

    A. randomized controlled trial

    B. case-control study

    C. ecologic study

    D. retrospective cohort study

5. A study finds that the risk of traumatic amputation in young men who drive intoxicated and experience a motor vehicle crash is 20% or .2. The risk of traumatic amputation in young women who drive intoxicated and experience a motor vehicle crash is 8% or .08. What is the relative risk of a young man having a traumatic amputation versus a young woman?

    A. 1

    B. 0

    C. 2

    D. 2.5

6. A study finds that ischemic stroke is 3 times more likely to occur in smokers as compared to nonsmokers. What is the relative risk of a smoker having an ischemic stroke compared to a nonsmoker?

    A. 3

    B. 0.3

    C. 0.33

    D. 30

7. You are reading a journal article describing a case-control study about use of Ritalin as a neurostimulant in pediatric patients with brain injury to increase alertness as measured on a particular scale. If the patient had an alertness score at or over a particular cut off score, he or she was considered as having "increased alertness." Given that the study is a case-control study, is it appropriate that the authors describe the measure of association using the odds ratio?

    A. yes

    B. no

    C. It depends on the prevalence of increased alertness in the study.

    D. It depends on the dosage of Ritalin used.

8. You are reading a journal article describing a case-control study about use of Ritalin as a neurostimulant in pediatric patients with brain injury to increase alertness as measured on a particular scale. If the patient had an alertness score at or over a particular cut off score, he or she was considered as having "increased alertness." In this study, there were 200 patients who were exposed to Ritalin and who were more alert. There were 100 patients who were exposed to Ritalin and were not more alert. There were 100 patients who were not exposed to Ritalin and who were more alert, and there were 100 patients who were not exposed to Ritalin and who were not more alert. What is the odds ratio for increased alertness of those exposed to Ritalin compared to those who were not exposed?

    A. 0.5

    B. 1

    C. 2

    D. 0.2

9. You are reading a journal article describing a case-control study about use of Ritalin as a neurostimulant in pediatric patients with brain injury to increase alertness as measured on a particular scale. If the patient had an alertness score at or over a particular cut off score, he or she was considered as having "increased alertness." In this study, those with increased alertness had 3 times the odds of exposure to Ritalin compared to those who did not have increased alertness. What is the odds ratio for exposure to Ritalin in those with increased alertness compared to those without increased alertness?

A. 30

B. 10

C. 3

D. 0.3

10. A study is designed to assess the relationship between the outcome of cerebral palsy in children and the exposure in maternal smoking. The study designers decide it is important to consider the effect of maternal age because they believe maternal age may be associated with the outcome and the exposure but is not in the causal pathway between the exposure and the outcome. Given this conceptualization, is maternal age a confounder?

A. No, maternal age is not a confounder.

B. No, maternal age is a mediator, not a confounder.

C. Yes, maternal age is a confounder.

D. A and B

11. A diagnostic test correctly identifies 80% of people as having a particular disease. What is the sensitivity of the test?

A. 80%

B. 8%

C. 30%

D. 98%

12. A diagnostic test correctly identifies 80% of people as not having a particular disease. What is the specificity of the test?

A. 80%

B. 8%

C. 30%

D. 98%

13. You are a patient's regular physician. Your patient has a workplace injury involving musculoskeletal strain. You treat the injury appropriately. Some time later, your patient requests that you perform an independent medical examination (IME) to determine disability. Is this appropriate?

A. Yes, because you treated the patient for the injury.

B. No, because you treated the patient for the injury.

C. No, because you have prior knowledge of the medical issue.

D. both B and C

14. Your patient experiences a workplace injury. He or she is undergoing therapy and showing steady improvement in his or her condition. Would it be appropriate that another physician evaluate his or her for maximum medical improvement (MMI) at this time?

A. No, because we do not know if 6 months has passed since the injury.

B. No, because the patient is still experiencing improvement in his or her condition.

C. Yes, because he or she has been evaluated by a physician and is participating in therapy.

D. Yes, because his or her condition is improving.

15. Define disability.

A. unable to finish an activity that most people at that age would be able to do

B. inability to complete a task

C. inability to work

D. inability to complete high school

16. What does FIM™ stand for?

   A. Functional Independence Method

   B. Functional Independence Measure

   C. Functional Individual Measure

   D. Formal Independence Measure

17. What level of independence does an overall Functional Independence Measure (FIM™) score of 5 entail?

   A. total assist

   B. complete independence

   C. moderate assist

   D. supervision

18. What condition was the Disability Rating Scale (DRS) developed for?

   A. heart attack

   B. stroke

   C. brain injury

   D. amputation

19. What federal disability law prohibits discrimination on the basis of disability in access to government programs (both local and state), employment, telecommunications, commercial facilities, public accommodations, and transportation?

   A. Rehabilitation Act of 1973

   B. Individuals with Disabilities Education Act

   C. Civil Rights of Institutionalized Persons Act

   D. Americans with Disabilities Act of 1990

20. How many impairment criteria are defined by American Medical Association (AMA) guides?

   A. three

   B. four

   C. five

   D. six

21. When determining an impairment rating, how many impairment classes are there?

    A. three

    B. four

    C. five

    D. six

22. What is an impairment grade?

    A. Impairment grade is the same as impairment class.

    B. Impairment grade is a higher level determination than impairment class.

    C. Impairment grade is a designation within impairment class.

    D. There is no such thing as impairment grade.

23. Impairment grades range from A to what letter?

    A. C

    B. D

    C. E

    D. F

24. Which of the following is not commonly used to describe frequency of activity for purposes of a functional capacity evaluation?

    A. bimonthly

    B. occasional

    C. frequent

    D. constant

25. How long do functional capacity evaluations usually last?

    A. half an hour

    B. a week

    C. 2 times a week for 4 to 6 weeks

    D. about 5 hours

26. Who typically performs a functional capacity evaluation?

    A. a physician

    B. a research scientist

    C. a nurse

    D. a therapist

27. What is maximal medical improvement?

    A. a point at which the condition has become stable as far as improvement

    B. the best outcome that could ideally be expected

    C. the patient's previous level of function

    D. the level of function at which on average, a patient of the same age would perform

28. At which time may it be appropriate to determine a permanent partial impairment rating?

    A. at the time of the injury

    B. within 24 hours of the injury

    C. as the patient is working in therapy

    D. once the patient has reached maximal medical improvement

29. A tool often used for measuring joint angles in physical medicine and rehabilitation (PM&R) is

    A. a ruler.

    B. a goniometer.

    C. a dynamometer.

    D. a compass.

30. Ergonomics is

    A. not a real thing.

    B. the study of the interaction between the body and the environment.

    C. the study of body movement.

    D. used to determine appropriate development.

31.   Persons with disability are

   A. more likely to be unemployed than similar individuals who are not disabled.

   B. as likely to be unemployed than similar individuals who are not disabled.

   C. more likely to be employed than similar individuals who are not disabled.

   D. always unable to work.

32.   Which federal disability law is most closely associated with requiring public schools to make free appropriate education in the least restrictive appropriate environment?

   A. Individuals with Disabilities Education Act

   B. Rehabilitation Act of 1973

   C. Architectural Barriers Act

   D. Americans with Disabilities Act of 1990

33.   What phrase describes a return to work that does not affect benefits, in order to evaluate ability to work?

   A. trial work period

   B. extended period of eligibility

   C. permanent disability

   D. family medical leave act

34.   You are investigating the relationship between smoking and heart disease. Another factor that is a known risk factor for heart disease and that is associated with smoking but is not a result of smoking is

   A. a confounder.

   B. a mediator.

   C. an unknown risk.

   D. an effect modifier.

35. You are reviewing a study for a colleague. You notice a generalized or systematic error in the study's proposed analysis. This systematic error would be a source of

  A. confounding.

  B. bias.

  C. effect modification.

  D. mathematical error.

36. If the disease being studied is very common, is the odds ratio a good estimate of the relative risk?

  A. no

  B. yes

  C. in certain circumstances

  D. The odds ratio and relative risk are not compatible concepts.

37. A medical test consistently producing results which are very similar and are also in line with the results produced by the gold standard. This test is

  A. accurate and reliable.

  B. accurate but not reliable.

  C. reliable but not accurate.

  D. neither accurate nor reliable.

38. Someone who tests as a "false negative," in general

  A. has the disease.

  B. does not have the disease.

  C. the designation "false negative" does not tell you anything about the person's disease status.

  D. may or may not have the disease.

39. The proportion of persons affected by a certain disease at a certain time can best be described as?

A. incidence of the disease

B. the mortality rate associated with the disease

C. prevalence of the disease

D. the case fatality rate associated with the disease

40. The proportion of the population affected by a disease at a certain point in time can best be described as?

A. the point prevalence

B. the period prevalence

C. the incidence

D. the mortality rate

41. A simple way to describe the relationship between prevalence and incidence might be

A. prevalence = incidence × disease duration.

B. prevalence = incidence + disease duration.

C. prevalence = incidence − disease duration.

D. prevalence = incidence + disease duration.

42. Limitations of data from hospital records might include which of the following?

A. hospital records have no limitations

B. generally do not include information on gender and age

C. generally are very inaccurate on basic facts such as gender and age

D. may not include details which would improve the quality of a research study

43. What is herd immunity?

   A. the resistance of a small group of people against a common disease

   B. the resistance of a small group of people against a rare disease

   C. the resistance of a group of people to a disease against which many people in the group are immune

   D. the resistance of a group of people to a disease against which most people in the group are susceptible

44. What is an incubation period?

   A. the time an animal or human needs to be born without significant medical problems

   B. the time period from start of infection to the presentation of clinical symptoms

   C. the time period that an animal or human needs to be free of an infection

   D. involves time in an incubator

45. New cases of a condition among persons at risk during a certain time period is best described as

   A. case fatality rate.

   B. mortality rate.

   C. prevalence.

   D. incidence.

46. Prevalence rate can be described as a

   A. measure of mortality.

   B. measure of morbidity.

   C. measure of determination.

   D. measure of causation.

47. Incidence rate can be described as a

A. measure of mortality.

B. measure of morbidity.

C. measure of determination.

D. measure of causation.

48. The attack rate for a disease can be described as

A. number of people at risk who develop disease/total number of people at risk.

B. total number of people at risk/number of people who develop the disease.

C. number of people at risk who develop the disease/total number of people in the population.

D. total number of people at risk/total number of people in the population.

49. Reliability of a test generally refers to

A. how much you trust the test.

B. how often the test is used.

C. the ability of the test to produce similar results with repeated uses.

D. the ability of the test to produce the result you wish to see.

50. A test always produces similar results, but they are quite different from those produced by the gold standard.

A. This test is reliable but not valid.

B. This test is valid but not reliable.

C. This test is both reliable and valid.

D. This test is neither reliable nor valid.

ANSWER KEY WITH EXPLANATIONS

1. The correct answer is D.
This is a retrospective cohort study because it uses preexisting data (precollected data) and compares groups that have been exposed and those that have not been exposed to a certain factor. In this scenario, the exposed group is composed of those patients with stroke who took the antidepressant. The nonexposed group is composed of those patients with stroke who did not take the antidepressant. The outcome of interest is cognitive function in patients with stroke.

2. The correct answer is C.
This is an ecologic study because it uses data from a group. The investigator is using group-level data, in this case population-level data. He or she does not have data from individuals.

3. The correct answer is A.
This is a randomized controlled trial because it uses the features of randomization and a control group. The term *randomization* means that study subjects are arbitrarily assigned to a group. This study includes a placebo, the *control*, and an active treatment, the antidepressant being studied. The presence of a control group allows the investigator to assess the difference in outcome between subjects who received the treatment of interest and subjects who did not receive the treatment of interest.

4. The correct answer is B.
This is a case-control study because the investigator identified patients who had the condition of interest, patients with stroke with poor cognitive function. These patients are the *cases*. Stroke with poor cognitive function is the disease state of interest (the outcome of interest). The investigator has identified a control group, patients with stroke without poor cognitive function. The exposure of interest is use of the antidepressant. The investigator will compare use of the antidepressant in patients with stroke with poor cognitive function (*the cases*) versus patients with stroke without poor cognitive function (*the controls*).

5. The correct answer is D.
The relative risk of a young man having a traumatic amputation versus a young woman having a traumatic amputation is $.2 \div .08 = 2.5$. The formula to calculate relative risk is risk in exposed $\div$ risk in unexposed. Here, we are calculating the relative risk of the outcome *traumatic amputation related to motor vehicle crash when driving intoxicated*. The "exposure" in this situation is gender, male or female.

6. The correct answer is A.
The relative risk of ischemic stroke in those who smoke versus those who do not smoke is $3 \div 1 = 3$, or to put it another way, $300\% \div 100\% = 3$. The formula to calculate relative risk is risk in exposed $\div$ risk in unexposed. Here, we are calculating the relative risk of the outcome *ischemic stroke*. The exposure in this situation is smoking status.

7. The correct answer is A.

Given that the study is a case-control study, yes, it is appropriate to use the odds ratio to describe the association between exposure and outcome. In a case-control study, one cannot directly calculate the relative risk because one does not have information about the incidence of the outcome in those with the exposure versus those without the exposure; one only has information about the cases and controls. As a separate issue, the odds ratio *may* be a good estimate of the relative risk when it meets certain conditions (described further in "Pearls" section).

8. The correct answer is C.

To calculate the odds ratio in a case-control study, the formula is odds ratio = odds of exposure in a case ÷ odds of exposure in a control.

One can create a two-by-two table to help determine this information:

	Cases (e.g., those with increased alertness)	Controls
Exposed (e.g., those that received Ritalin)	a 200	b 100
Unexposed	c 100	d 100

The odds that a case was exposed is the ratio of a to c, or a:c, or a ÷ c. The odds that a control was exposed is the ratio of b to d, or b:d, or b / d. The odds ratio for odds that cases were exposed to odds that controls were exposed is then:

a ÷ c divided by b ÷ d or (a ÷ c)/(b ÷ d), which is the same as ad ÷ bc. For this question, that is

$$\frac{200}{100} \times \frac{100}{100}$$

which is the same as 200 ÷ 100, or 2.

9. The correct answer is C.

To calculate the odds ratio in a case-control study, the formula is odds ratio = odds of exposure in a case ÷ odds of exposure in a control.
Here, this would be 3/1, or 3.

10. The correct answer is C.

In this question, maternal age is a *confounder* of the association between the exposure, maternal smoking, and the outcome of interest, cerebral palsy in a resultant child, because it is thought to be associated with both the exposure and the outcome of interest but is not part of the pathway of causation between the exposure and the outcome. Factors are particularly considered to be confounders when they are a risk factor for the outcome (and also meet the criteria of having an association with the exposure and are not in the causal pathway from the exposure to the outcome).

11. The correct answer is A.

The sensitivity of a test refers to the following: Of those individuals with the disease, what is the likelihood of the test correctly identifying those with the disease? This test correctly identifies 80% as having the disease, so the sensitivity of the test is therefore 80%.

12. The correct answer is A.

The specificity of a test refers to the following: Of those individuals who do not have the disease, what is the likelihood of the test correctly identifying those who do not have the disease? This test correctly identifies 80% of individuals who do not have the disease, so the specificity of the test is therefore 80%.

13. The correct answer is D.

The purpose of an IME is to provide an objective determination. The practitioner who performs the IME should not have previous involvement with the patient's medical condition. Therefore, it is not appropriate that one would perform an IME for one's own patient for whom one has treated the medical condition in question. The provider performing the IME should not be the treating physician.

14. The correct answer is B.

If the patient is still experiencing improvement in his or her condition, then it is not appropriate to make an MMI determination at this time. The definition of MMI is that the patient's condition has stabilized, such that he or she is not expected to change status in the near future.

15. The correct answer is A.

One may be considered disabled if one is unable to successfully complete tasks that most people one's age would be able to do. The definition of disability depends on contextual factors and involves one's role in the community or society. For example, one may be considered disabled if at 30 years old, one is physically unable to work in any usual working environment. Answer choices C and D could be true of a person who is disabled, but answer choice A would be more universally true. Consider, for example, a 3-year-old child unable to work would not be considered disabled.

16. The correct answer is B.

FIM™ stands for "Functional Independence Measure." The FIM™ provides a means to rate the severity of functional limitation in the areas of self-care, bowel and bladder function, transfers and general mobility, communication, and cognition.

17. The correct answer is D.

The FIM™ is a disability rating scale with levels 1 through 7. An FIM™ score of 7 would be a normal person requiring no assistance of any kind to go about usual daily activities. An FIM™ score of 5 indicates that the person requires supervision in activities.

18. The correct answer is C.

The DRS is a 30-point scale specific to brain injury. It provides information on ability to work inside or outside the home or as a full-time student within its "employability" subscale as well as information on responsiveness and functional independence in various areas.

19. The correct answer is D.

The "Americans with Disabilities Act of 1990" prohibits discrimination on the basis of disability in access to government programs (both local and state), employment, telecommunications, commercial facilities, public accommodations, and transportation. (Reference: United States Department of Labor. Americans with Disabilities Act. https://www.dol.gov/general/topic/disability/ada. Accessed September 8, 2017.).

20. The correct answer is B.

The AMA guides contain four impairment criteria including clinical history, physical examination, lab work/imaging/other tests, and functional history.

21. The correct answer is C.

When determining an impairment rating, there are five impairment classes, class 0 through class 4. This is a bit of a trick question because class 0's classification means there is no objective evidence of impairment; nevertheless, class 0 is one possible determination as far as assigning an impairment class.

22. The correct answer is C.

Impairment grade is a designation within impairment class. There are five impairment classes ranging from class 0 to class 4, with class 0 being defined as no significant evidence of objective impairment and class 4 indicating a very severe condition. Within the class assigned to the individual, the examiner also assigns an impairment grade with letter designation indicating the individual is significantly less impaired than most persons within the class up to being significantly more impaired than most persons within the class.

23. The correct answer is C.

Impairment grades range from A to E. An impairment grade is assigned within the assigned impairment class. The impairment grade indicates where the individual falls within the impairment class, with "A" indicating the individual is significantly less impaired than most persons within the class up to "E" indicating the individual is significantly more impaired than most persons within the class.

24. The correct answer is A.

When describing frequency of activity for purposes of a functional capacity evaluation, the commonly used categories are none, occasional, frequent, and constant. These four categories correspond to amount of time spent in the activity, with none being 0% of time, up to constant being 67% to 100% of time.

25. The correct answer is D.

A functional capacity evaluation usually lasts about 4 hours more or less in order to complete the assessment process including assessment of range of motion, strength, and endurance. The functional capacity evaluation provides objective information about abilities.

26. The correct answer is D.

A functional capacity evaluation is typically performed by a therapist with specialized training, either a physical therapist or occupational therapist.

27. The correct answer is A.

Maximal medical improvement refers to the time at which the condition has stabilized, such that the patient is not expected to change status in the near future.

28. The correct answer is D.

A permanent partial impairment rating determination may be appropriate once the point of maximal medical improvement has been reached, if the condition has not fully resolved.

29. The correct answer is B.

A goniometer is a tool used to measure the angle of joints and can provide information on restrictions in range of motion.

30. The correct answer is B.

Ergonomics involves study of the interaction between the environment and the body and may involve adjustments in workplace set up including changes to desks, seating, telephones, and computers.

31. The correct answer is A.

Persons with disability are more likely to be unemployed than similar individuals who are not disabled for a variety of different reasons including issues with transportation and other aspects of accommodation.

32. The correct answer is A.

The federal disability law most closely associated with requiring public schools to make free appropriate education in the least restrictive appropriate environment is the Individuals with Disabilities Education Act. Other federal disability laws do address education as well.

33. The correct answer is A.

A trial work period allows an individual to return to work in order to evaluate one's ability to perform in the work environment. This trial period does not affect disability benefits.

34. The correct answer is A.

Factors are particularly considered to be confounders when they are a risk factor for the outcome and also meet the criteria of having an association with the exposure and not being in the causal pathway from the exposure to the outcome. In this question, smoking is the exposure, and the outcome of interest is heart disease. If the other factor mentioned in the question is a risk factor for heart disease, is associated with smoking, and does not result from smoking, in other words is not in the causal pathway from smoking to heart disease, then you will likely want to consider it to be a possible confounder, and adjust your analyses appropriately.

35. The correct answer is B.

Bias is "any systematic error in the design, conduct or analysis of a study that results in a mistaken estimate of an exposure's effect on the risk of disease," attributed to Schlesselman JJ. *Case-Control Studies: Design, Conduct, Analysis.* New York, NY: Oxford University Press; 1982, quoted from Gordis L. *Epidemiology.* 4th ed. Philadelphia, PA: Saunders Elsevier; 2009.

   Of course, the bias you notice may result in mathematical error, choice D, but here, the best answer is B.

36. The correct answer is A.

In general, the odds ratio is only similar to the relative risk when the condition in question is rare. Because the relative risk cannot be calculated directly in a case-control study, the odds ratio is often used instead. The odds ratio is a legitimate measure of association in itself, but it should not be confused for the relative risk. In a case-control study, the odds ratio can be considered a good estimate of relative risk when the cases and controls exposure histories are representative of that of the whole population, and the condition being studied is not common.

37. The correct answer is A.

When a test consistently reproduces similar values, it is *reliable*. When those results are close to those produced by the gold standard test for the condition, the test in question is *accurate*. If a test produces results that are both consistently reproducible (reliable) and accurate, it can be considered a *valid* test.

38. The correct answer is A.

The concept of *false negative* implies that somehow one knows the true state of reality: who being studied really has the disease or does not have the disease in question regardless of what the test results show. In the real world, this would imply that one assesses the validity of a particular test with a gold standard test. Regardless, subjects are *false negative* when they do have the disease in question, but they test negative for it.

39. The correct answer is C.

The proportion of persons affected by a condition at a certain time is the prevalence of the condition. This use of prevalence can be further specified as point prevalence because one is concerned about the prevalence at a certain point in time.

40. The correct answer is A.

When one is interested in the prevalence of a condition at a certain point in time, one is interested in the point prevalence (as opposed to the period prevalence, the prevalence of the condition in a particular time period). Prevalence is the proportion of persons with the condition.

41. The correct answer is A.

In general, prevalence = incidence × disease duration. This equation takes into account both the rate of new cases of the condition as well as how long those with the condition survive when calculating prevalence.

42. The correct answer is D.

Hospital records are important for medical research but can be limited in the data they include as far as patient characteristics and details regarding care. The quality and condition of the data itself is also variable depending on the type of record and method of data collection, for example, handwritten notes, standardized report forms.

43. The correct answer is C.

Herd immunity refers to the situation in which, when most individuals in a population are immune to an infectious disease, those within the population who are not immune are also protected and are less likely to contract the disease because the condition is less likely to be spread within the population because it is less likely a susceptible individual will come into contact with someone capable of spreading the condition.

44. The correct answer is B.

The incubation period refers to the time from which one becomes infected with a disease to the time at which one starts showing clinical signs and symptoms of the condition. The incubation period varies for different conditions. A related concept is quarantine, a time period of isolation which should encompass the incubation period of the infectious disease of concern, to help prevent the spread of the disease.

45. The correct answer is D.

The incidence (incidence rate) of a condition is the number of new cases of the condition out of those at risk for developing the condition, during a certain time period. By contrast, prevalence refers to the proportion of persons with the condition.

46. The correct answer is B.

In general, the prevalence rate can be described as a measure of morbidity. It describes the amount of illness or morbidity, as opposed to measure of mortality which would account for deaths.

47. The correct answer is B.

In general, the incidence rate can be described as a measure of morbidity. It describes the amount of illness or morbidity, as opposed to measure of mortality which would account for deaths.

48. The correct answer is A.

The attack rate for a disease can be described as number of people at risk who develop disease/total number of people at risk. Usually, time is not included in the attack rate calculation.

49. The correct answer is C.

Reliability of a test refers to the ability of the test to be repeated with similar results consistently. In other words, the results of the test are reproducible. A test may be reliable and yet not produce accurate results, in which case it is not considered a valid test.

50. The correct answer is A.

If a test produces results that are consistently reproducible, it is reliable. However, if its results are not similar to the results of the gold standard test, then its results are not considered to be accurate and are therefore invalid. The test can be described as reliable but not valid.

Board Review Points ("Pearls") for Health Policy, Research, and Biostatistics

Disability Determination Terms

- MMI refers to the time at which the condition has stabilized, such that the patient is not expected to change status in the near future.
- IME provides an objective determination about the patient's condition with regard to disability status.

- Impairment class: There are five impairment classes, class 0 through class 4, with class 0 classification meaning there is no objective evidence of impairment and class 4 indicating a very severe condition.
- Impairment grade: Within the class assigned to the individual, the examiner also assigns an impairment grade with letter designation ranging from A to E. The impairment grade indicates where the individual falls within the impairment class, with "A" indicating the individual is significantly less impaired than most persons within the class up to "E" indicating the individual is significantly more impaired than most persons within the class.
- Impairment rating versus permanent disability rating: A permanent partial impairment rating determination may be appropriate once the point of MMI has been reached, if the condition has not fully resolved.

Disability Law

- The "Americans with Disabilities Act of 1990" prohibits discrimination on the basis of disability in access to government programs (both local and state), employment, telecommunications, commercial facilities, public accommodations, and transportation. (Reference: United States Department of Labor. Americans with Disabilities Act. https://www.dol.gov/general/topic/disability/ada. Accessed September 8, 2017.)
- Individuals with Disabilities Education Act is the federal disability law most closely associated with requiring public schools to make free appropriate education in the least restrictive appropriate environment. Other federal disability laws do address education as well.

Types of Research Studies

- An ecologic study uses data from a group, such as population-level data.
- A retrospective cohort study uses preexisting data (precollected data) and compares groups that have been exposed and those that have not been exposed to a certain factor.
- In a case-control study, the investigator identifies patients who have the condition of interest, these patients are the *cases*. The investigator also identifies a control group. The investigator will compare the distribution of the exposure of interest in the cases as compared to the distribution of the exposure of interest in the controls.
- A randomized controlled trial uses the features of randomization and a control group. The term *randomization* means that study subjects are arbitrarily assigned to a group. The presence of a control group allows the investigator to assess the difference in outcome between subjects who received the treatment of interest and subjects who did not receive the treatment of interest.

Basic Biostatistics

- Relative risk of a condition in the exposed versus the unexposed group is risk in exposed ÷ risk in unexposed.
- The odds ratio in a case-control study has the formula odds ratio = odds of exposure in a case ÷ odds of exposure in a control.

- In general, the odds ratio is only similar to the relative risk when the condition in question is rare. Because the relative risk cannot be calculated directly in a case-control study, the odds ratio is often used instead. The odds ratio is a legitimate measure of association in itself, but it should not be confused for the relative risk. In a case-control study, the odds ratio can be considered a good estimate of relative risk when the cases and controls exposure histories are representative of that of the whole population, and the condition being studied is not common.
- A confounder is thought to be associated with both the exposure and the outcome of interest but is not part of the pathway of causation between the exposure and the outcome. Factors are particularly considered to be confounders when they are a risk factor for the outcome (and also meet the criteria of having an association with the exposure and are not in the causal pathway from the exposure to the outcome).
- The sensitivity of a test refers to the following: Of those individuals with the disease, what is the likelihood of the test correctly identifying those with the disease?
- The specificity of a test refers to the following: Of those individuals who do not have the disease, what is the likelihood of the test correctly identifying those who do not have the disease?

Rehabilitation Research Outcomes

- Functional Independence Measure: The FIM™, Functional Independence Measure, is a disability rating scale with levels 1 through 7. An FIM™ score of 7 would be a normal person requiring no assistance of any kind to go about usual daily activities. An FIM™ score of 5 indicates that the person requires supervision in activities.
- DRS is a 30-point scale specific to brain injury. It provides information on ability to work inside or outside the home or as a full-time student within its "employability" subscale as well as information on responsiveness and functional independence in various areas.

REFERENCES & SUGGESTED READINGS

Braddom RL, Chan L, Harrast ME, et al, eds. *Physical Medicine and Rehabilitation*. 4th ed. St. Louis, MO: Saunders; 2011.

Centers for Disease Control and Prevention. *Principles of Epidemiology in Public Health Practice, Third Edition. An Introduction to Applied Epidemiology and Biostatistics*. Atlanta, GA: Centers for Disease Control and Prevention. https://www.cdc.gov/ophss/csels/dsepd/ss1978/. Accessed September 8, 2017.

Cuccurullo S. *Physical Medicine and Rehabilitation Board Review*. 3rd ed. New York, NY: Demos Publishing; 2014.

Frontera W, DeLisa JA, Gans BM, et al, eds. *DeLisa's Physical Medicine & Rehabilitation: Principles and Practice*. 5th ed. Philadelphia, PA: Lippincott Williams & Wilkins; 2010.

Gordis L. *Epidemiology*. 4th ed. Philadelphia, PA: Saunders Elsevier; 2008.

Rothman KJ, Greenland S, Timothy L. *Modern Epidemiology*. 3rd ed. Philadelphia, PA: Lippincott William & Wilkins; 2008.

Szklo M, Nieto FJ. *Epidemiology: Beyond the Basics*. 3rd ed. Burlington, MA: Jones & Bartlett Learning; 2014.

United States Department of Labor. Americans with Disabilities Act. https://www.dol.gov /general/topic/disability/ada. Accessed September 8, 2017.

Index